Gary Null's

POWER
AGING

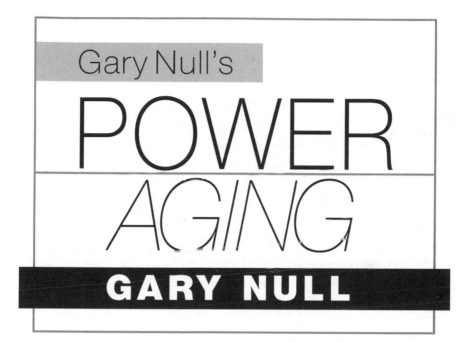

Gary Null's

POWER
AGING

GARY NULL

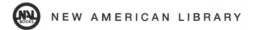

NEW AMERICAN LIBRARY

S

New American Library
Published by New American Library, a division of
Penguin Group (USA) Inc., 375 Hudson Street,
New York, New York 10014, U.S.A.
Penguin Books Ltd, 80 Strand,
London WC2R 0RL, England
Penguin Books Australia Ltd, 250 Camberwell Road,
Camberwell, Victoria 3124, Australia
Penguin Books Canada Ltd, 10 Alcorn Ave.
Toronto, Ontario, Canada M4V 3B2
Penguin Books (N.Z.) Ltd, Cnr Rosedale and Airborne Roads,
Albany, Auckland 1310, New Zealand

Penguin Books Ltd, Registered Offices:
80 Strand, London WC2R 0RL, England

First published by New American Library,
a division of Penguin Group (USA) Inc.

First Printing, December 2003
10   9   8   7   6

 REGISTERED TRADEMARK—MARCA REGISTRADA

LIBRARY OF CONGRESS CATALOGING IN PUBLICATION DATA
Null, Gary.
[Power aging]
Gary Null's power aging / Gary Null.
p. cm.
Includes bibliographical references and index.
ISBN 0-451-21050-6 (alk. paper)
1. Longevity. 2. Aging. I. Title.
RA776.75.N838 2003
613—dc21   2003012360

Set in Ehrhardt MT
Designed by Ginger Legato

Printed in the United States of America

PUBLISHER'S NOTE
Every effort as been made to ensure that the information contained in this book is complete and accu-
rate. However, neither the publisher nor the author is engaged in rendering professional advice or services to the individual reader. The ideas, procedures, and suggestions contained in this book are not
intended as a substitute for consulting with your physician. All matters regarding your health require
medical supervision. Neither the author nor the publisher shall be liable or responsible for any loss or
damage allegedly arising from any information or suggestion in this book.

Important Disclaimer—
Please Read

To people of any age who aren't afraid
to make conscious choices to be the best that they can be
and get the best from others.

Acknowledgments

Many months of research are necessary to create a book of this scope, and I had the good fortune of bringing together a team of skilled, dedicated, and determined people to assist me on this project. A very special thanks to Vicki Riba Koestler, Carolyn Dean, M.D., N.D., and Dr. Dorothy Smith; the editorial touch of all three is evident throughout the book. Thanks also to Ken Laufer and Gail Leinwall for their contributions to the initial manuscript; to Marcus Guiliano, whose culinary skills and knowledge were invaluable; and to Andre Turan, Pat Morgan, and Manette Loudon for covering all the bases on this project's journey to completion. Special thanks to Jennifer Armstrong for her administrative assistance.

Also, I want to express my appreciation to Saul Kent, Bill Faloon, and the editorial and scientific staff of the Life Extension Foundation for supporting this project with an enormous quantity of high-quality research on antiaging subjects. Their contributions and cooperation were invaluable to me.

For additional information on the Life Extension Foundation and antiaging support and research, visit the foundation's Web site at www.lifeextension.com, or call 1-800-544-4440.

Contents

PART II: WHAT YOU NEED TO KNOW NOW

CHAPTER 10: RECIPES FOR POWER AGING / 241
Jump-start Your Detox / 241

CHAPTER 11: COUNTERING COMMON CONDITIONS / 280
Specific Supplementation Plans / 280

PART IV: MORE HELP

PART I

BEGINNING THE PROCESS

CHAPTER 1

AN ANTIAGING OVERVIEW

*What We're Up Against, and
How We Can Beat It*

NEW MILLENNIUM, NEW MIND-SET

If you were to open your family album, you might be struck by the way your grandparents looked. Just decades ago, a fifty-year-old looked downright old, and a thirty-five-year-old looked more like a fifty-year-old of today. A lot of the reason has to do with how little people understood about the aging process. They believed that life after forty was a downward slide accompanied by a decline in energy, a decrease in muscle (which was then replaced by fat), cognitive difficulties, and a variety of minor health ailments. Over time, these minor ailments grew into full-blown disease and, thereafter, resulted in death—just a couple decades down the line. Limited by a scant knowledge base and a fatalistic belief system, Americans by and large allowed themselves to grow old before their time.

But as the saying goes, that was then and this is now—now being a new millennium in which the way we look at the human life span has wholly changed. When we entered the 2000s, many of us used that milestone as a chance to step back and ask, What's different now? and What's going to be different? about the way we live our lives. And what I saw in the field of aging was a conceptual shift—one that's actually been going on for about three decades now—in which Americans are exchanging a resigned attitude of "This will happen to me in my forties, and this will happen to me in my fifties, and this'll happen to me in my sixties . . ." for an assertive attitude of "*I'm* going to make this happen in my sixties . . ."—or seventies or eighties. And the kinds of things they're making happen run the gamut from running a marathon to starting a new business to becoming an accomplished ballroom dancer. In other words, the old limitations are being challenged, and the old "age-appropriate" labels are being thrown out the window.

This is an exciting time because along with people's willingness to discard old stereotypes about aging, modern science is making great strides in the effort to prolong healthful human life. Today, researchers are tracking natural substances and "smart" medicines that, if Ponce de León's fountain of youth were ever found, would probably prove the source of that storied spring. From the well-touted antioxidants, like vitamin C and beta-carotene, to lesser-known substances like trimethylglycine, numerous compounds are proving themselves as effective age-fighters through the rigors of clinical testing. What it all adds up to is that this millennium finds us on the brink of a new paradigm, wherein the natural expected life span may be extended from today's average of under eighty years to one hundred twenty years or more. That's over forty more years—almost a half century—of extra life.

Of course this increase will be gradual. And we have to remember that it all starts with individuals making physical changes to enhance their health and mental well-being, so that they're able to push the life span envelope. I've been advocating making such changes on my daily radio program for years, and I admit that sometimes it's been discouraging when I've found out about particular listeners who, although they've been *listening* for years, haven't actually *done* anything positive for their health. And you may have heard me speak of giving a lecture on health to an enthusiastic audience, only to leave and then see some of those same people heading into a fast-food place around the corner.

On the other hand, I know there are many who are conscientiously applying new life-enhancing information into their lives. A lot of these people are senior citizens. Today, I meet many older people who are eating wholesome foods and keeping their minds and bodies active by taking the time to regularly work out, read, socialize, and counter the daily stresses of life with meditation and yoga. Such individuals can remain active and healthy well into their seventies, eighties, and beyond, free from the crippling debilities of arthritis, macular degeneration, heart disease, and other infirmities. Putting all these factors together—incorporating scientific advances to increase the natural life span, improving the quality of life, and living an optimal lifestyle, will really pack a synergistic punch against aging.

UPDATING "OLD" IDEAS

By looking at the mass media, you wouldn't necessarily notice that a paradigm shift is occurring. On TV, for instance, there are still a lot of stereotyped "oldsters"—crotchety, annoying people who aren't very active and who like to sit around complaining about their ills. They're often depicted that way to add humor to a show, but after a while the joke wears thin. Also, both by TV and popular magazines, we're being bombarded by ads for prescription drugs—"Ask your doctor," the ads say—and a lot of them feature older people beset by various conditions, from arthritis to digestive problems. A viewer could get the idea that age and disease go hand in hand, and that disease is an inevitable part of growing older. What's worse, the substances being advertised generally have little to do with prevention or eradication of the condition. Instead, they are all about symptom control; the assumption being that the consumer can never get rid of the underlying condition. Granted, it all makes sense from the point of view of the marketplace: If you continue to be sick, you're going to keep buying the drug. Plus there's more profit in a patented drug than there is in, say, lycopene-containing tomatoes, or beta-carotene-rich carrots.

Another segment of society that hasn't caught up with new attitudes toward aging can be found in the medical establishment. Not all doctors, but a significant percentage, maintain the dismissive paternalism of the past century, when senior citizens were basically told, "There, there. Take these pills and you'll feel better." Most doctors don't try to get to the root of your condition and take nutritional measures to reverse it, nor do they think in terms of improving your health at a fundamental level. There are still too many physicians stuck in the mind-set that "senior equals symptoms."

And it always amazes me when I hear about older people who, *on their own,* used diet or supplements to reverse a condition, and then returned to their doctor's office to report on their success. The doctor is often not interested in the least. "Oh, that happens," he or she will say, as if the patient's experience was a fluke. But he doesn't really want to know about what the patient did because this patient's approach does not fit into the paradigm of healing that the doctor was taught in medical school. This is why I have to salute those seniors who are proactive about nutrition, supplements, exercise, and alternative therapies in optimizing their health. They're often not getting support from those who should be encouraging them—their own physicians. I hope this book empowers them further.

BABY BOOMERS DO IT AGAIN

Turning now to a generation with which I've been heavily involved—the baby boomers—I want to salute them too. You can say what you want about this group's sometimes obnoxious desire to have it all, but you have to hand it to them—as they've put their mark on so much else in our culture, the boomers are changing the very concept of what it means to get older. The fact is that today's aging baby boomers are yesterday's youth generation who do not passively accept the decline that goes with aging. They frequent gyms, eat lean foods, and use nutritional supplements, and their desire to maintain the vim and vigor of youth has set the stage for antiaging medicine.

I do have to mention, though, that sometimes the boomers' quest for an increased healthy life span is sabotaged by this group's tendency to want to do it all, so they can be very conflicted about their goals. I've seen this time and again.

I like to talk to people, ask probing questions, and then just listen to what they have to say about their lives. Recently, as I began work on this book, I did something interesting. I stood outside a New York City graduate school on Fifth Avenue and Thirty-fourth Street, where I teach, and asked baby-boomer types coming out the door how long they would like to live. Overall, most wanted to live a very long time. Some mentioned a hundred years of life. But they had issues that were troubling them, and many were willing to share their thoughts with me. While most were not plagued by serious illness, they were beginning to show signs of aging, such as increased levels of fatigue, stress, graying and loss of hair, and fat around the middle or bottom—and they were not ready to accept these. Many women seemed surprised to be growing old as quickly as they were.

This group was generally willing to do something to make a difference in their health status—provided they could make the time for it. In other words, they looked at the possibility of change pragmatically, weighing the pros and cons: "I already have a lot on my plate. Can I really fit what you're suggesting into my life when I've got a family, a career, many social responsibilities, and only so many hours in a day?"

It seemed as though these people had too much to do and too little time to get things done. The reality is that many baby boomers are severely stressed, starting the morning as if a gun going off was their signal to jump out of bed already dressed for the race of the day. Working two or more jobs to keep pace with the high cost of living, pushing themselves and their families toward ever bigger accomplishments, eating fast foods day in and day out because they have no time for wholesome, properly prepared meals, pushing down anxiety with drinking, overeating, and other destructive habits—all this and more leads to the stress that causes disease. People then start to rely on medication to get them through, as we are led to believe that being medicated equals health. Television ads say their miracle drugs are the answer for the millions of us who are suffering from arthritis, osteoporosis, depression, and the like. The trouble is, these endorsements quickly end with a long list of side effects that seem as bad as the condition itself. Plus, as we've mentioned, they are not claiming to cure conditions. They merely suggest that these drugs will diminish symptoms. Frequently, that translates into blocking pain receptors to help you feel better. The effect is temporary, causes a reliance on medication, and the drug does nothing to stop or reverse the progression of the disease. There has to be a better way.

In the conversations I had that day on Fifth Avenue, and in others, I've asked people to reframe the issue: What if, with some effort, you could make changes to give you the health and vitality to do more, feel better, and have less stress? Would you be willing to do so? To that, one person replied, "Gary, I don't want to end up with the diseases that so many people, just a little bit older than me, have. I do want to live a longer, quality life, and yes, I am willing to make some effort. It's just that this is all so new, and I don't know what it takes."

Here, from my point of view, is what it takes:

1. A willingness to set priorities in our lives, so that we're not constantly running a panicked race to get everything done.
2. A readiness to change our dietary and lifestyle habits, even if these changes are uncomfortable at first.
3. A curiosity about the science of optimizing health.

Incidentally, whether you're a baby boomer, Gen X-er, or senior, I know that you possess this third requisite. After all, you're reading this book!

There's a lot of promise and a sense of great expectations in the antiaging field. For instance, today more elders are plagued with Parkinson's disease than ever before, but antiaging researchers are discovering that Parkinson's patients have far lower than average levels of coenzyme Q10, a natural substance needed to promote energy production and fight disease-producing free radicals. Reintroducing coenzyme Q10, they find, may be a key component to slowing down the progression of Parkinson's, reversing symptoms, and even preventing the disease.[1]

This is not to say that substances such as Q10 are magic bullets. Because they are natural, their effects often take a while to be felt. Plus, in many instances, more research must be done before scientific breakthroughs can be confirmed. An example: Some scientists, swept off their feet by positive experiences with human growth hormone—they report increased alertness, fat loss, and renewed energy—are enthusiastically promoting its use, while others warn that more long-term studies are needed to confirm its safety and efficacy. Such controversies are inevitable in a new, rapidly developing field, and anyone considering an antiaging protocol, particularly one that incorporates hormones, should study the research to weigh the pros and cons, and work under the care of a knowledgeable and trusted physician.

Of course not every substance in the antiaging arsenal is controversial. Many substances are known to be safe in reasonable amounts; these include vitamins, minerals, enzymes, and herbs whose effects have been tested empirically for thousands of years and substantiated in multiple laboratory studies. The elderly usually require greater amounts of these substances—such as B vitamins, to improve memory function—and should utilize them as needed to promote healthful aging.

As we shall see, by promoting rejuvenation, nutrients can diminish or even eliminate a dependence on multiple medications, which has become a way of life for most senior citizens. The drugs on which elders rely on a daily basis have serious limitations: They do not correct the underlying cause of disease processes and, therefore, do not reverse illness; they may have dangerous side effects; they are also costly. In contrast, a nutritional analysis can help an individual determine the proportion of substances needed to correct an imbalance and return to health. For example, by understanding that high levels of blood fibrinogen are associated with a high risk of heart attack and stroke, and by knowing that such nutrients as vitamin C, fish oil, and bromelain lower fibrinogen levels, we can determine how much is needed to correct the imbalance so that our bodies once again function normally on their own.

Additionally, using these products should be only one facet of a healthy living plan that incorporates whole foods, regular exercise, and stress-management techniques. Improving our lifestyle habits may take effort, but the effort is well worth it, as the way we care (or don't care) for ourselves has a lot to do with the way we age. It is no secret that we live in an extremely toxic world. The problem is compounded for those with poor eating habits, particularly those who consume inordinate amounts of sugar and devitalized foods. Over a lifetime, these daily assaults cause an inevitable breakdown of our bodies, resulting in the diseases we associate with aging.

We've discussed senior citizens and baby boomers, but there's one more population group I want to mention: children. No, I don't think they're going to be interested in an antiaging protocol! But the example that their parents and grandparents set for them today will influence them long into the future, and have an impact on their health decades hence. Consider that as the pace of life quickens, poor habits and the diseases they promote trickle down to a much younger population. Just look at the many children today who consider fatty fast foods a dietary staple and who spend hours playing video and computer games rather than exercising. Never before have we seen so many disorders in children that are usually reserved for older populations—infirmities that include obesity, hardening of the arteries, and diabetes. This is scary, and it is a trend we must strive to reverse immediately.

WHAT'S HERE

So let's start our journey. We open our minds to allow for the possibility of change. In order to understand how to expand the human life span, both in length and quality, we must, in effect, see the challenge as a giant puzzle. In this book we will explore how various pieces of that puzzle fit together.

We'll begin, in Part I, by looking at what's working against us—at how our modern environment, as well as our own biological processes, contribute to aging. But if Part I is about the problem, the entire rest of the book will be about solutions.

In Part II, we'll take a "dive-right-in" approach to what you need to know about today's antiaging therapies. We'll look at hormonal keys to health, and then address specific concerns that many people have—maintaining cardiovascular function, facing the specter of cancer, and staying mentally sharp. And we'll go substance by substance down the list of today's antiaging armamentarium, explaining the benefits of each.

Part III is where we'll be putting it all together in a practical way so that you can start making positive changes. You probably have questions such as, How should I eat to maximize energy? What kind of exercise should I do to maintain flexibility? and What's the best way to lose weight? We'll have answers, and we'll be discussing everything from detoxification to strategies for each of the main meals of the day, to juicing, to exercising and liking it. By the way, I refer in this section to a "nondiet, no-exercise" program because I want to shake up the notion that a healthful life has to be lived as if it's a series of regimens. I want you to integrate such things as eating whole grains and moving aerobically into your routine so that they're not "dieting" or "exercising," but just living.

You'll be reading about a lot more in this "can-do" section. Chapter 10, on recipes for Power Aging, is both a program to jump-start your detox and a reference that will give you new ideas for how to prepare healthful soups, salads, main dishes, and more. As always, the emphasis is on the easy and great-tasting. For those particularly concerned about a specific common condition, I offer Chapter 11, a section on countering or preventing a variety of ailments; examples are allergies, colds, and osteoporosis. As in every book, I urge readers to consult their health care providers before making significant changes, but consider this volume a starting-off point in that process.

Part IV is a section providing additional help. There's a chapter on affirmations (meaning self-encouragement—check it out!) and another on what I call "Voices of Experience," in which people who have successfully used my antiaging strategies describe their journeys.

As you can see, there is a lot of information in this book that can help you improve your life. We'll be looking at beneficial changes you can make in your diet, your supplementation, and your environment, as well as in the areas of exercise and attitude. But this doesn't mean you must change everything right away. That would be overwhelming. Changes can be gradual but steady. After a while, you will begin to see life in a whole new way, and you will be able to make the changes you need to live longer, more healthfully, and more happily as well.

CHAPTER 2

IT'S THE ENVIRONMENT, STUPID!

*How the Environment Affects
Our Health*

NO, YOU'RE NOT STUPID, BUT THE ENVIRONMENT *IS* ALL-IMPORTANT

Most books about aging would start out with a discussion of the processes within your body that contribute to your getting old. We *are* going to do that—in the next chapter. What we're going to do in this one is look at how environmental factors— things that go on outside our bodies—can impinge upon what goes on within, and hence upon our health and longevity. The fact is that the environment we modern humans have made for ourselves is contributing to premature aging. I believe that this piece of the antiaging puzzle is so important that I want to start out with it.

In my view, the pollution in our bodies can be looked at as a microcosm of the pollution in our environments. You may never have thought about it, but imagine if you kept a journal for just a week to record all the different toxins that you encountered. What do you think would be on that list? First of all, you'd have to buy a pretty big notebook for the task. You'd have to include indoor and outdoor air pollution, such as motor vehicle and airplane exhaust, outgassing furniture and carpets in your office and home, thousands of industrial and agricultural chemical waste contaminants in our water supply, pesticide and fertilizer residues in both our fresh and processed foods, and synthetic additives and dangerous substances in everything from cosmetics to medicines—especially over-the-counter medicines, which require no prescription and hence are not thought to be dangerous.

And how about the caffeine that gets us started in the morning? The lunchtime cocktail to take the edge off the day? How about the cigarettes you smoke, or if you don't smoke, the secondhand fumes you breathe from those who do?

Is this picture familiar? It should be, because it's a broad sketch of our everyday exposure to harmful substances. And, sadly, it is a very wrong picture for our bodies. The reality is that we live in an extremely toxic world, far more toxic than that of our ancestors. And it's taking a toll on our bodies. In this chapter we'll survey the major ways environmental factors can affect us. The information is not meant to scare you, but rather to make you aware of possible roadblocks on the way to good health. In Parts II, III, and IV of this book, we'll be looking at ways to overcome them. But for now, let's take a step back to the world of our ancestors. . . .

A TRIP BACK IN TIME

Take a look at the life of someone living one hundred fifty years ago. What do you see? The majority of people live in an agrarian society, but do not use pesticides. They don't even have them. Nor do they have fungicides or genetically engineered crops. They don't use food irradiation, the equivalent of giving one hundred thousand chest X rays to a bunch of strawberries. And they don't give growth-stimulating hormones to their cattle to increase meat or dairy cow production (resulting in mastitis infections in the cows, which require antibiotic use, and produce pus in the milk).

Plus, look at the positive points in these people's lives. They generally eat lots of fruits and vegetables. The inhabitants of a typical farm in the U.S. work from sunup to sundown. It's a tough life, but they're exercising their bodies all day, and they have a purpose and meaning to their lives. They live in the midst of an extended family. They do things in balance and without extremes. They are patient, because they have learned the lessons of being impatient. They live for peace, harmony, and character development. Granted, this is an idealized picture of nineteenth-century life, and one not applicable to all Americans, but many people in the United States did live like this. So let's explore further.

By the time these nineteenth-century children reach sixth grade—likely in a little red schoolhouse—they are equivalent to today's eleventh graders. By necessity, people are more self-sufficient and interdependent. They share tasks. One person makes the quilts and does the mending. Another makes the candles or tends to the kerosene lamps so the family can read after sundown. One person runs the apothecary, grows herbs, and collects bee propolis, a natural antibiotic. They preserve perishables in honey because, while they don't know just *why*, they do know that honey doesn't go bad. Honey is also used to heal wounds and scratches. Someone has the job of drying fruit: Apples (of which there were two hundred varieties) are cut into thin slices, then strung on fishing wire to dry in the attic, or put out in the sun, covered with cheesecloth. After four days they have dried fruit that will last all year. Since grains, seeds, and nuts are easily stored, they generally always have them around, in giant barrels in storage areas together with dried fruit. In fact, many of the barns look a good deal like health food stores! They have a root cellar five feet underground where gourds, squash, potatoes, yams, rutabaga, kohlrabi, parsnips, carrots, and other root vegetables are stored. They have a cheese house containing many different cheeses, each aged in a wax casing and preserved on the outside by honey. They know that they can cut pieces off the cheese and have a good source of nourishment each day. Generally they do not kill their cows because they need them for plowing. Horses are used for hauling. They eat fish when they can be found, and if they're not consumed immediately, the entrails are removed, and they're salted and dried. They also dry a lot of vegetables. In the twenty-first century we might look at an old food dryer as a quaint technology, but one hundred fifty years ago it's a necessity in wintertime when people may not be able to get to a trading store. After all, there are no cars, and those living in the mountains, or even just in places like upstate New York, may be homebound for three or four months of the year. So they have to have everything they need for the winter ahead.

A typical day starts with a rich porridge, and later meals might include a hearty stew and, in summer, a fresh salad. While these people do not have the systematic workouts we design for ourselves today, they exercise vigorously every day. There is very little obesity. They use home remedies. And as long as they have good well water they have the potential to live long lives.

THE MOVE TO THE CITIES

It was when the Americans of one hundred fifty years ago moved to the cities that they ran into a whole set of problems. Unless they happened to have connections in that particular city, they lacked a support system. Most people who migrated had none. They were generally put into extremely harsh working conditions and given minimal pay. Children were forced to work for exploitative wages at industrial plants with none of today's safety standards. Families were under an enormous amount of stress, and malnutrition was rampant. The milk people drank came from multiple cows and was generally infected. The meat available to city dwellers was often vile. Tuberculosis, typhoid fever, chronic diarrhea—in short, many types of bacterial and viral infections—were common for those poor and stressed-out masses living in polluted areas and eating polluted foods. Naturally the affluent—those with clean water, decent sanitation, and variety in their diet, and those not under intense stress—were living longer lives. But still, it is interesting to see that generally the folks who lived longest also lived in the country.

A "GROWING" PROBLEM

The past century has seen some progress in raising people's awareness about the toxins in our lives. At the beginning of the century Upton Sinclair described the horrors of the meatpacking industry; his novel *The Jungle* told not only of contaminated meat, but also of the wrecked lives of impoverished workers in the industry. In the sixties, Rachel Carson's groundbreaking book *Silent Spring* warned of the dangers of pesticides and helped foster the burgeoning of a real environmental movement a decade later. But let's face it—when there are egos, power positions in society, and above all, monetary interests at stake, official policy change occurs at a glacial pace. At the same time industrialization and urban sprawl continue to grow, and it is unclear whether the environmental movement can meet the challenges of the future.

One thing is certain, though: What we don't know *will* hurt us. Here are just some examples of environmental realities we may not have known about. First, we have nearly one hundred thousand man-made chemicals today, and although some have been tested for safety singly, these have not been tested for safety in combinations. Yet we live in a world where everything is inhaled, eaten, and imbibed in combination. Water today can be contaminated with the medicines from AIDS, hepatitis, and chemotherapy patients. There is today so much excrement and toxic waste that it can't be totally contained. But it all has to go somewhere, and so microscopic amounts make it through the filters in our municipal water systems, come right back through the water we drink, and yes, end up in our bodies. True, these substances are present in very small amounts, but disease can result from as little as 100 parts per billion of a toxin. You don't need a large amount of a poison to cause injury to a cell.

And the problem is that no one is analyzing the damage toxins do to individual cells. Instead, researchers are looking for gross, obvious symptoms that can be tied to a single pollutant. And they're not necessarily going to find anything, because there could be a thousand different chemicals in a single glass of water, acting synergistically, and the research isn't sophisticated enough to pick up on this. Furthermore, in the single-pollutant studies, the researchers aren't looking specifically at the effects on people with weak immune systems, such as babies or senior citizens, who are already suffering from a disease. And these are the very populations that can be most impacted by pollutants.

Another little-discussed fact is that an extremely dangerous process has become a part of agriculture—the use of biosolids (human waste) for fertilizer. Such fertilizer can contain tiny amounts of toxic heavy metals, heat-resistant viruses, and chemicals from medications. Once these substances are in the soil they can enter the plants that we later eat.

A sad fact today is that many of the vegetables we eat have upwards of 60 percent fewer nutrients than their counterparts did just twenty-five to thirty years ago. So today, for example, when you buy a commercially grown lettuce, it doesn't have the same amounts of iron and magnesium—some of the very things you are eating it for—as lettuce did years ago. It is grossly lacking in these nutrients due to the growing methods of modern agribusiness. In short, our food gives us things we don't want and doesn't give us enough of what we do need. Could this have something to do with the increase in cancer, Hodgkin's disease, heart disease, stroke, and the other health calamities of modern life?

MESSING WITH MOTHER NATURE

In the past thirty years, Americans have finally had to start facing the grim results of our excessive messing with the natural order of things. Nature has let us know that the misuse of our air, water, and soil will not go unnoticed. On a large scale, the industrial revolution has brewed a heat-trapping mixture of carbon dioxide, nitrogen oxides, methane, and chlorofluorocarbons. The result is the worldwide greenhouse effect, in which the warming of the entire planet is causing the rapid melting of its polar ice caps, as well as unusual weather patterns worldwide, resulting in droughts and flooding.

Now, carbon dioxide is no villain: it is a naturally occurring gas that is not harmful when the ecosystem is in balance. We have managed, however, to make it a pollutant by releasing so much that its volume exceeds the earth's capacity to handle it. The burning of fossil fuels is a major contributor to this carbon dioxide buildup, and today we have a situation in which of the more than 5 billion tons of carbon dioxide being released worldwide, only half can be absorbed by the planet's oceans and forests.

Given that fact, the intentional burning of the rainforests of the Amazon to make way for cattle grazing is more than unacceptable—it's stupid! There's a double whammy with forest destruction, because, in addition to the carbon dioxide produced in the burning process, the trees destroyed would have taken up and used carbon dioxide, just as we use oxygen. Perhaps ten years ago people paid attention to this massive destruction, but now, typically, it's off the radar screen, as it is considered old news and there is so much else to grab our attention. Something new has taken its place. We're on to another idea; we want to watch reality shows! Well, in my view, a true reality show would present the international fast-food chains' need for more and cheaper hamburgers leading to the clear-cutting of Amazon hardwoods and the continued destruction of the land (to say nothing of our personal health) by raising cattle for the world's meat addiction.

Automobile emissions are another big contributor to atmospheric carbon dioxide. Not nearly enough attention is given to this today. Even people living in Los Angeles seem to accept their visibly dirty air with a shrug that says: "Okay, this environment is not good for us, but it's a good place to be because everyone wants to live next door to a movie star." They, and all of us, pay a big price for such indifference.

One aspect of that price is the phenomenon of acid rain. The very concept of acid rain should be enough to give you pause. It's like a curse: The by-products of our lifestyle—sulfur and nitrogen oxides from coal-burning power plants, as well as factory and automobile emissions—mix with precipitation in the atmosphere and then return to earth, sometimes thousands of miles from their source, showering an acidic solution onto our farmlands, forests, lakes, and oceans. (This could be in the form of rain, fog, snow, or dust.) The most common form of acid rain contains an acid that results from sulfur oxide emissions. It destroys the environment, an effect you can see if you fly over certain parts of some states, such as Connecticut and Maine. The land looks scorched, as if there has been a forest fire. This is the effect of acid rain on trees.

The aquatic ecosystem is altered too: when acid rain gets into freshwater lakes and streams, the bacteria and plankton at the bottom of the food chain are the first to die, followed by the insects, and finally the frogs and fish. While you might not care about the lives and deaths of individual insects, frogs, and fish, their demise should serve as a wake-up call that things are not going well with our stewardship of the earth.

THE ENVIRONMENT AND YOUR BODY

But what in the world does all this pollution have to do with aging? you might ask. After all, most of the pollutants and unhealthy foodstuffs in our lives are not going to cause acute, immediate reactions. And we've all heard of individuals who survived to a ripe old age while smoking cigarettes, eating additive-laced foods, and living in less than ideal environments. The point is that, in general, and over time, the pollutants we inhale or ingest are going to drag down our health. Our immune systems will be weakened, making us more susceptible to everything from colds to cancer. Toxins in food will inhibit the actions of our enzymes, resulting in less efficient action of our bodily systems. If we're interested in Power Aging—that is, in maximizing the power of our bodies and minds for as long as possible—anything that's going to lessen our efficiency is something to be guarded against.

In the final analysis, our bodies' efficiency is determined on the cellular level. The fight against aging is to a large extent the fight against oxidative stress that is undertaken by our cells as they are attacked by the unstable molecules called free radicals. You've probably heard of free radicals as factors that contribute to disease and aging—and this is true, because these oxidative culprits cause chromosomal damage and impair cellular function. On the other side of the battle lines are the antioxidants—substances such as vitamin E and selenium that we get from good food and that neutralize the damaging effects of free radicals. We run into trouble when the free radical–antioxidant balance in our bodies is tipped in favor of the former. Then we have the apoptosis, or programmed cell death, associated with the diseases and conditions of aging. And what environmental pollutants do, ultimately, is contribute to this harmful imbalance, either by actually containing free radicals or by impairing our antioxidant defenses against them.

Going back to the people who lived one hundred fifty years ago: they did not die of the same diseases we die of today. That's because they were not exposed to all the toxins that we are, which cause inflammatory responses and proliferation of DNA and chromosome damage; that is, they speed up the aging of the cell. They didn't have the artificial fertilizers, the pesticides, the adulterated food, and the contaminated water we have today. (Yes, there was polluted water, but people drank mainly well water, which, with the exception of limited incidents of arsenic and bacteria contamination, was healthy and clean.)

EVERY BREATH YOU TAKE

As animals with an innate mission to stay alive, our most immediate and constant need is air. We cannot survive without air for longer than three minutes. The oxygen we inhale enters our blood and is carried to all our cells so that they can create the energy that animates us. You would think that considering all this, we humans would have taken care to keep our air as pure as possible. But this has not been the case. During the past decade, for instance, researchers at Harvard

University estimated that air pollution from fossil fuel combustion was killing about 60,000 Americans every year.[1]

The major health threat from air pollution lies not in the kind of soot you can see, but rather in the fine-particle pollution that emanates from cars, trucks, fossil-fuel power plants, incinerators, and other sources. Fine-particle pollution has been related to a greater than 15 percent differential in death rates between the least-polluted cities and the most polluted. The mechanism of damage was examined in detail in the January 1995 edition of British medical journal *Lancet*, in which researchers described how particles lodged deep within the lung cause inflammation that leads to blood coagulation, to respiratory and circulatory diseases, and ultimately, death.[2]

Another major air-pollution problem is created when automotive exhaust fumes react with sunlight, producing ozone. Ozone is actually a form of oxygen; it differs in that its molecules each contain three atoms of the element instead of the usual two. In the upper reaches of the atmosphere this substance is actually protective, and you have no doubt heard of the ozone layer as a kind of shielding envelope that keeps excessive solar radiation from harming us.

In the lower atmosphere, though, it is excess ozone that is the problem. This colorless, odorless gas is a respiratory irritant, and can cause acute lung inflammation as well as decreased lung function. The very young, the very old, and people with preexisting respiratory conditions are particularly susceptible to ozone's damaging effects, which is one of the reasons why, on bad smog days, these people are advised to stay indoors. Ironically, though, retreating indoors is not always the answer when you want to breathe clean air, as we shall see in the next section.

INDOOR POLLUTION

You may think that your home is a safe oasis from environmental poisons, but the fact is that indoor pollution constitutes our largest exposure to toxins. Chloroform, formaldehyde, and benzene are some of the problematic fumes encountered indoors; they emanate from paints, building materials, and dry-cleaned clothes, among other sources. So while that suit you just picked up from the cleaner's may have a nice clean smell, it's actually toxic. Bleach is toxic, and if you're using it, you are breathing it in. At the workplace you can be exposed to all forms of outgassing fumes from copy machines, paint, carpeting, and furniture. The individual has more control over indoor pollution—as opposed to the outdoor type—and high-quality air purifiers are a means of protection from these fumes, although eliminating the sources whenever possible is obviously the best approach. In Chapter 9, we'll be talking more on how to detoxify your environment.

You should be aware that some dangerous indoor pollutants are totally odorless. Carbon monoxide, for one, can escape from space heaters, furnaces, stoves, and other appliances, especially when you're not ventilating them properly. Carbon monoxide poisoning from space heaters alone causes over two hundred people a year to die in the United States, and there have been many others who are exposed to carbon monoxide levels that exceed health standards and who are subtly sickened by the gas without realizing it. That's why every household should have a carbon monoxide detector. Then there is radon gas, another odorless and invisible pollutant. It is produced in the soil by deteriorating uranium, which then seeps indoors through cracks in basements. According to a National Academy of Sciences report, as many as 13,000 lung-related deaths each year can be attributed to radon exposure.[3] Kits are available to help you determine if your basement has a radon problem, and, if it does, protective sealants can be used to prevent contamination.

In recent years, Americans' drive to save energy has caused many of us to try to make our homes and offices as airtight as possible. The downside of this is that we're sealing ourselves in with pollutants, particularly volatile organic chemicals such as formaldehyde. Yes, this is the active ingredient in embalming fluid, but it's being used in a lot of other places besides dead bodies these days: in plywood, paneling, fiberboard, plastics, upholstery, carpeting, paper products, cosmetics, eye makeup, nail polish, and even in permanent-press clothing. It can be an extreme irritant to the lungs, sinuses, and liver. Low-level exposure to formaldehyde is associated with eye irritation, headaches, asthma, and depression.

Another problem for those living or working in sealed environments with closed ventilation systems is bacterial contamination. An extreme example is the Legionnaires' disease that felled thirty-four people in the 1970s; members of a veterans' club had been staying at a hotel with an inadequately maintained air-conditioning system in which lethal amounts of a deadly bacterium had been allowed to build up. Two hundred men fell seriously ill with a mysterious, pneumonia-like disease. Since then, we've realized that cooling and heating ducts can accumulate all sorts of debris, ranging from the microscopic to dead mammals, and the germs from these can then be recirculated ad nauseam (literally!) throughout the building.

THE GOOD EARTH

An important part of the puzzle of aging is our relationship with the soil in which we grow our food. If you're a city person, you may never have given it much thought, but soil is more than "dirt." It is where nutrition begins. It contains the raw materials that provide us with our amber waves of grain, and with all the other vegetable foodstuffs that nourish us. The topsoil, which serves as the growing medium for most plant foods, is a vibrant and active system. It consists, partly, of tiny rock particles and dust, made when water and wind break down larger chunks of rock. Another important component, known as humus, is a mixture comprised primarily of decaying vegetables and animal waste. Inside this rich topsoil is a complicated world of living organisms that help plants assimilate minerals from rock particles and other chemical compounds. Fungi, bacteria, earthworms, and insects are among the many forms of life that feed on humus. Thus these small life-forms slowly decompose plants left from the previous growing season, as well as animal carcasses and manure. They also aerate the soil so that gases can be exchanged and water absorbed. As a result both sulfuric and carbonic acid are generated, which further decays the rocks and releases their mineral contents, thus enriching the soil.

Out west, in unpolluted areas, this rich topsoil can sometimes go down to a depth of ten feet. However, in some midwestern states, such as Indiana and Kansas, it might go down only two inches. The sad fact is that, through mismanagement of the land, we have greatly reduced the quality of the topsoil left in some parts of the United States.

Let's look back into history again, to the 1830s. Then, each farm had a wide variety of crops growing on its land—and these were relatively small farms. A century later, in the 1930s, farms were larger, but now they grew only one crop. This crop was generally grown for feeding livestock that became meat for humans. Corn, soybeans, and wheat were the three primary crops grown in the United States. Corn is notorious for depleting the quality of the soil, and if you keep taking nourishment out of the soil without putting it back in, bad things begin to happen to it. In the wintertime the soil cracks after freezing, and water from melting snow carries remaining topsoil away, causing massive erosion.

That is what was happening in the "dust bowls" of the thirties. You may remember the tragic consequences of this chain of events depicted in John Steinbeck's novel *The Grapes of Wrath*. People had to give up their farms because they couldn't grow anything; their fields had become one big, dusty wasteland. This was a result of drought combined with poor soil management. Instead of growing a diversity of rotated crops, resting fields for a season, and putting in soybeans in the wintertime to protect the soil from erosion, farmers were just pumping out one harvest after another—and always the same crop—year after year. Not that they necessarily had a choice economically: they were being paid by the bushel, and as long as they could get their crop out they could meet basic expenses. But they could not control the price of the wheat or corn, and they didn't have enough money to rest their fields for a year or two. They were using every acre they had and mortgaging their houses and equipment. They worked hard, but they could not afford to work smart.

Today, we still live to some extent with the legacy of that time. We still have massive erosion, except we have used artificial fertilizers that were not available in the 1930s to give the impression that our topsoil is healthy when it is not. These fertilizers are in effect a disguise, used to hide the fact that we have not maintained an ecological balance.

WHAT'S WRONG WITH ARTIFICIAL FERTILIZER?

For most of the twelve thousand years since plants were first domesticated, farmers simply supplemented nature with organic fertilizers. They also learned to rotate crops or let fields lie fallow so that the soil's nutrients could be replenished. This was good soil management, since the earth was not forced to produce more than it is constitutionally able to bear.

The picture started to change in the early nineteenth century when a German chemist named Justus Liebig discovered that plants could be artificially fertilized with chemicals. He burnt numerous species of plants, analyzed the substances found in the ashes, and determined that the soil was merely a mixture of these substances. That was the beginning of artificial fertilizer. But his was not a scientifically sound conclusion. It failed to take into account that soil is more than its mineral content. Liebig all but ignored the organic, living components of soil that are contained in humus: the moles, mice, shrews, earthworms, and microorganisms—the indispensable life-generating part of our soil. Liebig was a reductionist. He dealt only with nitrogen, phosphorous, and potash, which he could create artificially. And the day the American farm started using this type of artificial fertilizer was the day the American farmer's fortune started to decline. Such poor soil management robbed our land of one-fourth of its topsoil.

It takes about seven hundred years to create one single inch of topsoil—and a small fraction of that time to lose it. Most of the early settlers and pioneers were not concerned with soil conservation because, after all, land was cheap or free. People could do what they wanted with their land—institute monocrop agriculture, cut down trees that would be better left to hold in moisture and hold back wind—and when the land didn't bear any more crops they could simply move west.

And what about today? Are we better off? Sadly, we are not. We have not replaced the topsoil. We simply use artificial fertilizers containing mainly nitrogen, phosphorous, and potash, which are not supportive of the organisms that create topsoil. In some soil, you can't find a worm. They simply cannot survive in the acidic environment created by these chemicals. In Australia, for example, nine-foot-long earthworms originally present in vast numbers were completely exterminated by sulfur phosphate fertilizer. And if a worm cannot survive in soil, that's a sign that the soil will not produce good crops worth eating.

A problem with chemical fertilizers is the nitrates contained in the water runoff from the fields. When too much of this runoff seeps into ponds and wells, it renders their water unfit for human or animal use. Animals that drink nitrate-containing water lose weight and are no longer able to utilize their food completely. Cows show the symptoms of nitrate poisoning by producing less milk. Humans also should not be ingesting nitrates from well water. In fact, many American farmers cannot drink from their own wells because of this pollution.

There is something that we can do to counter these destructive agricultural trends—we can buy organic produce. By doing so, we are supporting a return to natural, ecologically sound ways of managing soil. And, as an important bonus, we are getting higher nutrient value from these foods, a point we'll be discussing further in Chapter 9. You can think of it this way: a crucial part of your journey to health and longevity is buying produce. Is it going to be organic or nonorganic? If you think, "Well, I don't really care, it doesn't make that much of a difference," just remember the dust bowls of the thirties. Plus remember that you're not getting optimal nutritional content from food that hasn't been grown organically. It may look like a head of lettuce, or a pear, or a strawberry, but the nutrients are not there, because they were not in the soil. Why would you want to buy something that dishonors nature and does not nourish you the way it was meant to? And this is before we even consider the ever-increasing presence of pesticides!

WE'RE EATING *WHAT*?

Again, this chapter is not meant to be alarmist, but if you're going to embark upon a program of power aging, you have to understand your dietary choices. And, unfortunately, a lot of the choices available today are laced with pesticides.

The Problems with Pesticides

All pesticides have the potential to be health threatening; they can be extremely reactive with our central nervous system, and they can be carcinogenic. You may think that when you wash a vegetable or fruit you are getting rid of pesticide residues, but you can't wash off the substances that have entered the plant itself. So the nonorganically grown foods you eat—whether fresh, canned, or frozen—can present a health problem. This is especially true if you juice them, because then you're getting a higher concentration of pesticides. Note that the most heavily sprayed fruits are grapes and strawberries.

I find it scandalous how many Americans are poisoned by pesticides—as well as fungicides and herbicides—and how many people worldwide die from them: over 200,000 a year.[4] But agribusiness and the U.S. Department of Agriculture defend the use of these very toxic products. Why? Well, they're supposed to stop insect pests, fungi, and weeds. And they did at one time. But their effectiveness has diminished as pests and weeds have developed resistance to these chemicals. Before their advent, farmers were actually better off because pests could be controlled by the natural method of crop rotation. So one year, for instance, wheat was planted, the next, soybeans, and the next, cotton. That way a certain bug that liked one plant was at a disadvantage the next year. When they started planting nothing but cotton or nothing but wheat, the insects that favored that particular crop just took up house in the soil! Today, as we've mentioned, organic farmers, who by definition use no pesticides or herbicides, are perforce going back to such natural agricultural techniques as crop rotation. Again, eating organically pays off not just in a personal way; it helps the health of the earth as well.

It also helps those who work in the fields. As a reader of this book you may or may not have anything to do with agricultural fieldwork, but I believe we should all care about those who grow and harvest our food, and about the fact that pesticides put these workers at greater risk for leukemia, glioma (a brain cancer), Parkinson's disease, lymphoma, soft tissue sarcomas, tumors of the skin and prostate, and stomach cancer.

These chemicals are neurotoxins. And they are stored away in our fat tissues. The more fat you have, the more toxic pesticides you are carrying around—so overweight Americans, beware! To approach this problem from a positive angle, you should know that with proper weight loss and detoxification—subjects we'll be discussing in Chapter 9—you'll be able to remove from your body many of the accumulated toxins from the past, and then repair the damage done by them.

Our Overly Processed Food

In general, the more processed a food is, the worse it is for our health. Therefore there is yet another danger, even when we're dealing with organic food: additives. Most of the food you eat has been chemically treated at different stages of production. By the time it reaches the supermarket shelf, or even the health food store shelf, it has little in common with its original state. Most commercially grown, processed foods, whether of animal or plant origin, have their appearance, texture, and nutritional value manipulated and transformed by a lot of chemical wizardry. And these chemicals, which fall under the general category of food additives, range from reasonably benign food coloring to highly dangerous preservatives such as sodium nitrate and sodium nitrite, which contribute to the formation of cancer-causing toxins in our bodies. Other chemicals used include: degerming agents, artificial flavorings, synthetic dyes, flavor enhancers, stabilizers, mold inhibitors, aging agents, preservatives, bleaches, emulsifiers, and conditioners. In sum, we're eating fake and adulterated foods that have been stripped of much nutritional value.

This is why I believe many people who decide to be conscientious about their health start out by asking the wrong questions: Should I be on a high carbohydrate diet? they ask, or, What about a low carbohydrate, high protein diet? Such questions, having to do mainly with caloric content, are fine for a later stage of our journey, but more basic questions are, Is this food adulterated in any way? Is it denatured? Is it highly processed? Denatured foods are more likely to be concentrated in their sugars. They have no vital life energy. They have little or no enzymatic activity. They lack antioxidants. Eating some of them is practically like eating paper! For instance, processed cheese may be a combination of water, vegetable oil, powdered casein, and milk protein. Breads and cereals contain BHA and BHT, calcium proprionate, glycerides, conditioners, and emulsifiers. And the foods sold as substitutes, such as margarine, bacon bits, artificial whipped cream, and nondairy creamers, are filled with chemicals, colorings, and preservatives. Did you know that more than twenty-nine hundred food additives are currently available and being applied to your foods? Do you know whether these have been proven safe? The fact is that they have not been. Then why eat them?

Let's use BHA and BHT (butylated hydroxyanisole and butylated hydroxytoluene) as examples. These are petroleum products used to preserve fats and oils in foods, ranging from potato chips to cakes to meat to cottage cheese and to cereal, as well as in cosmetics and pharmaceuticals. They have never been proven safe. Some people have difficulty metabolizing BHT and BHA, experiencing physical and even behavioral effects.

Sodium nitrate and sodium nitrite are two additives used for curing meat and smoked fish. Neither is good for you! When you see processed meat that is kept red, it's frequently because this type of additive has been used as a color fixative. We don't want that, even if the meat industry does. A dead and decaying animal's flesh is not red; it's a color that would turn you off completely. And while nitrates and nitrites do serve to prevent botulism and enhance flavor, when they combine in your body with substances called amines, they become the carcinogenic chemicals known as nitrosamines. That's why I advise that foods with these additives be avoided completely.

Another problem category is the bromates, such as potassium bromate, used in flour and baked goods. These are supposed to improve baking results, but they're not needed, especially when you consider that they have been implicated as being causative of tumors. Look for "unbromated" on product labels to avoid this risk.

Let's proceed to food coloring agents, another additive that we don't really need. Why is it necessary to have our food colored? Even dog food is colored these days, and dogs are color-blind! Ninety percent of the colorings used by food manufacturers are synthetic, and most are coal-tar derivatives. They're put into soft drinks and wines, breads, cakes, and cereals. By using these dyes, manufacturers can make a food the color they think consumers want. For example, when you buy the most commonly available Atlantic farm-raised salmon, that pink flesh color you see is unnatural. A coloring agent has been added to the fish feed to make you think the salmon is good-looking. And the label "certified artificial color" means nothing substantial, because the USDA cannot certify something safe. In fact, of the nineteen dyes certified by the FDA under the Food, Drug, and Cosmetic Act, nine had to be decertified twenty years later when laboratory tests found them to be carcinogenic. Here are the names of colorings that used to be in all kinds of foods: Sudan 1; butter yellow 1, 3, and 4; red 1, 4, and 32; and orange 1 and 2. Although they are no longer used today, others have taken their place.

The coal-tar dyes are dangerous. When heated in the absence of air, coal is converted into coal gas and coal tar, which is a viscous black liquid. Ninety-five percent of synthetic colorings used in the U.S. are coal-tar derivatives. Red dye number 2 is the most infamous of these. But none of them should be used. Their health risks are beyond dispute. By the way, I would also stay away from other dyes, such as hair dyes.

Two thirds of the food additives used in the United States are synthetic flavorings. Do we need them? Well, you do if you're a manufacturer who wants to skimp on genuine ingredients and provide the public with flavor that is at least consistent. But there's a trade-off, and it involves the public's health. Example: the flavoring called safrole, used in root beer until 1960, was eventually found to cause liver cancer. But what about all the people who drank root beer in the fifties, when safrole was on the "generally recognized as safe" list? While there is no undoing the mistakes of the past, we can all make an effort, from our next meal forward, to avoid the artificial in our food, whether it be in the form of flavoring, coloring, or other additives.

If you start studying labels, you realize how much in our food is artificial. Are you familiar with diethylprocarbonate, or DEPC? It's a chemical that prevents the growth of microbes in fruit drinks and alcoholic beverages. DEPC has been found to combine with ammonia to form a potent carcinogen. And where do we get the ammonium? It's a by-product of a high-protein diet, the kind that's so popular for weight loss these days. There are many more agents: EDTA, glycerides, monosodium glutamate, probyl galate, sodium citrate, sorbitol, sulfiting agents, and disodium phosphate, a sequestering agent used in evaporated milk, macaroni, and noodle products. Two words to the wise: Avoid them!

Irradiated and Genetically Modified Foods

Did you know that the chicken you were planning on having for dinner could have been irradiated? That the fruits and vegetables on your table could have been as well? And here's a really perplexing question: Why would we want to use high-level nuclear waste, including the radioactive substances cesium 137, cobalt 60, strontium 90, and plutonium 238, to irradiate our food? One answer is that radiation kills bacteria and extends the shelf life of foods. But the negative side effects of this technology cannot be ignored. For one thing, sending ionizing radiation through foods results in chemicals that are known or suspected instigators of birth defects or cancer; these include benzene and cyclobutanones. Also, vitamins and essential fatty acids are destroyed in the process so that, once again, as with artificially fertilized foods, we are eating "less than meets the eye." Further, we do not know the long-term effects of eating irradiated foods. Americans—especially those interested in healthful aging—should be asking more questions about what's happening to their food before it reaches their supermarket shelves.

The genetic engineering of food is another area that we should be examining closely, and, in my view, soundly rejecting. Traditional methods of breeding combine two animals or two plants in an effort to produce a new strain that offers the good points of each. But genetic engineering goes way beyond this by cutting and splicing genetic material between two totally different types of organisms. So today we have GM (genetically modified) food plants that contain genes from bacteria, for instance, and we may soon have insect, fish, or other animal genes in the plants we eat.

There are so many problems here that it's hard to know where to begin. Perhaps first we should mention the fact that this audaciously unnatural experiment is invisible to American consumers. That's because our laws do not require labeling of GM food. Already, genetically modified ingredients are being added into the processed food we buy, without our knowledge, even though surveys have shown that the vast majority of Americans favor such labeling. There's an ethical problem with consumers being kept in the dark about the true nature of the food they are buying, eating, and feeding their children; it is particularly troubling for vegetarians, who can now no longer be sure that a seeming plant food does not contain animal genes.

We should never lose sight of the fact that genetic engineering is not a time-tested practice; it is an experiment. Some of the questions this experiment may eventually answer are: Will cross-species and cross-kingdom genetic transfers result in unforeseen diseases and weaknesses, both in the plants created and in those who consume them? Will the inserted genes produce toxins? Will some people prove to be seriously allergic to these new foods? Some plants are being genetically engineered to produce their own pesticides; will these unintentionally destroy beneficial insects and bacteria? The list of possible problems is longer still, but the main point is that this is a risky experiment that is being conducted on our food supply, on our health, and on our ecosystem—all without our approval.

Two other important points must be made about this technology. One is that we do not need it in order to feed the world, a task that could be accomplished by making the right geopolitical and economic changes. So this form of "progress" is something that is being carried out for the benefit of companies—not humanity. Second, once health-damaging effects caused by genetic engineering occur, there is no cleaning them up. Genetic mistakes are passed down in perpetuity, and this is yet another reason society should think twice before accepting this vast modification of agriculture as we've previously known it.

The Danger in Sugar

To return to the relatively controllable sphere of our dinner table, let's look at one of the really dangerous single items in our diet—sugar. This is a crucial piece of the aging puzzle. High up on my list of things that will cause cells to be attacked, cause disease, and cause premature aging is this white poison (and sugar substitutes as well). I strongly urge you to take action vis-à-vis this "drug of choice," before it is too late! Sugar is denatured, devitalized, and shouldn't be consumed at all. Yet Americans, on average, consume 140 to 160 pounds of sugar yearly. Picture this in terms of thirty 5-pound bags of the stuff, and know that these are truly empty calories. The typical American diet can easily give you 50 teaspoons per day, when you take into account both the sugar in prepackaged foods and that added at the table. And these 50 teaspoons represent more than 800 calories, approximately one third of the body's total daily requirement of food energy! This dulcet danger is going to adversely affect blood sugar, and here's the bad part: when you have an elevated blood-sugar level, you're going to elevate your insulin level. You're also going to elevate your stress hormones, which follow right behind your blood sugar. These are all capable of causing inflammatory responders to go into high gear in the body, and this can damage the mitochondria of the cells, which are their main energy-producers. When the mitochondria are damaged by constant elevation of blood sugar, especially if you are overweight, this may constitute a prediabetic or diabetic condition. More often than not, this causes the opening of what is known as the mega-channel in the mitochondria. The mega-channel is like the doorway that allows the cell to function properly. Once you've allowed the energy of that cell to be depleted through this mega-channel, the cell deteriorates and dies. This may not happen in a straightforward or orderly fashion, but it is responsible for the fatigue felt by so many sugarholics.

Ask baby boomers or senior citizens "What are the two most common problems you face?" and they'll be very likely to answer "Fatigue and pain." Well, an elevated blood sugar level contributes to both. It prematurely ages the cells. Plus scientific studies show that, in general, you can shorten your life span by increasing your caloric intake. And conversely, by decreasing caloric intake you can lengthen the life span by preserving cells. Thus, it is high time to stop our national bingeing on refined carbohydrates such as sugar!

Any simple, or refined, carbohydrate can contribute to dysinsulinism. So in addition to sugar, white-flour baked goods, such as pastries, breads, and bagels, and white-flour pastas, are going to disrupt the body's metabolism and hormone levels because they provide the cells with pure energy and little else in terms of nutrients. The body's engine doesn't work that way. It needs a full spectrum of nutrients in order to thrive, and refined carbohydrates do not provide this. So the body takes these nutrients out of healthy cells, leeching precious vitamins, minerals, and enzymes from itself. The advice "eat sugar for quick energy" has become one of the most successful techniques to lure the nutritionally ignorant into a form of sweet suicide. What happens when you follow this advice is that you get a rebound or yo-yo effect: First, the sugar is absorbed much too rapidly into the bloodstream. (And this is when you do get a brief rush of energy.) As a result, the pancreas releases a lot of insulin in an attempt to bring the blood sugar level down again. Then, though, when the level goes down, it plummets, you are fatigued, and you have a hunger for more sugar! So you indulge again, your blood sugar level goes way up again, and the up-and-down cycle continues, with the down part of it leading very possibly to hypoglycemia and its associated fatigue, headaches, depression, and irritability. Think of the people in this country who have been tired, irascible, or overweight, and who have gone to their doctor and been given a prescription for a psychotropic medication, when all they had was a self-inflicted sugar habit.

Refined sugar is actually a poor energy source. Sucrose, or white sugar, consumption lowers performance levels in children. Still, their most common reaction is to reach for something sweet and repeat the process. Actually, since sugar in its natural state is a vital component of plants, such as the sugar beet or sugar cane, the raw material of sugar does contain valuable nutrients. It's the refining process that destroys them. I recommend that if your children or you want something sweet, use raw, unfiltered, organic honey, and use it sparingly. Another wholesome sugar alternative, good in home baking, is pure maple syrup.

Other problems with sugar are that its overconsumption challenges the immune system, reducing antibody activity. And eating sugar makes one less hungry for more nutritious food. This substance's lure, of course, is that it is quick and convenient as a "feel good" food and it is cheap for the food industry. And, sure enough, when the industry wants to make you quickly feel good—and increase profits—they add sugar, in one or more of its many forms. Glucose, corn syrup, sucrose, and fructose are all very inexpensive. These substances can be found in dozens of foods, including canned corned beef hash, ketchup, canned and powdered soups, salad dressings, peanut butter, boxed casserole "helpers," and frozen dinners. So avoiding this health compromiser is more than just avoiding cookies, cakes, and the like. You have to be really diligent about reading labels,

and, when possible, preparing your meals from scratch. We'll be looking at how to do this—deliciously—in Chapter 10.

You might be thinking at this point that artificial sweeteners
are the way to go. Actually, they're the way to go wrong. Don't use
them. It is common for people to have neurological problems—
headaches, migraines, and attention and cognition difficulties—after
using these sweeteners. Also, the sugar substitute aspartame is particularly dangerous for those with the metabolic condition called PKU
(phenylketonuria).

More Bad News about the Sweet Stuff

A serious risk for people who chronically overindulge in sugar is type II
diabetes. Diabetes is the opposite of hypoglycemia, and it is amazing
how widespread this condition is. We're now seeing it in children,
where previously it has been a disease of the middle-aged and older.
Diabetes results from an inadequate supply of insulin, too much
sugar in the blood, improper cell utilization of insulin, or a combination of these factors. When the pancreas becomes exhausted by the
constant demand of producing insulin to convert all that sugar into
heat and energy, it finally malfunctions and the excess sugar then
pollutes the bloodstream. And without sufficient insulin to process
glucose, the body is deprived of an essential food and the diabetic remains hungry no matter how much he or she eats. Sugar accumulates
in the bloodstream faster than the body can excrete it through the
urine, and the victim is literally poisoned. He becomes tired, weak,
nauseated, and depressed. Holistic doctors attempt to counter this
condition with a multifaceted approach, as opposed to relying too
much on insulin. With lifestyle changes, some type II diabetics can
reduce or eliminate their insulin requirements altogether. Components of this are exercise, weight control, eating healthful complex
carbohydrates and quality protein, and taking the right supplements.

Sugar also plays havoc with our teeth. It feeds the bacteria normally present in the mouth, causing them to multiply. This leads to
plaque formation, cavities, and gum disease. Tooth enamel is the

strongest material in the body, and yet the bacteria inside plaque are able to eat through the enamel and attack the dentine inside, then the pulp that feeds the tooth, and finally the root canal, causing a toothache and eventually destroying the tooth. Meanwhile, the excess sugar inside the stomach depletes the body's calcium supply, further weakening the tooth's ability to protect itself. The gums suffer as well because the soft, sticky nature of overrefined foods does not supply sufficient friction during chewing to keep the gum margins hard, stimulated, and tight around the teeth. Periodontal disease results when the plaque collects at the base of the teeth and forms into a hard deposit called tartar. In this case bacteria attack the gums and bones that support the teeth, causing bleeding and swelling. Periodontal disease is endemic in our society, and one more problem for which we can accurately blame sugar.

The list of sugar-related problems goes on. It leads to obesity because surplus sugar gets stored in the body as fat. And this then makes sugar a contributor to coronary heart disease, because the more overweight you are with stored fat, the more susceptible you'll be to clogged arteries and free radical pathology.

Sugar can cause gastrointestinal trouble. And I believe it's also a primary contributor to hyperactivity in children. Sending your kids off to school with a lot of sugar in them makes them more prone to the kind of "bouncing off the walls" activity that leads to an ADHD diagnosis. And it matters not if the sugar is in the form of corn syrup, glucose, fructose, or sucrose. In all these forms it is bad for your children and bad for all of us. Let's keep our cells young and healthy by never using refined sugar. That will be an important achievement in our journey to longevity and a disease-free life.

OUR WATER

Another important aspect of maintaining health is drinking lots of pure water. Since up to 74 percent of your body's tissues are water, it's really your number-one nutrient. Do you know what's in the water you drink? Have you been led to believe it's clean because municipalities put chlorine into it? This is not the case. While chlorine does kill some germs, it does not affect other harmful microorganisms, including parasites, to say nothing of industrial pollutants and drug residues.

There are five major categories of harmful substances in our water supply. The first is, ironically, the additives that are put into it with the intention of helping us. Chlorine itself is one; although it disinfects water to some extent, its prolonged ingestion has been associated with cancer. Another widely used additive is fluoride, which is supposed to prevent tooth decay. In truth, fluoride is a poison when overconsumed, and it's hard to control the level at which people ingest it, since it's in other sources. Too much fluoride can cause the discoloration of the teeth—called fluorosis—skin rashes, and a variety of other problems, some as serious as bone cancer.

Waterborne microorganisms such as bacteria and viruses constitute a large class of pollutants, and while chlorine does kill many, others of these disease-causers—particularly protozoan parasites such as giardia and cryptosporidium—can live in a chlorinated environment. Toxic minerals and metals are a third class of water pollutant. These include aluminum, asbestos, cadmium, and mercury. A toxic metal that can leach into water from old pipes is lead, which will accumulate in the body until it causes health problems.

Organic chemicals from fertilizers, pesticides, and fuels are a tremendous problem in water supplies. We've already mentioned volatile organic chemicals, or VOCs, in relation to air pollution, but they're in water too. Benzene, from such sources as paint removers and plastics, is a common example of this type of pollutant, which can cause harm to the nervous system, among other bodily systems that are extremely important to our functioning. Other organic chemicals, the polychlorinated biphenols, or PCBs, are notorious carcinogens that have been illegally released by industry into our waterways. Lastly, our water can be contaminated by radioactive substances that come from mining, nuclear power plant discharge water, and other sources.

While we can't clean up the nation's water supply at this moment, the good news is that you can screen out these pollutants from your own personal supply. Home filtration systems are effective. Distilled water is an excellent alternative to tap water, and spring water, if you know the spring and have a list of the minerals present, is good too. We'll be mentioning this again in Chapters 9 and 10, to remind you of the importance of making sure your primary beverage is as clean as possible.

. . . AND WHAT ABOUT YOUR EMOTIONAL ENVIRONMENT?

I've saved it for last, but I actually feel that the most important aspect of any person's environment is not a physical factor, but rather the individual's emotional environment. By this I mean the attitudes she or he carries around all day, the kinds of interactions that person has with others, and the general tenor of his or her lifestyle. All of this is going to have a big impact on how successfully that individual ages, because when there's a lot of stress in a person's emotional environment, it takes a toll. When you're constantly stressed, your body is full of "fight-or-flight" hormones, which over time weaken the immune system.

Let's Ask Questions

I'm always advocating that people ask themselves questions. "Are we missing something?" is a good one to start with. Our society fosters a great deal of stress, and it's my opinion that in our constant search for a higher standard of living we really are missing something. What we're missing is the fact that a high standard of living is not synonymous with a good quality of life.

When I've asked people in my surveys, "If you could do anything right now, what would you like to change?" they've responded with answers like the following.

"Live a less complicated life."

"Slow it down, spend more time with what I really enjoy—my family, a relationship, my pets, going to museums, reading."

"I like to catch up on stuff, and so I look forward to my vacations, but even those are stressful since I've got to cram it all into a few weeks."

"Everything is just too fast!"

Here's a question: What is "fast" for? Ultimately the quick, unrelenting pace of modern life is deemed necessary so we can afford things in order to support a certain standard of living. We assume we are just going to reach into that standard of living and pull out a good quality of life. But what we pull out is everything that stresses us to the max.

So you might want to ask yourself the following: "Do I have to keep making this amount of money just to support the house and lifestyle I've become used to?" And the answer is probably yes. "Have I thought about changing my standard of living, reducing it, deconstructing it?" That's probably a no. "Do I pride myself on being able to afford an expensive dinner?" "Have I really thought about the necessity of buying a high-priced cappuccino every day?" "Have I thought about the long-term true cost (to my health) of repeated fast food indulgences?" "Why am I living in New York City?" To afford to live in a decent-sized apartment in New York is extremely expensive. In one building, for example, monthly rent for a two-bedroom apartment averages five thousand dollars, and how many people can afford that without working themselves into an early grave?

Of course I don't know how you're going to answer all these questions. I don't even know if you live in a city or drink cappuccinos, or if I have a right to make assumptions about you or tell you how to live. I don't, actually. But my point is simply this: However you choose to live, make sure it's a conscious choice, and that it's your own choice—not the choice of some voice from your upbringing, or the Joneses' choice, or your coworkers' choice, or Gary Null's choice. If you make conscious choices based on your own needs, chances are, your emotional environment will be a nontoxic one. We'll be talking more about these issues, particularly in relation to stress-reduction, in Chapter 13, on affirmations.

CHAPTER 3

WHY DO WE AGE?

The Biological Processes of Aging

W hat causes aging? The easy answer to that question is the uncontrollable passage of time. But aging is also the result of a number of biological and pathological processes that vary from person to person and that *are* controllable to some degree, with existing therapies. Consider that some people retain a good appearance and abundant health well into their senior years, while others start to fall apart soon after thirty. Depending upon the rate at which a person's body ages, that individual's chronological age, or age in years, can differ markedly from his or her biological age. So understanding the biological processes involved can really pay off. To the extent that we can effectively counter these processes, we can prevent or postpone the diseases that cripple and kill us. What's more, by forestalling age-related diseases, we put ourselves in a position to take advantage of future medical breakthroughs that could result in dramatic extensions of the healthy human life span.[1]

The Life Extension Foundation is a group dedicated to using science to address the problems of disease, aging, and death, and the following information on the mechanisms of aging is based largely on their synthesis of what is known in this field at the present time.

WHAT TELOMERES TELL US

Some of the most exciting research going on in the antiaging field involves a new understanding of what goes on deep inside the human cell. It has long been known that our DNA will facilitate only about sixty to eighty cell replications, with variations depending upon the particular organ involved. As they approach the end of their programmed life spans, older cells divide less rapidly and less efficiently. Today, scientists are furthering our understanding of this process of cell senescence by taking note of structures called telomeres; these are small fragments, composed of DNA, that form the protective ends of chromosomes. What scientists are seeing is that with each new cell division, the telomeres are shortened, and that after these structures shrink down to a certain size, cell division stops. In other words, telomeres are a kind of biological clock, with decreasing length indicating a decreasing amount of cell lifetime left.

But what if we could replenish shrinking telomeres? A recent development leads some researchers to think that this might be possible. A naturally occurring enzyme called telomerase has been discovered, and what it seems able to do is copy the telomeres' RNA in the form of DNA, and then put it on the ends of chromosomes, thereby extending cell life. The down side of telomerase is that it plays a role in the unchecked cell growth that is cancer. However, experiments with yeast telomerase show some promise in the area of genetic manipulation of the enzyme in order to stop cancer cell division. A really intriguing question is whether it will be possible to use telomerase to increase the life span of cells—without causing cancer. This has actually already been accomplished experimentally. The telomerase gene was introduced into human cells that then went on to divide more times than they ordinarily would, and thus live longer, without becoming cancerous.

Additional research into the telomere clock, and how to reset it, may provide real help in countering the conditions and diseases of aging. If telomerase could be induced to help keep cells dividing at youthful levels, we could someday be adding a whole new facet to the fight against aging.

FREE RADICALS

At present, though, there is one factor that is pervasive in the diseases and conditions of aging that we do understand—and know how to combat. If your skin is aging prematurely and you are suffering from cataracts—both common conditions associated with advancing years— the culprit could be the free radical. We touched on free radicals in the last chapter. They are dangerous molecules in our bodies that impair cells through a process called oxidation, which is the human body's equivalent of rusting. Oxidation begins when a molecule loses one of its electrons, particles that orbit an atom's nucleus. This causes that molecule to become unstable. It is now in a new, highly reactive energy state called a free radical.

After a free radical is formed, it seeks to rebalance itself by taking an electron away from another molecule. Sometimes it can accomplish this within a harmless chemical reaction. But sometimes, in its quest to get an electron from another molecule, the free radical will inflict molecular damage. Thus normal enzymes, proteins, and cells are destroyed. The process can cascade swiftly, much like a multivehicle automobile accident, with one car crashing into another, and with the end result being a wrecked transportation system, or, on the bodily level, an impairment of normal functioning. When DNA is attacked by free radicals, for instance, genetic mutations result, and are passed down, a situation that can result in cancer.

OXIDATIVE STRESS

Free radical damage, or oxidative stress, has been implicated in most of the diseases associated with aging, and it intensifies from continual exposure to harmful stimuli. For example, breathing in cigarette smoke just once will probably not cause injury, but repetitive exposure to smoke and smog certainly will. Unfortunately, as we discussed in Chapter 2, most of us come into contact with toxins on a daily basis. Auto exhaust is especially detrimental as one of its components, ozone, lodges in the lungs, where it becomes highly reactive with the oxygen molecules that are so vital to all body processes.

Brain cells appear particularly vulnerable to oxidative destruction. Their high-level energy production encourages free radical activity. As a result, we see many neurological diseases in the elderly, including Alzheimer's and Parkinson's diseases.

It is important to note that free radical formation accompanies normal and essential biological processes and, thus, can never be fully eliminated. For example, when our immune system is called into action to fight off bacteria or viruses, a by-product of that activity is the generation of free radicals. Moreover, aerobic exercise, so essential to keeping young, has its down side because vigorous exercise increases the body's use of oxygen, and in the process, may form unstable oxygen molecules. But while we cannot eradicate the free radical, we can control it. This is where antioxidant foods and supplements come into play. Antioxidants can latch on to free radicals and neutralize them. Unfortunately, few people eat enough antioxidant foods or take the proper combination of antioxidant supplements to adequately compensate for age-induced loss of endogenous antioxidants (those that originate within the body), such as the enzymes superoxide dismutase, catalase, and glutathione peroxidase. Furthermore, most of us in this society eat foods that speed up the production of free radicals, such as saturated fats. Plus in the process of consuming more calories than we need, we are producing more free radicals than we need to.

CHRONIC INFLAMMATION

Another factor that you could call both causative of aging and associated with it is chronic inflammation. We all know that aging people suffer an epidemic of outward inflammatory diseases, such as arthritis. But chronic inflammation also does interior damage—to brain cells, arterial walls, heart valves, and other structures in the body. Heart attack, stroke, heart valve failure, and Alzheimer's disease have been linked to the chronic inflammatory cascade that so often afflicts aging people.

Many scientific studies reveal the factors contributing to these inflammations and how to lessen them. We can, therefore, take constructive measures to prevent unexpected death from a heart attack, paralysis from a sudden stroke, or slow downfall from Alzheimer's disease. The first step is to take a blood test that identifies whether or not we have elevated markers of inflammation. Here are the substances we should be checking:

Fibrinogen. Fibrinogen, also known as Factor I, is a protein used in the blood-clotting process. High levels can contribute to a heart attack by raising platelet aggregation, literally thickening the blood, so the fibrinogen may give rise to a blockage in your heart or your brain. Elevated levels of fibrinogen increase one's risk of a heart attack or stroke two- to three-fold.

C-Reactive Protein. Too much of this inflammatory marker promotes abnormal arterial clotting and destabilized atherosclerotic plaque (a deposit of fat and other substances that accumulate in the lining of the artery wall). Destabilization can result in plaque bursting open and blocking an arterial pathway, causing an acute heart attack or stroke. Once a heart attack or stroke occurs, individuals with high levels of C-reactive protein have a significantly greater chance of experiencing another one shortly afterward. The substance is also associated with autoimmune conditions that predispose individuals to a variety of degenerative diseases.

Pro-Inflammatory Cytokines. Cytokines are proteins our bodies manufacture to trigger activity in other cells. Both fibrinogen and C-reactive protein are produced in the liver by harmful pro-inflammatory cytokines called interleukin-1b, interleukin-6, and tumor necrosis factor-alpha. Cytokines, by themselves, can contribu to increased heart attack risk, even after inflammatory markers are corrected. So suppression of pro-inflammatory cytokines through supplementation is also necessary.

Homocysteine. Physicians rarely check for elevated blood levels of homocysteine, but this could be a fatal mistake, as studies correlate raised homocysteine levels with increased risk of heart attack or stroke.

Homocysteine forms from the amino acid methionine found in red meat and chicken. Sometimes this substance is elevated due to inadequate levels of folic acid and vitamins B_6 and B_{12}. The problem may also be the result of a genetic defect. Some doctors recommend taking a multivitamin or B_6 supplements to lower elevated homocysteine, but this advice may prove insufficient. Specific protocols (to be discussed in Chapter 5) and periodic blood tests are needed to ensure that your treatment is actually working.

According to some life extension experts, the allowable norms that most doctors use for inflammatory markers in the blood are dangerously high. Instead, these experts recommend that fibrinogen should be under 300 mg/dl, C-reactive protein less than 2 mg/l, and homocysteine below 7 micro mol/l.

HORMONE IMBALANCES

The trillions of cells in the human body are delicately synchronized in their functioning by chemical modulators called hormones. Hormonal imbalances are often a contributing cause of many conditions associated with aging, ranging from new patterns of fat distribution, loss of libido, and increased fatigue to depression, osteoporosis, and coronary artery disease. Antiaging physicians often attempt to retune body systems with hormone replacement therapy.

In Chapter 4, we'll be looking at the most important hormonal keys to health, and at the most current ideas about how to best maintain them. Here, we'll introduce a few of the hormones that commonly go astray.

DHEA. Dihydroepiandrosterone, or DHEA, is a hormone vital in protecting the body against the ruinous effects of aging, and it is underproduced in most people over thirty-five. When DHEA levels are insufficient, levels of destructive inflammatory cytokines increase, setting the stage for a number of serious conditions. These include heart disease, stroke, cancer, osteoporosis, Alzheimer's disease, and autoimmune diseases such as rheumatoid arthritis.

While all inflammatory conditions may benefit from DHEA supplementation, of particular interest is the crippling infirmity rheumatoid arthritis. New research indicates that female patients—women most often fall victim to the disease—demonstrate low DHEA serum levels and that DHEA's replacement may be an important aspect of treatment and prevention.

Researchers also report that declining levels of DHEA are responsible for neurological impairments, and may contribute to memory loss and to brain changes that lead to Alzheimer's disease, as well as depression, anxiety, and loss of libido.[2]

Insulin. It is common knowledge that too much fat contributes to disease, yet despite repeated attempts at dieting, over 75 percent of Americans remain overweight or obese. Aging populations, in particular, have great difficulty diminishing their bulging waistlines, even though they may be consuming fewer calories than they did in their younger years. In numerous instances, the reason is traceable to an insulin imbalance whereby people become saturated with high blood levels of the hormone.

Normally, insulin allows cells to take in food particles through points on cell membranes called cell receptor sites. In some people, the process goes awry as the cells become insensitive and fail to respond, a condition known as insulin resistance. As a result the insulin is forced to remain in the bloodstream where it starts to build tissue, including fat tissue.

Too much insulin in the bloodstream contributes to weight gain in other ways as well. Excess insulin depletes glucose in the blood, creating a condition known as reactive hypoglycemia. In an attempt to replace the used-up glucose, the individual experiences constant cravings for sugar. Eating does not resolve the problem, though, as the insulin continues to feed off the sugar. Additionally, too much insulin in the blood prevents the release of fat stores. Thus, people may find themselves unable to lose weight, even with caloric restrictions and exercise.

Being overweight, particularly the abdominal obesity associated with an overabundance of insulin, is a risk factor for several diseases associated with aging, such as type II diabetes, heart disease, stroke, atherosclerosis, and cancer.

Testosterone. Testosterone, the male sex hormone, has a variety of important functions. In addition to promoting libido (in women as well as men—women do produce small and necessary amounts of the hormone) and facilitating sexual performance, testosterone sites throughout the body function to maintain muscle mass and form bone. Important to the heart, this hormone builds cardiac muscle, promotes coronary artery dilation, and helps regulate cholesterol. Testosterone receptor sites in the brain ward off depression, improve memory, and may even protect against Alzheimer's disease. Moreover, the hormone increases the uptake of oxygen throughout the body, helps to control blood sugar, and supports healthy immune function.

Levels of testosterone and DHEA (a precursor hormone for the manufacture of testosterone) diminish after age forty. These deficiencies increase risk factors for a heart attack or stroke. Cholesterol, fibrinogen, triglyceride, and insulin levels rise, for example, while human growth hormone, a substance associated with strong heart function, decreases. Blood pressure becomes elevated and the coronary arteries lose their elasticity.

Inadequate testosterone levels may also cause feelings associated with clinical depression, such as the inability to concentrate, moodiness, irritability, fatigue, and lack of interest in one's surroundings. A misdiagnosis could result in antidepressant therapy, when upping testosterone to youthful levels is all that's really needed.

Groundbreaking research is linking low testosterone levels to Alzheimer's disease. Testosterone has been shown to play a protective role in limiting secretions of a destructive substance called beta-amyloid, deposits of which are the hallmark of the Alzheimer's brain.[3]

As testosterone levels fall in males, estrogen levels rise, throwing the delicate testosterone–estrogen relationship out of balance. This occurs for a number of reasons. With increasing age, males manufacture more of the aromatase enzyme, which changes testosterone into estrogen. Obese males produce even more of this enzyme because fat cells manufacture the aromatase enzyme. Additionally, one of the liver's multiple functions is to get rid of excess estrogen, and liver function weakens with age. Alcohol and some medicines further hamper this liver function.

Small amounts of estrogen are normally present in all males, but an overabundance can "fool" the brain into thinking that the body is producing enough testosterone when it's not. Instead, estrogen is taking over testosterone receptor sites. When this occurs, the brain shuts off its testosterone-producing signal so that even less testosterone is produced. As testosterone signals shut down, so does the libido. Other problems that manifest are an increased risk of heart attack or stroke, and benign prostatic hypertrophy (enlarged prostate). Anti-aging experts say restoring testosterone to youthful levels is an essential part of helping aging men achieve renewed strength, stamina, sense of well-being, sexuality, and cardiac health. But care must be taken to restore testosterone properly, as external replacement therapies will only cause testosterone to aromatize (turn into estrogen with the help of the aromatase enzyme). The key is to eliminate estrogen excess by replacing testosterone in a way that blocks its conversion to estrogen.

DNA MUTATIONS

All cellular processes are directed by genes, which are composed of DNA. Indeed, our very existence depends upon precise genetic control. Strong, young cells have reasonably perfect genes. As we age, however, our DNA repair mechanisms lose their punch. As their efficiency decreases, a never-ending onslaught of natural and artificial substances has the opportunity to wreak genetic damage, through the mechanism of free radicals that we've described. Too often, the end result of such mutation is the out-of-control proliferation of cells that becomes cancer.

Most genetic mutations are the result of environmental factors—exposure to smoke, radiation, chemical pollutants, and, most commonly, what we eat. The worst culprits are foods cooked at high heat, such as well-done burgers, barbecued chicken, and even grilled salmon. Heat breaks up amino acids and creatinine to form undesirable chemicals called heterocyclic amines (HCAs). There are several types of HCAs, but they all have one thing in common—they predispose the body to cancer; in most cases, cancer of the colon, liver, and breast.

Grilled and fried foods are more detrimental than broiled foods in this regard. Also, longer cooking produces larger numbers of HCAs, as a University of Minnesota study clearly demonstrated when it reported that women who ate well-done hamburgers were at greater risk for breast cancer than women who ate their burgers less well done. Eating well-done hamburgers, as opposed to lesser-done ones, significantly increased breast cancer risk in women.[4]

IMMUNE SYSTEM DYSFUNCTION

The thymus gland, important as a source of infection-fighting T-cells, shrinks as we get older, partly in response to assault by free radicals. This is one of the reasons the aging immune system loses its ability to attack bacteria, viruses, and cancer cells. Moreover, as we get older, the body produces high levels of dangerous cytokines that can cause the body's immune system to attack healthy tissue, thus giving rise to the autoimmune diseases, like rheumatoid syndrome, associated with aging.

GLYCOSYLATION

It is well known that diabetics age prematurely, but even nondiabetics suffer from a devastating chemical reaction called glycosylation, wherein protein molecules bind to glucose molecules in the body to form nonfunctioning structures. If we want to age healthfully, our goals should include reduction of both blood glucose and insulin; we will thereby reduce glycosylated protein levels. Glycosylation is most evident in senile dementia, stiffening of the arterial system, and degenerative diseases of the eye.

METHYLATION DEFICIT

DNA requires constant enzymatic actions (remethylation) for maintenance and repair. Aging is associated with the impairment of methylation metabolism, causing DNA damage that can manifest as cancer, liver damage, and brain cell degeneration.

MITOCHONDRIAL ENERGY DEPLETION

The cell's energy factories are tiny structures called mitochondria. The mitrochondria generate energy for all cellular activities, transport nutrients through the cell membrane, and purge the cell of toxic debris. They are major generators of free radical activity, but they also produce potent antioxidants such as coenzyme Q10 and alpha-lipoic acid, which work to counter free radical activity. In order to function properly, the mitochondria require the presence of a complex series of chemicals, and when this system breaks down the result is mitochondrial energy depletion, a condition associated with congestive heart failure, muscle weakness, fatigue, and neurological disease.

EXCESSIVE CALCIFICATION

As a person ages, it is common for the transport of calcium in and out of cells to become less efficient. As a result, calcium can migrate from the bones, contributing to osteoporosis, and into the arteries, contributing to arteriosclerosis.

FATTY ACID IMBALANCE

The body requires essential fatty acids to maintain cell energy output. Aging causes alterations in enzymes required to convert dietary fats into the essential fatty acids the body requires to sustain life. The effects of a fatty acid imbalance are wide-ranging, and include an irregular heartbeat, joint degeneration, low energy, excessive blood coagulation, dry skin, and a host of other common ailments associated with aging.

DIGESTIVE ENZYME DEFICIT

The aging pancreas often fails to secrete enough digestive enzymes, while the aging liver does not secrete enough bile acids. The result: the chronic indigestion that so many people complain about as they grow older.

NONDIGESTIVE ENZYME IMBALANCES

Aging may cause enzyme imbalances, primarily in the brain and liver. Brain imbalances contribute to severe neurological diseases such as Parkinson's or to the persistent memory loss often experienced by aging people. Imbalances in the liver can impair liver function, and cause toxic damage throughout the body.

EXCITOTOXICITY

This describes a process in which brain cells are literally "excited to death" as the aging brain loses control over the release of neurotransmitters (the chemicals that transmit messages between one nerve and another in the brain). Excitotoxicity can lead to devastating brain cell damage and destruction.

CIRCULATORY DEFICIT

Decreased circulation to the tiny capillaries in the eye, brain, and skin is part of normal aging. The result is that disorders of the eye (such as cataracts, macular degeneration, and glaucoma) are the number-one type of aging-related degenerative diseases. Major and mini strokes are common problems associated with circulatory deficit to the brain, and the skin of all aging people shows the effects of inadequate circulation of nutrient-rich blood.

AGING'S A "THOUGHT THING" TOO

In addition to all of the foregoing physical mechanisms of aging, we should not forget the mental or emotional component. It's not that you can "think yourself old" or "think yourself young." But science has shown a link between what goes on in our brains and the state of our health. That link is the immune system, which can be affected by mental and emotional factors—e.g., stress—and which in turn affects how well we fight illness. The study of the brain's effect on physical conditions is called psychoneuroimmunology, or PNI.

How do we know that PNI is a valid field of medicine, and not merely a product of New Age wishful thinking? There are a lot of ways we know, and psychologist Robert Ader, a pioneer in the field, summarizes some of them. For one thing, we now know that the nervous system and the immune system are linked: there are nerve endings within the tissues of the immune system; i.e., in the bone marrow, the thymus, the spleen, and the lymph nodes. For another, changes in the central nervous system, that is, in the brain and spinal cord, have been shown in animal experiments to alter immune responses. And increased levels of stress hormones have been shown to decrease immune response. Chronic or intense stress, in particular, is correlated with lessened immune system effectiveness. An interesting experiment was done by Ader himself, when he and a colleague showed that rats could actually learn to suppress their own immune response. Initially, the researchers gave the rats saccharine-flavored water in conjunction with an immune-suppressing drug. The immune system of the animals was thus rendered less effective every time they got the saccharine water. But then, when the saccharine water was given without the immune suppressant, a funny thing happened: The rats' immune systems continued to respond, by working below par, to the now harmless water. The animals had learned to associate the sweet water with an immune deficit. Sickness and death were the result of this mental connection that the rats had made.[5]

Now, nobody really wants to force rats to think themselves to death. The point is that these experimental animals helped show us an important fact—that the mind and the body work as one. We sense this happening all the time, although rigorous scientific studies do help us to believe it. And many more studies have been done, not just with rats, but with people.

In 1991, for example, the *New England Journal of Medicine* published a report on the strong correlation between psychological stress levels and susceptibility to the common cold. A fascinating long-range study known as the Harvard Study of Adult Development found that optimism is good for our health. Harvard men from the classes of 1942 through 1944 were followed for thirty-five years. At the outset of the study, psychological tests and interviews were used to determine how optimistic or pessimistic each individual was in the way he explained life events that befell him. As the men aged, higher optimism ratings were shown to have exerted a positive effect on health, particularly as the subjects reached age forty-five.[6]

How, exactly, does the brain influence immunity? When we are under stress, catecholamines, or stress hormones, are released. These do good things for us in terms of activating the kind of fight-or-flight response we might need to save ourselves in a true crisis situation. So for instance, if we had to escape from an attacking bear, these hormones would increase our muscle tension, blood pressure, and heart rate, to help us run, and concomitantly decrease the energy we're expending on nonpressing tasks, such as digesting dinner. But most of the stresses we experience in the modern world are not of the acute bear-attack variety, but are, instead, chronic. Our bodies, though, don't know the difference. Thus we may have catecholamines coursing through our bodies over long periods of time, and since one of their effects is immune system suppression, this is not a good thing. Other stress hormone effects are heightened blood pressure levels, which over the long term can become chronic hypertension, the "silent killer"; and increased muscle tension, which can translate to headaches, chronic pain, and fatigue. Numerous studies have borne out the stress–disease connection. Just one example: A Canadian researcher showed that heart disease patients who were given stress-reduction guidance and then monitored for stress levels were half as likely to die from cardiac problems compared to a similar group that was not given such help.

No one is saying that we must eliminate stress from our lives in order to be completely healthy. But we can try to lessen chronic stress through such means as exercise, meditation, and affirmations. We'll be looking at these in Part III of this book.

PART II

WHAT YOU NEED TO KNOW NOW

CHAPTER 4

HORMONAL KEYS
TO HEALTH

*How Our Hormones Affect the
Aging Process*

Scientists are on the verge of radically extending the healthy human life span. The question is, will we live long enough to benefit personally from these discoveries? Here's my answer: We will—*if* we are willing to take the steps necessary to slow and reverse our rate of aging.

One way we can do this is through safe hormone modulation, which will prevent and treat many common diseases of aging. Who can benefit from hormonal modulation? I'd say that, in general, for people over forty, hormones can really make a difference. It is at this stage of life that many folks just don't feel as young as they used to. This is not true of everyone, but in our society it is often in our forties that our energy levels start to decline, minor health ailments develop, and we experience a noticeable loss of the sense of well-being. As the aging process progresses, vitality can deteriorate rapidly unless the individual takes aggressive steps to restore the body's biochemistry to its youthful profile.

HOW DOES THE HORMONAL SYSTEM WORK?

Your body manufactures hormones, which are chemical messengers—such as adrenaline, DHEA, human growth hormone, and dozens of others—that help regulate your body's functions. Most hormones are produced by glands, but some are made by organs, such as the heart, the stomach, and the small intestine. Some hormones appear to be responsible for controlling levels of other hormones. Many hormones released by the pituitary gland, for instance, signal other glands, such as the thyroid or adrenals, to release other hormones.

Just as your legs work together, many hormones work in pairs to create balance, according to the principle of opposing forces, with one hormone opposing the action of the other. The pancreas produces the insulin-glucagon pair, for example—a pair in which insulin reduces blood-sugar levels, while glucagon increases blood sugar. By the pancreas adding first a little of one hormone and then a bit of the other, the sugar concentration in the blood is kept nearly constant. It is evident that such a system must be precise in order to maintain a healthy balance. A breakdown in such a sensitive system—one that depends upon one reaction triggering a second reaction that in turn triggers a third, and so forth—could result in shifts that could be catastrophic to your body.

WHAT CAUSES THE HORMONAL SYSTEM TO BREAK DOWN?

The hormonal system may become imbalanced in the presence of environmental toxins, such as the ones we discussed in Chapter 2—e.g., lead, mercury, cadmium, the amalgam fillings in your teeth, fluoride or chlorine in your water, bacteria, viruses, or even electromagnetic stressors. Hormonal dysregulation can result and it may be subtle, with no obvious symptoms, but if your metabolism changes, you may see a corresponding decline in your energy level, with weight gain that could lead to obesity, a risk factor for major diseases.

Metabolic rate changes may trigger a pernicious cycle. As the body stores more fat, you may feel more fatigued, and then you may lose some of your enthusiasm for everyday activities. You may begin to skip exercising, but since exercise dispels depression, you may then get more depressed. And since depression itself may cause hormonal imbalances, as well as the release of stress hormones, the effects can spiral.

After a number of years, the body adapts to a reduction in the central hormones and/or an imbalance in how they are used. A sign of a possible hormonal imbalance is the inability to lose weight no matter what you do (although you must remember to take into account the fact that after age forty, the metabolism naturally slows down). High protein diets, vitamin supplementation, counting calories, or skipping meals will not correct an underlying hormonal imbalance. Determining whether you are out of balance is done by careful examination and testing of your hormone system. If you do in fact have a hormone-related problem, then by going through a comprehensive detoxification program and then a hormonal rebalancing, you may be able to lose weight without dieting, and regain energy.

Not everyone suffers from a hormone imbalance, but it is a good idea to rule out such a condition before embarking on any rejuvenation program. Hormone problems are actually more common than you might think. See an endocrinologist who can perform a simple hormone test to determine if you are producing adequate levels of melatonin, estrogen, thyroxin, and other critical hormones. If your tests come back normal, clearly your problem is not related to hormones. If an imbalance is identified, the treatment you receive may improve both your weight and your overall health.

Let's look at the most important hormones, and at how you might optimize their benefits in an antiaging plan.

DHEA

It's got a long name: dehydroepiandrosterone. But you can call it DHEA, and you should know that this is one hormone that is deficient in almost everyone over the age of thirty-five.

A wealth of data indicate that DHEA is a vitally important hormone in the human body. In fact, it appears to protect every part of the body against the ravages of time. A variety of published studies link low DHEA levels to aging and disease states; specifically, a DHEA deficiency correlates with:

- Chronic inflammation
- Immune dysfunction
- Depression
- Rheumatoid arthritis
- Type II diabetic complications
- Greater risk of certain cancers
- Excess body fat
- Cognitive decline
- Heart disease in men
- Osteoporosis

DHEA replacement therapy involves supplementation of the hormone to restore serum (meaning blood) levels to those of a twenty-one-year-old. This is really helpful because DHEA is the precursor building block that allows your body to create other hormones more easily, even if you are in decline because of age, disease, prescription medications, or other factors. Levels of hormones such as testosterone, estrogen, and serum DHEA begin to decline between twenty-five and thirty years of age and by age eighty-five, they may be reduced by 95 percent of youthful peak levels.

DHEA Suppresses Inflammatory Cytokines

Chronic inflammation, as we explained in Chapter 3, is an epidemic disease of aging. Inflammatory chemicals known as cytokines increase with age, and contribute to many degenerative diseases. Rheumatoid arthritis is a classic autoimmune disorder in which excess levels of cytokines (examples of which are tumor necrosis factor-alpha, interleukin-6, interleukin-1b, and leukotriene B_4) prompt the immune system to attack the body's own joint tissues.

Studies find that adrenal hormones, including DHEA, are of special importance in the treatment of rheumatoid arthritis. There is some evidence pointing to adrenal hypofunction—meaning underachieving adrenal glands—before the onset of rheumatoid arthritis, especially in women with low serum DHEA levels, who form the overwhelming majority of rheumatoid arthritis patients. DHEA replacement does in fact appear to be especially important for female rheumatoid arthritis patients.

Male rheumatoid arthritis patients show low plasma and synovial fluid testosterone. Androgens—male hormones—generally appear to be protective against the development of autoimmune diseases, and DHEA is an important precursor of various androgens.

Moreover, by lowering our levels of pro-inflammatory cytokines and protecting against their toxic effects, DHEA plays an important role in the prevention of conditions associated with chronic inflammation, including atherosclerosis, congestive heart failure, heart valve dysfunction, diabetes, cancer, and Alzheimer's.

DHEA's ability to inhibit interleukin-6 (IL-6) and tumor necrosis factor is of special interest. As we have learned, levels of these pro-inflammatory cytokines rise with age, and they are especially high in patients with inflammatory diseases. IL-6 plays a role in promoting bone loss and possibly also joint destruction. It also promotes the production of certain immune cells that attack the body's own tissue in autoimmune conditions, such as rheumatoid arthritis. Conditions associated with abnormally high IL-6 also include atherosclerosis, Alzheimer's disease, osteoporosis, and certain cancers. Because DHEA is a precursor to sex hormones, the deficiency of DHEA observed in people with inflammatory diseases suggests that they may also have a corresponding deficiency in sex hormones. These estrogenic and androgenic hormones have beneficial effects on muscle, bone, and blood vessels, as well as other tissue.

DHEA's Antiaging Properties

Research shows that DHEA improves neurological function, memory, and mood, helps alleviate stress disorders, and works to normalize EEG readings and immune function. Perhaps the most remarkable discovery on DHEA comes from a study in which 50 mg a day of DHEA given to people over a six-month period restored youthful serum levels of the hormone in both men and women. According to S.S.C. Yen and associates at the University of California, where the study was carried out, this translated into an increase in perception of physical and psychological well-being for both men (67 percent) and women (84 percent). Men taking 100 mg a day of the hormone reported increases in lean body mass and muscle strength, although this dose appears to be excessive in women.

DHEA at 50 or 100 mg a day was also shown to significantly elevate insulin growth factor (IGF). Why is this important? Aging causes a decline in IGF levels that contributes to loss of lean body mass, as well as to excess fat accumulation, neurological impairment, and age-related immune dysfunction.

Some DHEA proponents point to studies showing that this hormone protects against atherosclerosis and heart disease. A study using coronary artery angiography shows that low DHEA levels predispose people to more significant coronary artery blockage. Other research shows that DHEA inhibits abnormal blood platelet aggregation, a factor in sudden heart attack and stroke.

DHEA and the Brain

The neurotransmitter acetylcholine transmits nerve impulses from one brain cell to another. Acetylcholine protects brain cells against age-associated atrophy, and it is crucial for short-term memory. But with age, the release of acetylcholine into regions of the brain where it is needed for learning and memory declines.

Again, DHEA seems to offer help. A 1996 study in the journal *Brain Research* showed that compared to a control group, rats administered DHEA had a fourfold increase in acetylcholine release in the hippocampus of the brain, a critical area for the storage of memory. A 1997 study published in *Behavioral Brain Research* traced DHEA's interaction with certain neuronal receptors involved in the storage of short- and long-term memory. The results showed an improvement in both short- and long-term memory in mice. Further, a 1996 study in *Life Sciences* shows that DHEA can protect against early changes in brain cells associated with Alzheimer's disease. This hormone's ability to protect the hippocampus and enhance its activity is particularly important with regard to Alzheimer's disease. Studies generally find an increase in levels of the stress hormone cortisol and lower DHEA in patients with Alzheimer's disease. We know that excess cortisol damages the hippocampus and is associated with the formation of amyloid plaque, an abnormal structure that is one of the hallmarks of Alzheimer's disease.

DHEA and Immune Function

Scientists in a 1997 study proposed that oral administration of DHEA to elderly men would activate their immune systems. Then they did a controlled experiment to prove it. Nine healthy men averaging sixty-three years of age received a placebo for two weeks, followed by twenty weeks of treatment with DHEA (at 50 mg/day). After two weeks on oral DHEA, serum DHEA levels increased by three to four times. And here is what they found in terms of health effects: Compared with the placebo, DHEA administration results in

- A 20 percent increase in IGF-1. IGF stands for insulin-like growth factor, a substance thought to be responsible for some of the antiaging, anabolic effects that DHEA has produced in previous human studies. Many people take expensive growth hormone injections to boost IGF levels.
- A 35 percent increase in the number of monocyte immune cells

- A 29 percent increase in the number of B immune cells, and a 62 percent increase in B-cell activity
- A 40 percent increase in T-cell activity, although the total number of T-cells was not affected
- A 50 percent increase in interleukin-2 , a protein made by the body that makes infection-fighting cells multiply and mature

And there were no adverse effects noted with DHEA administration. The scientists concluded that, while further studies were needed, DHEA seemed to be of benefit to people needing immune system help.

DHEA and Women

The importance of DHEA, a precursor of estrogen and testosterone, has been emphasized in a number of studies on psychological and sexual health. A German study, for example, finds that when women who are deficient in DHEA supplement with 50 mg a day of the hormone for four months, their symptoms of depression and anxiety decrease, and their libido improves.

TESTOSTERONE

Turning now to men, if you are a man over the age of forty, you may be experiencing hormonal changes that noticeably limit you physically, sexually, and mentally. Your abdominal fat and shrinking muscle mass, a sign of hormone imbalance. A lessening of your sense of well-being is a common psychological complication of hormone imbalance that may deepen into clinical depression.

These changes have classically been ascribed to "growing old," and you are expected to accept the fact that destiny is irrevocably coaxing your body into a long degenerative process that culminates in death. Recently, however, a remarkable amount of data has been compiled proving that many of the conditions of middle-aged men— including abdominal weight gain, depression, fatigue, alterations in mood and cognition, decreased libido, erectile dysfunction, prostate disease, and heart disease—are directly related to hormone imbalances that are correctable with currently available drug and nutrient therapies. These symptoms usually manifest between the ages of forty and fifty, although with smokers the onset is significantly earlier.

Some doctors might be surprised to learn that adjusting patients' hormone levels to fit the profile of a healthy twenty-one-year-old male could eliminate many of their patients' problems. They may wish to check their male patients' blood levels of estrogen, testosterone, thyroid hormone, and DHEA, as an alternative to prescribing drugs to treat symptoms.

Aging Men and Estrogen Overload

The most critical hormone imbalance in aging men is the decrease in free testosterone, while estrogen levels either remain the same or increase precipitously. As men grow older, the dangerous combination of low testosterone and excess estrogen gives rise to a variety of insidious biochemical shifts. The result is a testosterone–estrogen imbalance that directly causes many of the debilitating ailments associated with aging. One report shows that estrogen levels of the average fifty-four-year-old man are higher than those of the average fifty-nine-year-old woman!

Estrogen is an essential hormone for men, but too much of it causes many health problems. The most dangerous acute effect of excess estrogen, without enough testosterone, is an increased risk of heart attack or stroke. High levels of estrogen may cause benign prostatic hypertrophy (enlargement of the prostate), although we can note that nettle root extract blocks the binding of growth-stimulating estrogen to prostate cells.

When there is not enough free testosterone available, estrogen attaches to testosterone cell receptor sites throughout the body and creates many difficulties for aging men. As a regulator in youth, small amounts of estrogen turn off the powerful cell-stimulating effects of testosterone. As estrogen levels increase with age, testosterone cell stimulation may become locked in the "off" position, reducing sexual arousal and sensation, the loss of libido so common in aging men.

High serum levels of estrogen also trick the brain into thinking that enough testosterone is being produced, further slowing the natural production of testosterone. This happens when estrogen saturates testosterone receptors in the hypothalamus region of the brain. The saturated hypothalamus then stops sending out a "make more testosterone" message, and in some cases, shuts down the normal testicular production of testosterone.

The Critical Need for Free Testosterone

Testosterone is much more than a sex hormone. There are testosterone receptor sites in cells throughout the body, most notably in the brain and heart. Testosterone is required for healthy protein synthesis to maintain muscle mass and bone formation. Testosterone improves oxygen uptake throughout the body, helps control blood sugar, regulates cholesterol, and maintains immune surveillance. The body requires testosterone to maintain youthful cardiac and neurological function. Testosterone is also a critical hormone in the maintenance of healthy bone density, muscle mass, and red blood cell production. Numerous studies show that maintaining youthful levels of free testosterone can enable the aging man to restore strength, stamina, cognition, heart function, sexuality, and a positive outlook on life, and to combat depression.

Indeed, psychiatrists are currently concerned with studies showing that men with depression have lower levels of testosterone than do control subjects. Elevation of free testosterone levels could prove to be an effective antidepressant therapy for some men. There is, thus, a basis for measuring free testosterone levels in men with depression, and if free testosterone levels are low, for initiation of replacement therapy. Unfortunately, testosterone is one of the most misunderstood hormones, and so therapy with this hormone is considered to be controversial. Bodybuilders tarnished the reputation of testosterone by overloading their young bodies with synthetic testosterone drugs. Synthetic testosterone abuse can be detrimental, but this has nothing to do with the benefits that a man over age forty can enjoy by properly restoring his natural testosterone to the levels of his youth.

Conventional doctors do not recommend testosterone replacement therapy because of an erroneous concern that testosterone causes prostate cancer. But as we will show later, fear of prostate cancer is not a scientifically valid reason to avoid testosterone modulation therapy.

Skeptical physicians are also dubious about prescribing testosterone replacement therapy (TRT) because some poorly conducted studies show TRT to be ineffective in the long-term in the treatment of aging. These studies record antiaging benefits when testosterone is first given, but the effects often wear off. What physicians fail to appreciate is that exogenously administered testosterone (testosterone from outside of the body) can convert to estrogen in the body, and the higher estrogen levels may then negate the benefits of the exogenously administered testosterone. The solution to the estrogen overload problem is not to cease testosterone therapy, but to block the process of aromatization, the conversion of testosterone to estrogen in the body.

Further ammunition against TRT was presented in a 1999 study in the journal *Drugs and Aging*. This study suggested that androgen therapy could result in polycythemia—increased numbers of red blood cells—that can cause an increase in blood viscosity and risk of clotting. Many aging men, however, find that borderline anemia is a greater concern than the overproduction of red blood cells. When men are deprived of testosterone during prostate cancer therapy, anemia frequently follows. Polycythemia rarely develops in men replacing testosterone to youthful ranges. Of course, too much testosterone can cause problems, but replacing testosterone to the level of a healthy twenty-one-year-old should not produce the side effects that some doctors are concerned about.

Medical Testing Is Required

Before anyone embarks on a program of hormone modulation, he or she must be thoroughly tested by a qualified physician. Testosterone replacement therapy is no exception. First, you must have a baseline blood PSA measurement taken to exclude existing prostate cancer. A digital rectal exam is also recommended to eliminate the possibility of prostate cancer.

In addition, you'll want to have your blood tested to determine liver and kidney function, as well as levels of testosterone, estradiol (estrogen), DHEA, thyroid hormone, glucose, minerals, lipids, free and total DHT, and homocysteine. Follow-up monitoring for testosterone, estrogen, and PSA is required during the therapy program.

Why Testosterone Levels Decline

Testosterone production begins in the brain. When the hypothalamus detects a deficiency of testosterone in the blood, it secretes a hormone called gonadotropin-releasing hormone to the pituitary gland. This prompts the pituitary to secrete luteinizing hormone (LH), which then prompts the Leydig cells in the testes to produce testosterone.

In some men, the testes lose their ability to produce testosterone, no matter how much LH is being produced. This type of testosterone deficiency is diagnosed when blood tests show high levels of LH and low levels of testosterone. In other words, the pituitary gland is telling the testes (by secreting LH) to produce testosterone, but the testes have lost their ability to do so. So the pituitary gland continues, in vain, to secrete LH because there is not enough testosterone in the blood to provide feedback to tell the pituitary to shut down.

In other cases, the hypothalamus or pituitary gland is the problem, because it fails to produce sufficient amounts of LH, and thus prevents healthy testes from secreting testosterone. The appropriate therapy is determined by testing the blood to see if sufficient amounts of LH are being secreted by the pituitary gland. If serum (blood) testosterone levels are very low, it is important to diagnose the cause, but no matter what the underlying problem is, therapies exist today to safely restore testosterone to youthful levels in any man who does not have prostate cancer. (Most prostate cancer patients should avoid any substance that increases testosterone.)

Testosterone and Libido

Sexual stimulation and erection begin in the brain when neuronal testosterone receptor sites are prompted to ignite a cascade of bio-chemical events involving testosterone receptor sites in the nerves, blood vessels, and muscles. Free testosterone promotes sexual desire and then facilitates performance, sensation, and the ultimate degree of fulfillment.

The quality of a man's sex life is adversely affected and his genitals atrophy without adequate levels of free testosterone. When free testosterone is restored, positive changes can be expected in the structure and function of the sex organs. (Note that sexual dysfunction can be also caused by factors that are unrelated to hormone imbalance. An example of such a factor is arteriosclerotic blockage of the penile arteries. Plus there are many other physical and psychological causes of dysfunction, including stress.)

The genital-pelvic region is packed with ultra-sensitive testosterone receptors that facilitate free-testosterone-induced sexual stimulation. Clinical tests on testosterone injections, creams, and patches often fail to show a long-lasting, libido-enhancing effect in aging men. Now we know why—the testosterone can be converted to estrogen. And as we described earlier, testosterone receptor sites in cells throughout the body then take up the estrogen. Estrogen molecules occupying testosterone receptor sites on cell membranes block testosterone's ability to induce a healthy hormonal signal. It does not matter how much free testosterone is available if excess estrogen is competing for the same cellular receptor sites.

Estrogen can also increase production of sex-hormone-binding globulin (SHBG) to bind any active free testosterone into inactive "bound testosterone." Testosterone receptors on cell membranes cannot pick up bound testosterone. Testosterone must be kept in the "free" form (not bound to SHBG) in the bloodstream in order to produce long-lasting, libido-enhancing effects. Thus we see that excess estrogen must be suppressed because it competes with testosterone for testosterone receptor sites in the sex centers of the brain and in the genitals.

Testosterone and the Prostate Gland

Many doctors will tell you that testosterone causes prostate disease, but the published scientific literature indicates otherwise. Estrogen, however, *is* a primary culprit in the development of benign prostatic hypertrophy.

Fear of prostate cancer is the major concern that stops men from restoring their testosterone to youthful levels. The theory is that it is better not to replace testosterone that is lost with age because most prostate cancer cell lines use testosterone to proliferate. The problem with this theory is simply that most men who develop prostate cancer have low, not high, testosterone levels, and most published studies show that serum testosterone levels do not affect risk for developing prostate cancer.

Because there is such a strong perception that any testosterone augmentation can increase the risk of prostate cancer, I conducted an on-line search, using MEDLINE, of all published studies on serum testosterone and prostate cancer. You can do the same thing yourself, and you'll probably get results similar to my own: MEDLINE revealed twenty-seven studies, five of which indicated that men with higher testosterone levels have a greater incidence of prostate cancer, but twenty-one of which showed that testosterone is not a risk factor for prostate cancer. (One study was essentially neutral.)

As stated earlier, you must have a serum PSA test and a digital rectal exam to rule out prostate cancer before you start a testosterone replacement program. Then you should have continuing PSA monitoring as you begin your hormone augmentation program. The reason for this is that nothing is risk-free. Small minorities of men with low testosterone have prostate cancer without an elevated PSA or palpable lesion detectable by digital rectal examination. These men risk an acute flare-up of their disease if they use supplemental testosterone. That is why it is so important to have PSA monitoring every thirty to forty-five days during the first six months of any type of testosterone augmentation therapy. If an undiagnosed prostate cancer is detected because of testosterone therapy, it is usually treatable by nonsurgical means.

Please remember that testosterone does not cause acute prostate cancer, but if you have existing prostate cancer and you do not know it, testosterone administration is likely to boost your PSA sharply. (By the way, you should be aware that elevated PSA does not automatically mean that you have prostate cancer. Noncancerous conditions, such as an infection or benign enlargement of the prostate, can give a higher PSA reading than normal, which is why the digital rectal exam is used in conjunction with a PSA test.) You would have the benefit of early detection if your doctor diagnoses prostate cancer after you receive testosterone therapy, with an opportunity to receive very early treatment. And we do acknowledge that some aging men will not wish to take this risk.

Once a man is diagnosed with prostate cancer, testosterone therapy cannot be recommended or continued because most prostate cancer cells use testosterone to promote growth. Regrettably, this denies prostate cancer patients the wonderful benefits of testosterone therapy. Men with severe benign prostatic hyperplasia (BPH) should approach testosterone replacement with caution. If you have BPH and you are taking testosterone replacement therapy, it would be judicious to also use the drug Proscar (finasteride), in order to suppress the formation of dihydrotestosterone (DHT). This is a substance ten times more potent than testosterone in promoting prostate growth, and so DHT suppression is a proven therapy for treating benign prostate enlargement. Saw palmetto extract suppresses some DHT in the prostate gland, but saw palmetto's effectiveness in alleviating symptoms of BPH probably has more to do with the fact that saw palmetto:

- Blocks alpha-adrenergic receptor sites on the sphincter muscle surrounding the urethra (this is how the drug Hytrin works)
- Inhibits the binding of estrogen to prostate cells (as nettle does)
- Inhibits the enzyme 3-ketosteroid (which causes the binding of DHT to prostate cells)
- Has an anti-inflammatory effect on the prostate

Note: Men with severe BPH can also use the drug Arimidex to suppress excess estrogen levels. Estrogen can worsen BPH, and supplemental testosterone can elevate estrogen unless an aromatase-inhibiting drug, such as Arimidex, is used.

Testosterone and Depression

A consistent finding in the scientific literature is that testosterone replacement therapy produces an increased feeling of well-being. As stated earlier, published studies show that low testosterone correlates with symptoms of depression and other psychological disorders. Conversely, one study shows that patients with major depression receiving testosterone therapy experience improvement equal to that achieved with standard antidepressant drugs.

The suppression of libido is a common side effect of prescription antidepressant drugs. Those with depression must either accept this drug-induced reduction in the quality of life, or get off the antidepressant drugs to have at least a somewhat normal sex life. This is where testosterone replacement is superior, because it often enhances libido. The need for libido-suppressing antidepressant drugs could be reduced or eliminated if more psychiatrists would test their patients' blood for free testosterone, and prescribe natural testosterone therapies for men with low free testosterone.

Androderm, an FDA-approved drug, is one of several natural testosterone replacement therapies that doctors prescribe. The results of a twelve-month clinical trial using Androderm show a statistically significant reduction in depression as measured on a scored test. There are also highly significant decreases in fatigue—from 79 percent before the Androderm patch to only 10 percent after twelve months.

Jonathan Wright, M.D., coauthor of *Maximize Your Vitality & Potency*, reports that the following effects are reported in response to low testosterone levels:

- Loss of ability to concentrate
- Moodiness and emotionality
- Touchiness and irritability
- Timidity
- Feelings of weakness
- Inner unrest
- Memory failure
- Reduced intellectual agility
- Passive attitudes
- General tiredness
- Reduced interest in surroundings
- Hypochondria

The above can all be clinical symptoms of depression, and testosterone replacement therapy has been shown to alleviate these conditions. Testosterone thus shows exciting therapeutic potential for the treatment of depression in men.

Testosterone and Mental Decline

New evidence indicates that low levels of testosterone may contribute to memory impairment and increase the brain's vulnerability to Alzheimer's disease and related disorders. Beta-amyloid, a toxic peptide that may accumulate in certain regions of the aging brain, is implicated in the development of Alzheimer's. Researchers have found that testosterone decreases secretion of harmful beta-amyloid and increases secretion of a substance called sbetaAPPalpha; the end result is a neuroprotective effect. The conclusion of this work indicates that testosterone supplementation in elderly men may be beneficial in the treatment of Alzheimer's.

Hormone Imbalance and Obesity

A consistent finding in the scientific literature is that obese men have low testosterone and very high estrogen levels. Central or visceral obesity (a "pot belly") is a recognized risk factor for cardiovascular disease and type II diabetes. New findings shed light on subtle borderline hormone imbalances in obese men that often fall within the normal laboratory reference range. Boosting testosterone levels appears to decrease abdominal fat, reverse glucose intolerance, and reduce lipoprotein abnormalities in the bloodstream. Further analysis also shows a regulatory role for testosterone in counteracting the accumulation of visceral fat, or fat surrounding internal organs. Along with this, epidemiological data demonstrate that relatively low testosterone levels pose a risk for the development of visceral obesity.

One study shows that serum estrone and estradiol (both kinds of estrogen) were elevated twofold in one group of morbidly obese men. Male hormones convert into estrogens when fat cells synthesize the aromatase enzyme. Fat tissue, especially in the abdomen, has been shown to literally "aromatize" testosterone and its precursor hormones into potent estrogens.

One study that measured serum levels of sex steroid hormones after ingestion of different types of food suggests that eating high-fat foods may reduce free testosterone levels. A meal containing fat reduced free testosterone levels for four hours, whereas high-protein and high-carbohydrate meals had no effect on serum hormone levels.

Testosterone deficiency in obese men is caused by the production of excess aromatase enzyme in fat cells as well as in the dietary fat. The resulting hormone imbalance (too much estrogen and not enough free testosterone) partly explains why so many obese men are impotent and have a wide range of premature degenerative diseases.

Causes of the Estrogen–Testosterone Imbalance in Men

If your blood tests reveal high estrogen and low testosterone, here are the common factors involved:

Excess Aromatase Enzyme. As men age, they produce greater quantities of the enzyme aromatase, which, as we've said, converts testosterone into estrogen in the body. Inhibition of the aromatase enzyme results in a significant decline in estrogen levels, often boosting free testosterone to youthful levels. Thus an agent designated as an aromatase inhibitor may be especially helpful to aging men who have excess estrogen.

Impaired Liver Function. A healthy liver eliminates surplus estrogen and sex-hormone-binding globulin. Aging, alcohol, and certain drugs impair liver function and can be a major cause of hormone imbalance in aging men. Heavy alcohol consumption increases estrogen in both men and women.

Obesity. Fat cells create aromatase enzyme and especially contribute to abdominal fat buildup. Low testosterone allows abdominal fat to form, which then causes more aromatase enzyme to form, resulting in even lower levels of testosterone and higher levels of estrogen (by aromatizing testosterone into estrogen). It is especially important for overweight men to consider hormone modulation therapy.

Zinc Deficiency. Zinc is a natural aromatase enzyme inhibitor. (Adequate daily zinc consumption is generally 30 to 90 mg; we'll be considering this important mineral further in Chapter 11.)

Some Natural Solutions to Male Hormone Imbalances

Chrysin. The bioflavonoid, or plant pigment, chrysin shows potential as a natural aromatase inhibitor. Chrysin is extracted from various plants. Body builders use it as a supplement to boost testosterone, since by inhibiting the aromatase enzyme, less testosterone is converted into estrogen. One problem with chrysin is that its poor absorption into the bloodstream does not produce the testosterone enhancement users expect. However, it's been shown that a pepper extract called piperine may significantly enhance chrysin's function. Pilot studies find that when chrysin is combined with piperine, reductions in serum estrogen (estradiol) and increases in total and free testosterone result in thirty days.

Aromatase-inhibiting drugs are also used to treat women with estrogen-dependent breast cancers. The rationale for this therapy is that if they can halt the aromatasation process, and hence the production of the estrogen, they can slow the course of the cancer.

A 1993 study published in the *Journal of Steroid Biochemical Molecular Biology* compares chrysin and ten other flavonoids to an aromatase-inhibiting drug (aminoglutethimide). Chrysin was not only shown to be the most potent of these aromatase inhibitors, it was found to be similar in effectiveness to the aromatase-inhibiting drug. The scientists conducting the study conclude that the aromatase-inhibiting effects of certain flavonoids may contribute to the cancer-preventive effects of plant-based diets.

The advantages of using plant extracts rather than drugs to boost testosterone are twofold: plant extracts have ancillary health benefits and minimal, if any, side effects. Chrysin, for one, is a low-cost potent antioxidant with vitaminlike effects in the body.

It is also an anti-inflammatory. Now that aging is viewed as a pro-inflammatory process, it follows that substances that control or prevent chronic inflammation may protect against diseases as diverse as atherosclerosis, senility, and aortic valve stenosis. Chrysin is one of many flavonoids currently being researched as a phyto-extract, or plant extract, that may prevent some forms of cancer. If tests on chrysin bear out their promise, men would have an inexpensive natural supplement that would:

• Increase free testosterone
• Decrease excess estrogen
• Produce a safe antianxiety effect

Chrysin is sold to bodybuilders by commercial supplement companies that do not know whether or not their product is modulating testosterone and estrogen levels favorably in men. The Life Extension Foundation, on the other hand, has conducted studies to evaluate chrysin's effects (when it is combined with piperine to enhance absorption) on aging men.

Nettle. Concentrated nettle root can be useful in increasing levels of free testosterone. The testes produce about 90 percent of testosterone; the adrenal glands produce the remainder. Testosterone functions as an aphrodisiac hormone in brain cells, and as an anabolic hormone in developing bone and skeletal muscle. Testosterone that becomes bound to serum globulin is not available to cell receptor sites and fails to stimulate libido. It is, therefore, necessary to increase free testosterone levels to ignite sexual arousal in the brain.

A hormone that controls levels of free testosterone, as previously discussed, is called sex-hormone-binding globulin (SHBG). Testosterone loses its biological activity when it binds to SHBG, and it becomes "bound testosterone," as opposed to the preferable "free testosterone." As men age past forty-five, SHBG's binding capacity increases dramatically—by 40 percent on average—which coincides with the age-associated loss of libido.

Some studies show that the decline in sexual interest with advancing age is not always a result of the amount of testosterone produced but is, rather, due to the increased binding of testosterone to globulin by SHBG. This explains why some older men who are on testosterone replacement therapy fail to report a long-term aphrodisiac effect. The artificially administered testosterone becomes bound to SHBG and is not "available" to cellular receptor sites, where it would normally enhance libido.

This is where nettle root can be helpful. A highly concentrated extract of nettle root provides a unique mechanism for increasing levels of free testosterone. Constituents of nettle root that bind to SHBG in place of testosterone, thus reducing SHBG's binding of free testosterone, have been identified in European research. The authors of one study state that these constituents of nettle root "may influence the blood level of free, i.e., active, steroid hormones by displacing them from the SHBG binding site."

Nettle root also benefits the prostate gland. The substance has been used in Germany for decades as a treatment for benign prostatic hyperplasia (enlargement of the prostate gland). Enlargement occurs when dihydrotestosterone (DHT), a metabolite of testosterone, stimulates prostate growth. Nettle root inhibits the binding of DHT to attachment sites on the prostate membrane.

Nettle extracts also inhibit enzymes, such as 5 alpha reductase, that may give rise to benign prostate enlargement, excess facial hair, and hair loss at the top of the head.

Muira Puama. An herbal extract identified by French scientists shows libido-enhancing effects in two human clinical studies. Muira puama, which comes from the stems and roots of the *Ptychopetalum olacoides* plant, is in wide use as an aphrodisiac, tonic, and cure for rheumatism and muscle paralysis in the Amazon region of South America.

INSULIN

Another hormone we'll discuss is one that's not just the concern of diabetics. It is common knowledge that too much fat contributes to disease, yet despite repeated attempts at dieting, a high percent of

Americans remain overweight or obese. Aging populations, in particular, have great difficulty losing weight. The reason for this, in many cases, is traceable to an insulin imbalance in which people become saturated with high levels of the hormone in their blood.

After eating, the body produces the hormone insulin to carry food particles to the cells. Normally, insulin allows cells to take in food particles through points on cell membranes called cell receptor sites. This process goes awry in some people, as the cells become insensitive and fail to respond, a condition known as insulin resistance. As a result, the insulin is forced to remain in the bloodstream, where it starts to build tissue, including fat tissue.

Excess insulin in the bloodstream contributes to weight gain in other ways as well. It depletes glucose in the blood, creating a condition known as reactive hypoglycemia. The body generates constant cravings for sugar in its attempt to replace the used-up glucose. Eating does not resolve the problem, however, as the insulin continues to feed off glucose. Also, too much insulin in the blood prevents the release of fat stores. Thus, people may find themselves unable to lose weight, even when they reduce their calorie intake and exercise.

Several factors precipitate insulin resistance. Just gaining ten or fifteen pounds above normal throws your hormonal system off balance. The condition is also related to a lack of trace minerals, such as chromium and zinc; overconsumption of refined carbohydrates; genetics, when there is a family history of diabetes; and a sedentary lifestyle.

Being overweight, particularly the abdominal obesity associated with an overabundance of insulin, is a risk factor for several diseases and conditions associated with aging, such as type II diabetes, heart disease, stroke, atherosclerosis, impotence, and cancer.

How can you work to normalize your insulin situation? Begin by eliminating alcoholic beverages, sugar, white flour, and white rice from your diet. Then add in some whole grains, beans, and legumes and lots of nonstarchy vegetables. Increase your daily exercise level. All these measures will help you to rebalance your insulin levels, lose weight, restore your energy, and rejuvenate your system.

MELATONIN

Melatonin is a pineal hormone that is best known for its role in promoting sleep. The studies regarding its potential in ameliorating sleep disorders continue to increase, but research on the aging process now suggests that melatonin may have a much wider range of potential benefits.

Data indicates that melatonin can be a potent free-radical scavenger that acts as a primary defense against cell destruction caused specifically by hydroxyl free radicals. Hence, melatonin can slow aging and even postpone the onset of age-related diseases, including cancer. Animal studies support these findings.

Results of animal studies also indicate that melatonin has cardioprotective, antidiabetic, antiglucocorticoid, anticonvulsant, anticataract, and immuno-enhancing effects. It improves adrenal function, and can reduce the severity of colitis, seizures, brain injury, and gastric lesions. It can delay disease onset and death due to viral encephalitis. Melatonin has also exhibited cytoprotective (meaning cell-protective) and antioxidant activity in laboratory situations (outside of animals).

Jet lag is a common problem for which melatonin can provide an answer. A double-blind placebo-controlled study found that 5 mg of melatonin taken once a day for three days prior to a flight, once during the flight, and once a day for three days after the flight alleviates jet lag and fatigue in healthy travelers. This information may be especially helpful if you're traveling and must make a business presentation at your destination, or entertain, or even just plan to sightsee.

The ideal daily dose of melatonin varies according to each individual, but experts believe 1 to 3 mg taken at night will produce positive effects in most people.

GROWTH HORMONE

The secretion of growth hormone by the pituitary gland gradually declines as you age. This slowdown is your body's way of telling you that you've reached the end of your reproductive years. In addition to a diminished libido and sexual performance, you see changes in your body's composition. Most notably, fat increases and lean muscle mass decreases. In fact, each year after the age of forty, a pound of fat replaces a pound of muscle. This means that by the time you are fifty, ten pounds of your muscle have been replaced with ten pounds of fat.

Experts disagree on the benefits of supplementing with growth hormone. Some are excited about the antiaging benefits seen in scientific studies. In these studies, senior citizens given growth hormone show an increase in lean muscle mass, a decrease in body fat, increased energy, stronger immune systems, sharper eyesight, and better mental acuity. Other experts, however, caution that more research into safe amounts is needed. We certainly need to stay informed about new studies on this potential youth hormone.

THYROID HORMONE

Hypothyroidism (Underactive Thyroid Gland)

Every cell in your body needs thyroid hormone to function properly. Hypothyroidism, or low thyroid function, slows down all body processes, including metabolism. Symptoms of hypothyroidism can include: weight gain; fatigue; even chronic fatigue syndrome; loss of appetite; cold intolerance; cold hands and feet; lethargy; weakness; thinning hair; dry, coarse skin; a puffy face or hands; loss of the outer third of the eyebrow; cramping; infertility; absence of periods or, conversely, excessive menstrual bleeding; swelling of the neck or abdomen; constipation; arthritis; fibromyalgia; and allergies.

When the brain is affected, you might have depression, poor memory; an inability to concentrate; a loss of appetite; or slow speech. Long-standing hypothyroidism can be an underlying factor in diabetes, hyperlipidemia (elevated cholesterol), heart disease, stroke, or kidney failure. Hypothyroidism depresses the immune system, so it can cause chronic infections and set the stage for cancer later in life.

Your thyroid gland sets your body's temperature. When your thyroid is not functioning properly, your body temperature drops, disturbing homeostasis, your body's natural state of balance. Every cell must be within a very narrow range of temperatures to function optimally. Your enzymes control every function, and they are all temperature-sensitive. When your body temperature is too low because of a low thyroid, then everything starts to slow down and every cell can start to malfunction.

Most doctors rely on two types of tests to detect hypothyroidism. Standard blood tests check levels of thyroid hormone, an iodine-containing compound released by the thyroid gland as thyroxine (T4) and a more powerful component, triiodothyronine (T3). A more sensitive test also checks levels of thyroid stimulating hormone (TSH), a substance released by the pituitary gland that regulates T4 and T3. Unfortunately, both tests detect only severe deficiencies. Many people have subclinical levels of hypothyroidism, which these tests do not detect.

Doctors then tell people that nothing is wrong when searching for answers to chronic illness. One unfortunate result is that Prozac and similar medications are prescribed for growing numbers of depressed patients when correct diagnosis and treatment of hypothyroidism may be all that are needed. Fatigue is often due, at least in part, to an underactive thyroid, and it can be missed with the standard diagnostics.

Causes of Hypothyroidism

Mineral deficiencies are common causes of hypothyroidism. People tend to associate the condition with an iodine deficiency, but the widespread use of iodized salt means most Americans have enough iodine. Two of the primary minerals involved in thyroid metabolism are selenium and zinc. A deficiency of either of these can prevent proper conversion of T4 to T3.

Stress and excessive intake of refined carbohydrates are also major contributors to this condition. Refined carbohydrates raise blood sugar levels and increase cortisol, and then stress impacts on cortisol activity as well. High cortisol levels can overwork and exhaust the thyroid.

Excessive fasting or low caloric intake can lead to slow metabolism and a decrease in the body's ability to burn fat and calories. Food allergies and caffeinism, a "toxic condition caused by excessive ingestion of caffeine-containing substances," can also contribute to hypothyroidism.

Thyroid hormone remains inactive until it is broken apart by intestinal enzymes. Repeated antibiotic therapy, poor diet, or intestinal problems may cause an intestinal microflora imbalance, resulting in a decrease in intestinal ability to reabsorb, or reuptake, the active thyroid hormone.

Metal and chemical toxicity from secondhand smoke or organic compounds, such as softeners in plastics and food wrap, may lead to a thyroid problem. Mercury from dental amalgam fillings and pesticide exposure can tax the thyroid. Tap water with fluoride and chlorine additives may negatively affect thyroid function as well. And any exposure to radiation can harm your thyroid gland.

A healthy thyroid gland depends on a healthy liver. The liver must turn absorbed toxins into soluble substances that your body can eliminate as waste. The enzymes that break down many environmental toxins also break down thyroid chemicals. An overworked liver processing poisons can speed up its enzymes and too much thyroid hormone may then be destroyed.

Antidepressants are toxins that can block thyroid function. This is not a common scenario, but it can happen. Surprisingly, eating too much of certain foods, such as broccoli, cauliflower, and cabbage, can contribute to hypothyroidism. These are cancer-preventing foods, so they're good to eat—but in moderation, because an overdose of these cruciferous vegetables can be a problem for some people. The bottom line is that you should not believe the commonly accepted medical line that the cause of hypothyroidism is unknown.

Treatment for Hypothyroidism

Orthodox medicine treats hypothyroidism with doses of thyroxine to substitute for the hormone your gland is not able to produce.

Alternative treatment includes detoxification, diet improvement, and stress reduction. Some holistic physicians may give patients a natural form of thyroid hormone replacement therapy.

Acupuncture is considered to be an excellent therapy for hypothyroidism; it's often administered along with Chinese herbal preparations. Another alternative treatment to help regulate thyroid function is infusions of the herb bladderwrack. Homeopaths generally prescribe *Arsenicum albicans* for this condition, with a required consultation first.

Hyperthyroidism (Overactive Thyroid Gland)

Hyperthyroidism is a medical condition caused by the effects of excess thyroid hormone (thyroxine) on body tissues. All cells in the body respond to an increase in thyroid hormone by increasing their rate of functioning. Our hormones are interconnected. High or low thyroxine, for example, can affect secretion of insulin. There are different causes of hyperthyroidism, but the symptoms tend to be similar in everyone with this problem. Metabolism increases, so patients typically feel hotter than others around them. Patients feel tired at day's end, but they have trouble sleeping. Hands tremble and palpitations may develop. Nervousness, irritability, and easy upset may prevail. Bowel movements may increase. Bulging eyeballs, a thin physique, and fits of energy characterize hyperthyroidism, which is easier to treat than hypothyroidism because it is easier to reduce the amount of hormone than to produce more of it.

In severe cases, shortness of breath, chest pain, and muscle weakness may occur. Hyperthyroid symptoms are usually so gradual in onset that patients don't notice them until they become more severe. Warm moist skin, hair loss, and a staring gaze may occur. It may be weeks or even months before patients realize they are ill. In older people, some or all of the typical symptoms may be absent; the patient may simply lose weight or be depressed.

Causes of Hyperthyroidism

The most common cause of hyperthyroidism is Graves' disease, which is an autoimmune condition. What happens is your own immune system turns against your own thyroid gland. Graves' disease is characterized by overactivity of the enlarged thyroid gland, inflammation and swelling of the tissues around the eyes, and skin thickening on the lower legs. Graves' disease affects about eight times more women than men. It's actually uncommon over age fifty; those in their thirties and forties are more apt to have it.

Hyperthyroidism can also be caused by a single nodule in the thyroid, not the entire gland. Thyroiditis (thyroid gland inflammation) can trigger release of excess thyroid hormones. Hyperthyroidism may occur in patients taking excessive doses of any form of thyroid hormone, especially those containing T3. Your doctor must determine which form of hyperthyroidism you have in order to find the best treatment options.

Treatment of Hyperthyroidism

The only conventional treatment for hyperthyroidism is to take a chemical to reduce the hormone's activity in your body.

Herbal medicine for hyperthyroidism focuses primarily on the herb bugleweed taken as an infusion by pouring a cup of boiling water onto one teaspoonful of the dried herb and steeping for ten to fifteen minutes three times a day. One to two milliliters of tincture may be taken instead three times a day. Bugleweed is prescribed by practitioners of alternative medicine as a way of checking production of thyroxine, especially when the symptoms of hyperthyroidism include strained breathing, palpitations, and shaking. Bugleweed may be used with nervines, such as skullcap. Lemon balm, motherwort, and skullcap are other herbs that may be used in a tonic prescribed by an herbalist, or as a tincture diluted in tea. Hyperthyroidism is a serious condition, so you should be sure to see a qualified medical herbalist for supervision of these treatments. Remember that herbs, like antithyroid drugs, must not be abruptly withdrawn. Herbs must be slowly tapered off after you achieve remission.

Some herbs may react with your medications. Please consult your physician before starting any herbal therapy if you are taking prescription medicine.

Homeopathic preparations, especially Kelpasan, Coffea, Natrum muriaticum, and Thyroidinum, may be useful, or homeopaths may prescribe Iodum 30C twice a day for two weeks. Homeopathy can yield excellent results.

Acupuncture is recommended to restore health to your immune system. Stress causes changes in your immune system that promote autoimmune disease. Stress reduction techniques, such as meditation, yoga, or tai chi, can all be effective. Laughter is said to be particularly beneficial in managing autoimmune diseases. Dr. Norman Cousins managed to reverse his own autoimmune disease using Marx Brothers humor and biofeedback, as he describes in his book *Anatomy of an Illness.*

Iodine, an essential component of thyroid hormone, triggers hyperthyroidism. Dietary changes include limiting iodine to less than 150 mcg per day, and replacing iodized salt with a good quality sea salt. Add cruciferous vegetables such as broccoli and cabbage to your diet, along with almonds and peanuts, to help block iodine absorption. Avoid wheat, dairy products and meat containing hormones and antibiotics, saturated fats, sugar, and the sugar substitute aspartame. Add seaweeds and algaes to your diet.

Other steps that may be helpful with this problem: Use dietary supplements to alleviate symptoms by correcting nutrient deficiencies that cause them; for example, place emphasis on vitamins C, E, A, D, B_2, B_1, B_6, as well as the essential fatty acids, and copper. And finally, be sure to get sufficient rest to promote healing.

CHAPTER 5

THE HEART OF THE MATTER

*Understanding and Reversing
Cardiovascular Disease*

HEART DISEASE IS A PROCESS

More people suffer from cardiovascular disease than from any other condition. Cardiovascular disease, including stroke, is an ongoing process. You don't wake up one day and suddenly have a heart attack. Similarly, the underlying reason you have a stroke is not something that happened ten minutes ago. No, both of these events represent a terrible breakdown in your system. An accumulation of toxic and inflammatory reactions has reached the state at which your body can no longer defend itself. That is when you end up going into crisis. When that happens, you'll want to investigate every major way to fortify and protect your body, and use the most appropriate ones.

But here's the question I'm always asking: Why not take up the task of educating yourself and correcting your habits *before* a crisis occurs? After all, by the time you have a heart attack or stroke, you've probably been doing the wrong things for twenty, thirty, or forty years. If you suspect that last sentence applies to you, I recommend a change of course right now. It makes so much more sense than waiting for an unpleasant health event.

A FRESH APPROACH TO HEART DISEASE

The first thing you should know is that a lot of what we call heart disease has been misdiagnosed. Why? During the 1950s and '60s, the "big thing" was cholesterol. At that time, medical authorities were looking into blocked arteries. They saw that an artery could be 80 to 90 percent blocked, causing high blood pressure, since it took greater pressure from the heart to push blood through this ever-narrowing tube. The person with this blocked artery was a candidate for a heart attack, with kidney problems looming up ahead as well.

The researchers took tissue samples from these narrowed arteries and said that the primary ingredient was cholesterol, and they called for a cholesterol-lowering diet. They made cholesterol the primary risk factor for heart disease (along with cigarette smoking). This was a premature and only partially correct answer.

We now know that cholesterol is not a risk factor per se, and that this substance is, in fact, vital to the health of every cell in your body. However, the LDLs, or low-density lipoproteins, are the real danger. They contain high levels of cholesterol, and when they are elevated, they become a major risk factor for building up plaque in the arteries.

Today we know that a safe level of cholesterol is around 150, and an unsafe level is 200. If you have normal blood chemistry with no inflammatory processes going on—no fibrinogen, homocysteine, or C-reactive protein—you have a chance of living a relatively normal life. If you have a cholesterol level of 200, together with inflammatory processes, you then have a great chance of dying prematurely. So the true risk is the entire chemical picture of your body, not just cholesterol by itself.

In the 1990s, we discovered that cholesterol was building up where there were tiny little lesions, little scabs, on the arterial wall. Why were the lesions there? Doctors learned that they were caused by oxidative stressors, such as free radicals and other factors that cause inflammation. But cholesterol was still seen as the culprit. The situation was analogous to the following: You cut yourself, and as part of the recovery process a scab soon develops. However, someone then diagnoses the scab—rather than the sharp object that cut you—as the cause of your problem. This is the fallacious reasoning that was put forth when cholesterol buildup in the lesions was blamed, instead of the free radicals that caused the lesions.

Today we find that oxidative stress, due to inflammations from nutritional and environmental hazards, is the primary cause of cancer, Alzheimer's disease, Parkinson's disease, arthritis, and all forms of heart disease. Here is an example: Heterocyclic amines are the by-products of deep-frying, barbecuing, or grilling something. Well-cooked meat is loaded with heterocyclic amines. These are extremely destructive. When you eat a hamburger, those heterocyclic amines are released into your system. Then they cause damage to the arterial wall. The body tries to repair this damage, but if the immune system is not strong enough, and if you have not been giving the body as many tools for immune repair as for immune destruction, the body will not have what it needs to fully repair the damaged arterial walls. The lesions thus remain partially unhealed, and plaque starts to build up in them.

That is when Dr. Dean Ornish and others observed that free-radical scavengers, including the antioxidants vitamin C, green tea, and garlic, stop the accumulation of plaque. By taking in phytonutri-ents (beneficial chemicals naturally found in plant foods and juices), especially in concentrated amounts, we speed up the healing process to the point at which we have actually reversed heart disease. We have reversed occlusion. We have lowered high blood pressure. And we have lowered elevated cholesterol.

And this brings up an important concept: What reverses a disease will also prevent a disease. So our dietary and lifestyle recommenda-tions for people not yet suffering from heart disease are based on our protocols for reversing heart disease. And here is another concept that now seems correct: Just as one disease process can create multi-ple illnesses, a counter protocol can help avoid those many diseases.

For example, giving up heterocyclic amines from highly cooked foods does more than just protect your heart. It protects your joints, your brain, your intestines, and your liver.

We have made the mistake of not looking at the body as a dynamic whole. We have looked at it as a series of separate broken-down parts that each needs a specialist. So you have doctors working on one little part of the body—the ear, the eye, the nose, the groin, the heart, the muscle, the lung, the spleen—without understanding the dynamic of the whole. We never think that something as relatively simple as a dietary, exercise, or environmental factor could cause a myriad of body conditions, but it does. Once we accept this reality, we can adjust our approach to all types of heart disease.

CHRONIC INFLAMMATORY SYNDROME

As we've mentioned, there is a growing consensus among scientists that common disorders such as heart attack, stroke, and other vascular-related diseases are all caused, in part, by a chronic inflammatory syndrome. Numerous studies demonstrate that the presence of blood indicators of inflammation are strong predictive factors for determining who will develop coronary artery disease and suffer cardiac-related death. The good news is that lifestyle changes and certain dietary supplements can suppress these insidious inflammatory blood components.

You'll recall that one of these dangerous inflammatory markers has been identified as a coagulation protein called fibrinogen. High fibrinogen levels can induce a heart attack via several mechanisms, including increased platelet aggregation, hypercoagulation, and excessive blood thickening. Published scientific studies show that those with high levels of fibrinogen are more than twice as likely to die of a heart attack compared to those with normal levels.

Another inflammatory marker is C-reactive protein. This marker indicates an increased risk for destabilized atherosclerotic plaque and abnormal arterial clotting. When arterial plaque becomes destabilized, it can burst open and block the flow of blood through a coronary artery, resulting in an acute heart attack. Some studies show that people with high levels of C-reactive protein are almost three times as likely to die from a heart attack as are others.

CORRECTING INFLAMMATORY RISK FACTORS

Cardiovascular risk factors such as fibrinogen and C-reactive protein are produced in the liver by the destructive, inflammatory cytokines interleukin-1b, interleukin-6, and tumor necrosis factor alpha. Supplements, such as highly concentrated DHA fish oil and DHEA, suppress excess production of some of these dangerous cytokines.

One recent study shows that interleukin-6 alone increases the risk of heart attack, even after adjustment for the elevation in C-reactive protein induced by interleukin-6 itself. Both vitamin K and DHEA suppress interleukin-6, which helps explain why these supplements have been shown to protect against such a wide range of age-related diseases. Nettle leaf extract appears to be the most effective dietary supplement for suppressing the dangerous tumor necrosis factor alpha and interleukin-1b cytokines.

Protecting Against Fibrinogen-Induced Heart Attack

Agents that inhibit platelet aggregation (thin the blood) reduce the risk that fibrinogen will cause an abnormal arterial blood clot. Such platelet aggregation inhibitors include aspirin, green tea, ginkgo, garlic, and vitamin E. It also makes sense, for optimal protection against heart attack, to use therapies that directly lower elevated fibrinogen levels.

High serum vitamin A and beta-carotene levels have been associated with reduced fibrinogen levels in humans. Animals fed a vitamin-A-deficient diet have an impaired ability to break down fibrinogen. On the other hand, when animals are injected with vitamin A, they produce tissue plasminogen activator, a substance that breaks down fibrinogen.

High doses of fish or olive oil have been shown to lower elevated fibrinogen levels. Excessive homocysteine blocks the natural breakdown of fibrinogen by inhibiting the production of tissue plasminogen activator, but folic acid, trimethylglycine (TMG), vitamin B_{12}, and vitamin B_6 can help by reducing elevated homocysteine levels.

Also, the ever-helpful vitamin C, in large doses, has been shown to break down excess fibrinogen. In one study, heart disease patients were given either 1,000 or 2,000 mg a day of vitamin C to measure the fibrinogen breakdown effect. At 1,000 mg a day, there was no detectable change in fibrinogen or cholesterol. But when C was given at 2,000 mg a day, there was a 27 percent decrease in the platelet aggregation index, a 12 percent reduction in total cholesterol, and a 45 percent increase in fibrinogen breakdown activity.

Some of the nutrients that can lower fibrinogen include at least 2,000 mg a day of vitamin C, 1,000 mg of flush-free niacin, 2,800 mg of EPA/DHA from fish oil, and 2,000 mg a day of bromelain. Some practitioners suggest low-dose aspirin, vitamin E, and garlic, along with ginkgo and green tea extracts to protect against a fibrinogen-induced arterial blood clot, which could cause a stroke.

Detoxifying Homocysteine

Conventional medical journals have published hundreds of studies in recent years that unequivocally link elevated homocysteine to a greater risk of heart attack and stroke. As a result of these findings, some cardiologists suggest that coronary artery disease patients take a multivitamin supplement to lower their homocysteine levels. Patients who follow this advice, but fail to have their blood tested for homocysteine, could be making a fatal mistake.

The clear message from new scientific findings is that there is no safe "normal range" for homocysteine. While commercial laboratories state that normal homocysteine can range from 5 to 15 micromoles per liter of blood, epidemiological data reveal that blood levels of homocysteine levels above 6.3 cause a steep progressive risk of heart attack. One study found that each 3-unit increase in homocysteine equals a 33 percent increase in myocardial infarction (heart at-tack) risk.

People taking vitamin supplements think they are being protected against the lethal effects of homocysteine when, in reality, even supple-ment users can have homocysteine levels far above the safe level of 6.3.

Elevated homocysteine can be controlled in two ways. The most common is via the remethylation (or detoxification) process, whereby methyl groups are donated to homocysteine to transform it into me-thionine and S-adenosylmethionine (SAMe).

Trimethylglycine (TMG) is a potent remethylation agent. The "trimethyl" means there are three methyl groups on each glycine mole-cule that can be transferred to homocysteine to turn it into methionine and SAMe. The detoxification process of homocysteine requires ade-quate levels of folic acid and vitamin B_{12}, in addition to TMG.

Another approach to lowering homocysteine levels is the conver-sion of this substance into cysteine, and eventually into glutathione, through a process called transsulfuration. This process depends on sufficient amounts of vitamin B_6. The precise dose of vitamin B_6 re-quired to lower homocysteine varies with each individual. You should know that if you eat foods that are rich in methionine, such as red meat and chicken, you may need more vitamin B_6, because methio-nine is the (only) amino acid that creates homocysteine. Homocysteine can rise when you have a weak supply of the vitamin cofactors —such as folate and vitamin B_6—that are needed to fight toxic levels of me-thionine in your diet.

There is a genetic defect that blocks the transsulfuration pathway by inducing a deficiency of the B_6-dependent enzyme cystathionine-synthase. Again, powerful doses of vitamin B_6 can counter this de-fect, allowing the transsulfuration pathway to limit homocysteine accumulation. Homocysteine blood testing can monitor whether or not you are taking enough B_6 to keep homocysteine levels in a safe range without overdosing. Excessive doses of vitamin B_6 are more than 300 to 500 mg a day, long-term. Some people lack an enzyme to convert vitamin B_6 into its biologically active form, pyridoxal-5-phosphate. In this case, if low-cost vitamin B_6 supplements do not sufficiently lower your homocysteine levels, a more expensive pyridoxal-5-phosphate supplement may be required.

Many people find that the daily intake of 500 mg of TMG, 800 mcg of folic acid, 200 mcg of vitamin B_{12}, 250 mg of choline, 250 mg of inositol, 30 mg of zinc, and 100 mg of vitamin B_6 will keep homocysteine levels in a safe range. The only way to really know is to have your blood tested to make sure your homocysteine levels are under 7.

Controlling C-Reactive Protein

One of the best-documented ways of determining who will have a stroke is to measure levels of C-reactive protein in the blood. One study shows that elevated C-reactive protein doubles or triples the risk of stroke. Other research shows that in those who have had a major stroke, higher levels of C-reactive protein predict a much greater likelihood of having another vascular event, such as a heart attack or another stroke, or of dying within the year following the initial stroke. In this study, stroke patients with the highest C-reactive protein levels had nearly a 2.4 times greater chance of experiencing a second vascular event or of dying within the next year, compared to patients with the lowest levels of C-reactive protein.

High levels of C-reactive protein indicate a potentially destructive inflammatory autoimmune condition that could predispose you to a host of degenerative diseases. C-reactive protein can be suppressed by aspirin or vitamin E. Some of the pro-inflammatory immune cytokines that cause elevated C-reactive protein include interoleukin-6, interleukin-1b, and tumor necrosis factor alpha. Supplements such as DHEA, vitamin K, nettle leaf extract, and highly concentrated DHA fish oil can help suppress these dangerous inflammatory cytokines that can cause C-reactive protein elevation.

Lowering Your Stroke Profile

Doctors have been concentrating for the past fifty years on controlling blood pressure as the primary method of preventing stroke. Prevention of even borderline hypertension is critical in reducing stroke risk, but there are also factors in the blood that can be tested to further determine your risk of having a stroke. If you are over age forty, have your blood tested to make sure that your homocysteine, fibrinogen, C-reactive protein, LDL-cholesterol, and other factors are in the safe range.

If any of these risk factors for stroke are elevated, they can be safely lowered with therapies that are proven to work. These same risk factors also predispose you to heart attack and other diseases, so anyone concerned about living a long and healthy life would do well to take action to stay at the optimal levels.

Blood Tests Recommended for Cardiovascular Care

Blood Test	What the Standard Reference Range Allows	Optimal Level (Your Goal)
Fibrinogen	Up to 460 mg/dL	Under 300 mg/dL
C-reactive protein	Up to 4.9 mg/L	Under 2 mg/L. Below 1.3 mg/L in some studies
Homocysteine	Up to 15 micro mol/L	Under 7 micro mol/L
Glucose	Up to 109 mg/dL	Under 100 mg/dL
Iron	Up to 180 mg/dL	Under 100 mg/dL
Cholesterol	Up to 199 mg/dL	150–80 mg/dL
LDL cholesterol	Up to 129 mg/dL	Under 100 mg/dL
HDL cholesterol	No lower than 35 mg/dL	Over 50 mg/dL
Triglycerides	Up to 199 mg/dL	Under 100 mg/dL
DHEA	Males: No lower than 80 mcg/dL	400–560 mcg/dL
	Females: No lower than 35 mcg/dL	350–430 mcg/dL
Fasting Insulin	6–27 :IU/mL	0–5 :IU/mL

HOW EXCESS INSULIN
CAUSES HEART ATTACKS

Despite aggressive use of weight-loss therapies, far more Americans are fat today than ever before. According to a recent report, nearly 80 percent of Americans are overweight or obese. Doctors predict that obesity will become a greater health hazard than cigarette smoking. Weight gain is most often associated with cardiovascular disease, but new studies reveal that other age-related disorders, such as cancer, occur at sharply higher rates in overweight individuals. As a result, the government is now encouraging us to lose weight to protect our health.

As we age, we tend to accumulate excess body fat, even though we may be consuming fewer calories now than when we were young. The insidious culprit responsible for these bulging bellies is the hormone insulin. We are not talking about normal insulin secretion. It is, rather, the overproduction of insulin that causes so many of us to gain weight uncontrollably.

Excess insulin is a primary risk factor in the many diseases associated with obesity. First of all, if you are overweight, you face a significant risk of developing type II diabetes. The treatments of obesity and type II diabetes are so remarkably interrelated that if you manage to treat either one of these diseases effectively, it is likely that you are improving the outcome of the other disease.

Diabetes sharply increases the risk of heart attack and stroke. It is critical for you to reverse the diabetic process if you are concerned about cardiovascular disease. Loss of excess fat is a must if you are trying to control a type II diabetes condition.

There are serious misconceptions about why we accumulate so much fat as we age. A fact that is often overlooked is that corpulent people have startlingly high levels of insulin in their blood. When the blood is saturated with insulin, the body will not release significant fat stores, even if you restrict your calorie intake and do exercise.

Hyperinsulinemia is the medical term for the condition in which too much insulin is produced. One way in which excess insulin makes us gain weight is that high insulin levels rapidly deplete blood glucose, triggering chronic hunger. Reactive hypoglycemia is the name for this state in which the blood becomes deficient in glucose because it contains too much insulin.

The May 8, 2002, issue of the *Journal of the American Medical Association* (*JAMA*) features an article on the effects of consuming high glycemic-index foods and the subsequent hyperinsulinemia, hunger, and weight gain that ensue. Here is how the authors of this *JAMA* article summarize their position: "It is possible that the hunger incident to hyperinsulinemia may be a cause of overeating, and therefore, the obesity that so often precedes diabetes."

A plethora of studies show that excess serum insulin (i.e., hyperinsulinemia) is a major health problem. Excess insulin suppresses the release of growth hormone, in addition to preventing fat from being released from cells in people trying to reduce body fat. High serum insulin is associated with the development of abdominal obesity and a number of health problems this induces, including atherosclerosis and impotence.

TESTOSTERONE AND YOUR HEART

Normal aging gradually weakens the heart, even if there is no significant coronary artery disease. The heart of the elderly male just stops beating at some point, if nothing else kills him.

The hormone testosterone builds muscle, and the heart has many testosterone-receptor cites. A testosterone deficiency can weaken heart muscle. Testosterone supports heart muscle protein synthesis, as well as coronary artery dilation, and it helps maintain healthy cholesterol levels.

An ever-increasing number of studies establish an association between high testosterone levels and low cardiovascular disease rates in men. In most patients, symptoms and EKG measurements improve when low testosterone levels are increased. One study shows that testosterone therapy increases blood flow to the heart by almost 70 percent. Doctors in China use testosterone therapy to treat angina successfully.

The effects of low testosterone on cardiovascular disease are as follows:

- Blood pressure rises
- Coronary artery elasticity diminishes
- Cholesterol, fibrinogen, triglycerides, and insulin levels increase
- Abdominal fat increases (raising the risk of heart attack)
- Human growth hormone (HGH) declines (weakening heart muscle)

If you have cardiovascular disease, you should have your blood tested for free testosterone and estrogen. You may be able to correct a testosterone deficit or a testosterone-estrogen imbalance and (with full cooperation from your physician) stop taking risky, expensive drugs to lower your cholesterol, stimulate cardiac output, and keep your blood pressure under control.

A recent study of eleven hundred men presents compelling evidence that those with serum DHEA-S in the lowest quarter (<1.6 :g/mL) are significantly more likely to develop heart disease, and other research confirms this association. DHEA, which is a hormone produced by the adrenal gland, is a precursor for the manufacture of testosterone.

Many studies substantiate the beneficial effects of testosterone therapy in treating heart disease, yet conventional cardiologists continue to overlook the important role this hormone can play in keeping their cardiac patients alive.

THE RIGHT DIET IS CRUCIAL . . .

If your heart is always beating very quickly, that crucial muscle is aging prematurely. All tissue in the body has only a finite length of time that it can live. Anything that speeds up that process is, unfortunately, accelerating the death process. The further along your body is in this death process, the less integrity your cells will have. For example, an eighteen-year-old has greater strength and resiliency in the legs than a thirty-eight-year-old has. Similarly, heart rate can vary with age. The hearts of a fifty-year-old, a forty-year-old and a seventy-year-old are all different. However, the common needs at any age are to slow down the heartbeat, improve circulation, and clean the arteries, veins, and capillaries.

Historically, we were told you could not help heart conditions with nutrition and complementary treatments. We were told we need balloon angioplasty, coronary bypass operations, beta-blockers, calcium blockers, and all kinds of drugs. A lot of what we now know is based upon the work of Dr. Dean Ornish, whose findings were published in peer-reviewed mainstream medical journals. He has also written several popular books.

Dr. Ornish worked with a group that had advanced degeneration of the heart, capillaries, and other vessels; in other words, they had atherosclerosis and arterial sclerosis. They were able to reverse their own arteriolosclerosis, thereby saving themselves and their hearts, by using a vegetarian diet with fish, supplements, exercise, and stress management. So we have a model that demonstrates to the world that this can be done. The fact that the average physician has not yet implemented this model does not mean that there is not good science behind it. There is.

At this point, I think it is necessary to address the problems of a very popular type of diet. High-protein diets are dangerous for cardiovascular health. It is true that you can lose weight on such a diet, but you would be doing so at the cost of flooding the body with toxic protein that can increase your LDL cholesterol, your homocysteine, your fibrinogen, and your C-reactive protein. When you have an elevated C-reactive protein level, you increase the likelihood of a deadly heart attack by up to 500 percent, and of a stroke by up to 700 percent. Is there a point to losing a few pounds on a high-protein diet and dying of a heart attack in the process? Is there a point to losing weight, but increasing inflammatory processes, flooding the body with antibiotics and growth stimulating hormones and toxic debris, creating so much by-product within the system that the liver and kidneys cannot flush all of it out? This is for you to decide.

Moreover, although it is not widely talked about, kidney disease is on the rise. From being a relatively obscure condition at the beginning of the twentieth century, it is now among the top five major diseases in the United States. Why? We are eating more protein, and "fast," highly processed foods than our kidneys and livers can handle. And if we lose our ability to clear our body of these toxins, our hearts will pay the price.

In general, we should be consuming nutrients that feed, strengthen, and protect the cells, and heart cells are no exception. The heart needs to be nourished. When you strengthen your heart, it doesn't have to work so hard to pump blood through your arteries. And the arteries themselves will be less clogged and more resilient, as well.

A diet packed with living, vital foods is widely recognized for its ability to:

- Lower your blood pressure
- Lower your triglycerides
- Lower your LDL cholesterol
- Increase your HDL (the good cholesterol)
- Turn off the flame of cytokines, homocysteine, fibrinogen, and C-reactive protein

In short, a vital diet turns off inflammatory agents all over the body, and turns on the healing agents.

. . . AND SO IS EXERCISE

Exercise is supremely important for cardiovascular health. This fact is so well known that it ought not be necessary to mention it. And yet many people in our busy, complicated world never take the time to exercise at all, to say nothing of exercising properly for an effective period of time.

Senior citizens and baby boomers, the people who need exercise the most, are getting it the least. Every single muscle in your body needs exercise each day. Americans tend to exercise only occasionally, but the notion that we are lazy or indifferent stems from a wrong assumption. We are just not programmed to do regular exercise, and thus we automatically seek the most comfortable route. But you can alter that through awareness. Start walking instead of riding, for a change; climb stairs instead of taking the elevator all the time. I'm not telling you to overdo it; proceed gradually, but steadily, to make wiser choices every day.

In point of fact, when you are sedentary, you are doing yourself a great deal of harm. Exercise increases your body's lymphatic drainage. (Note that the lymph system, unlike our circulatory system, does not have a pump to keep it moving.) Exercise relaxes your body. Aerobic exercises increase circulation, stimulate the release of toxins, and help the arteries to heal. I'm an advocate of yoga, as well, because it stretches the body, stretches the muscles, increases our deep rhythmic breathing, and aligns our posture.

Although the benefits of exercise are many and rich, before you start any exercise program, take the time to have the proper medically supervised tests to make sure you have no underlying heart condition that would contraindicate the exercise. Get a cardiovascular stress test and receive a diagnosis before starting the program. You do not want to drop dead because your body has been keeping a deadly secret! In addition, initially, your exercise program can be medically directed. As with anything new, start the amount and intensity of exercise on the low side and increase the exertion gradually.

I have been training athletes since 1976 when I started my Natural Living Running and Walking Club. I have trained thousands of people who have gone on to run in the New York City Marathon and other races. They've lost weight, reduced their blood pressure and cholesterol levels, improved their immune systems, and in general increased their health. It's been an exciting and rewarding process all around.

Exercise is a missing link for most Americans who are overweight with heart disease and high blood pressure. Exercise, done properly, can help many disease states, even arthritis. But you must do it gradually. It is a bad idea to start off just running, or even walking, as fast as you can. Warm up. Stretch properly before and after the exercise period. Cool down. Make sure you have proper hydration, and most important, take lots of antioxidants afterward because exercising increases oxidation, thereby increasing free radicals, which increase destruction to the cells and inflammatory processes. In this way, you will get the benefits of the exercise but none of the side effects. We'll be talking more about exercise in Chapter 9.

WHAT YOU CAN DO: THREE SPECIFIC PROTOCOLS FOR HEART HEALTH

First, a word of caution. When it comes to protocols, or specific programs, it is important to remember that they are designed to be done in an incremental fashion, under medical supervision. It is stated here in the strongest possible way that you must, you simply *must* follow this protocol under a holistic physician's supervision, ideally a board-certified cardiologist.

A CARDIOVASCULAR PROTOCOL

Supplements

The following nutrients are needed for the cardiovascular system. It is not suggested that all of these be taken at once. That would be too much for the body, so take only a few at a time over the course of the day.

Coenzyme Q10 is a superstar in protecting the heart. It feeds the cell. It allows the transport of fatty acids to the cell so that the cell's mitochondria have the energy needed to function properly. This is especially important for the heart muscle, for obvious reasons!

I believe that if every American took between 100 to 300 mg of coenzyme Q10 a day, and if people with cardiovascular disease took between 300 to 500 mg of this wonder-nutrient daily, we could be saving hundreds of thousands of lives a year. If you're taking a large amount of coenzyme Q10, do so in divided doses. For example, if you are taking a total of 500 mg of coenzyme Q10, you should take 100 mg five times a day.

Calcium and magnesium from citrate (always taken together) in the amount of about 1,500 mg a day are a crucial pair of nutrients for the heart. There will be more information about magnesium, the most important but sadly neglected heart nutrient, below.

Other important substances include garlic (1,000 to 5,000 mg), onion (a raw onion a day helps keep strokes and heart attacks away), and L-carnitine (500 to 1,000 mg). L-carnitine increases energy by burning fat within the cell's mitochondria. This helps the body to recover quickly from fatigue. And L-carnitine is especially good when combined with vitamin E, another superstar heart disease fighter, phosphatidylcholine (500 mg twice a day), DMG (dimethylglycine) (100 mg once a day), TMG (trimethylglycine) (200 mg twice a day), Maxepa (fish oils) (1,500 mg), potassium (500 mg), selenium (200 mcg), melatonin (1–3 mg), B complex (50 mg), vitamin C (2,000–10,000 mg), DHEA (25 mg; do not use DHEA if you have cancer), chromium picolinate (200 mcg), chondroitin sulfate (500 mg two times a day), evening primrose oil (generally at 1,500 mg in divided doses), polycosinol (10 mg), and N-acetyl cysteine (1,500 mg). Alpha-lipoic acid (300 mg) is very important as a free-radical scavenger.

Also very important for heart disease is natural (not synthetic) vitamin E (with tocotrienols and the gamma fraction) generally at 400 IU with tocotrienols at 100 mg. Bioflavonoids are also quite helpful. Make sure you have what are called methylating agents, namely vitamin B_{12}, folic acid (800 units), and TMG. The essential fatty acids are just that—essential! The two types are called omega-3 and omega-6. Fish oils are a source of omega-3 and evening primrose oil is a source of omega-6. Generally, 3,000 mg of omega-3 and 2,000 mg of omega-6 should be divided into three doses, daily.

L-arginine facilitates the body's production of nitric oxide, which has an antiangina and antistress effect upon the arteries, enabling the muscles in the arterial walls to relax. This amino acid is generally taken at 2,000 to 3,000 mg per day.

Lecithin can reduce arterial plaque, lower blood pressure, and lessen angina pectoris. Take lecithin granules in one teaspoon in the morning (they can be sprinkled over cereal). Taurine, an amino acid that acts as an antioxidant, can help fortify cardiac contractions and consequently enhance the outflow of blood from the heart. Take it generally at 500 mg. Niacin (vitamin B$_3$) has been shown to help prevent heart attacks. It also helps prevent people from dying from them.

Mineral for the Heart

Magnesium is the single most important mineral for the heart. Generally, people don't realize that a magnesium-deficient heart is almost always more susceptible to heart attack. This brings up the ever-important concept of the preventive approaches. Logic suggests that if filling a specific nutrient deficiency in a sick person ameliorates the condition, then giving a healthy person that nutrient in more than adequate amounts should prevent the condition from developing in the first place. In the case of heart disease, we see certain nutrients, such as magnesium, that are deficient in all patients. Common sense would then dictate that giving more than adequate amounts of these nutrients to people will help prevent or reverse heart disease.

Herbs for Heart Health

There are some herbs that are excellent for promoting cardiovascular health. Cayenne is a superstar because it contains the active ingredient capsaicin. Capsaicin lowers blood pressure and cholesterol and prevents heart attacks and strokes. It is a natural blood thinner. However, it is not safe for everyone to take this herb, because for those taking certain medications, such as Coumadin (warfarin), there could be contraindications. So you have to ask your physician if any prescription drug you are taking may prohibit the use of cayenne. This is very important.

Otherwise, cayenne, best known as the spice cayenne pepper, should definitely be used, but carefully, because it is very hot! If you use this as a spice, do not cook the pepper with the food but sprinkle it on food only after cooking the food, to avoid irritation.

Hawthorn berry improves arrhythmias, angina, blood pressure, and arterial hardening. It can enhance circulation. It treats valve insufficiencies, irregular pulse, and abnormal acid levels in the blood. In short, it is a really terrific herb! Hawthorn is generally taken at 100 mg twice a day. Bugleweed helps alleviate heart palpitations and lowers blood pressure. Ginkgo biloba, the well-known multipurpose herb, gets more blood flowing into the small blood vessels. It's suggested at 300 mg in divided doses. Motherwort helps secure cardiac electrical rhythm. Tansy is another herb used for heart palpitations, and it can be ingested as a tea. Wild yam enhances the body's production of DHEA, and DHEA is crucial in helping to prevent heart attacks. Arjuna is an Ayurvedic herb that enhances circulation and lowers blood pressure. Indian snakeroot also has anti-hypertensive qualities. Black cohosh, an American herb, helps lower blood pressure.

We've said this before, but let's restate the warnings: It is not at all advisable to take all these substances at the same time. Instead, take one or two of these for a month, as professionally directed. Record the results. Then, under continued guidance, repeat or increase the dosage, or move on to different substances. Do not self-medicate. These supplements are not meant as medicines. These are not meant to treat diseases, but only to augment the body's internal biochemistry, to help strengthen it, so that whatever else you are doing can be better applied.

Intravenous Treatments for Cardiovascular Health

There are several intravenous treatments that have proven very effective in the cardiovascular arena. EDTA chelation therapy is crucial, I believe, for treating coronary artery disease and arterial sclerosis. I have seen many people who were about to receive coronary bypass operations, or some other drastic treatment, improve tremendously, even dramatically, using chelation therapy. If you already have a heart condition, you have to be patient and courageous, because it may take some time, probably upwards of two years, to do this properly, but your life is worth it. We have seen from the literature that this therapy definitely works and that you can reclaim your life!

Vitamin C, taken intravenously, is another extremely important therapy given at a practitioner's office. This lifesaving treatment has been able to help people with cancer and heart disease, among many other conditions.

A PROTOCOL TO LOWER CHOLESTEROL

Stressed-out baby boomers worry about (among other things!) their cholesterol level. And well they might, since stress tends to elevate cholesterol. Having elevated blood sugar can also contribute to high cholesterol. Generally, most people don't have their cholesterol level checked. They should. This is done as part of a blood lipid profile.

You cannot eliminate cholesterol from the diet, and, indeed, you should not do so, because, as mentioned previously, cholesterol is important. But it must be kept in check.

We know that high-fiber foods, and the pectin found in apples, will lower cholesterol. Blueberries are very good at this, too. Hot grain cereals such as oats, barley, and buckwheat are also good. Therefore, having some apples and blueberries in your cereal is exceptionally helpful. Other anticholesterol foods are polyunsaturated oils (in small amounts only!) and linoleic oils from cold fish (but do not eat shellfish), walnuts, almonds, sunflower seeds, and nut butters.

Supplements That Lower Cholesterol

L-carnosine can help rejuvenate the cell and protect it from prematurely aging, going into apoptosis (programmed cell death), and dying, because it protects the chromosomes. (Note: Do not confuse this substance with L-carnitine, another helpful supplement taken at 1,000 mg a day.) Additional recommendations are L-glutamine (2,000 mg a day), vitamin E (400 IU), bromelain as directed, maitake and shiitake mushrooms (generally at 100 mg each), as well as ganoderma (reishi) mushrooms, and bioflavonoids.

Herbs That Lower Cholesterol

The most helpful herbs for lowering cholesterol and triglycerides are ginger, cayenne, raw garlic, and onions; also take ginkgo biloba, gotu kola as directed, and red clover as directed.

Mineral That Lowers Cholesterol

Potassium is the superstar mineral for lowering hypertension and cholesterol. Generally taken at 500 mg a day, it will help significantly.

Phytochemicals That Lower Cholesterol

The healing phytochemicals in fruits and fruit juices are also very important. For people with high blood sugar, there are now concentrates on the market without the fruit sugar in them, so everyone can get the benefits of drinking a lot of fruit juice. Remember that red fruits and their concentrates repair damage to your DNA. This is crucial because once you repair the damage to the DNA, the cell can regain much, if not all, of its previous functioning.

Exercise to Lower Cholesterol

When you exercise aerobically for up to an hour a day, you are increasing the good HDL cholesterol and reducing the bad LDL cholesterol. It may take three, four, or five months, but you will see a noticeable change.

A PROTOCOL TO LOWER HIGH BLOOD PRESSURE (HYPERTENSION)

Hypertension is one of the top killers. It is estimated that 60 million Americans suffer from it. Stress is a major cause. Being under pressure on the job, or trying to do too much, or any of the hundreds of tension-filled situations in life may cause elevated blood sugar and stress hormones. And the unfortunate fact is that elevated blood sugar plus elevated blood pressure is a deadly combination, if ever there was one. One is bad enough. Two together can be catastrophic. If you have these two conditions, you are probably in for some serious consequences. In addition, inflammatory responses are the frequent accompaniment. A heart attack or stroke is just waiting to happen.

Supplements to Reduce High Blood Pressure

When your goal is reducing hypertension, the following will help: the superstar mineral potassium (500 to 800 mg); 1,500 mg of calcium magnesium citrate; vitamin C (5,000 to 10,000 mg); vitamin B_6 (100 mg); coenzyme Q10 (generally 300 to 500 mg); the omega-3 fatty acids from fish (1,500 mg); L-carnitine (1,500 mg); L-glutamine (1,000 mg); vitamin E with tocotrienols and gamma tocopherol (400 to 800 units); red clover; and again, our tried and true friend garlic.

Remember, Please . . . The following caution has been given several times before, but it is extremely important. It will be given in the form of an example: If you have high cholesterol, heart disease, and hypertension, and each has a protocol calling for garlic at 1,000 mg, this does not mean that you are to take 3,000 mg. You take only the amount called for in one protocol. In other words, these protocols are not additive.

Generally, you would follow the protocol for the primary condition. Let us say you have five illnesses. Take the illness that seems to be the most threatening, and follow that protocol. Once you have followed this protocol for a year, and you see the condition improving, chances are very great that the other conditions are improving as well.

Your whole body, at this point, should be stronger and healthier, and your immune system should be working better. The energy-enhancing vitality of one protocol will, no doubt, help you with your other conditions. However, if you still find you need help, go to the second protocol (the one for the next most troublesome condition). Try that one for a year as well. Never take three protocols for three conditions at once. That would overwhelm the system.

I also want to stress again that in suggesting alternative treatments, I am not claiming that these treatments are absolute cures, only that they can have a major, beneficial effect on the conditions. I am not asking you to give up whatever your doctor is suggesting, if you decide to go with any of these protocols. These are complementary, augmentative treatments. That is why they should be followed under medical supervision.

Phytochemicals to Reduce High Blood Pressure

What can be done about this situation? The advice here is short, but good: First, we have to thin our blood. Green vegetable juices naturally do this.

Stress Management for Lowering Blood Pressure

Keeping all the foregoing in mind, we can end the chapter on a positive and constructive note. Stress management techniques are very important for bringing down your blood pressure. Meditation can play a role here, as can destressing exercises and techniques, prayer, listening to calm music, going for walks, playing with your companion pets, spending quality time in your relationships without arguing, and pursuing hobbies or anything that can bring you joy during the day—or night, for that matter!

Bring your energy to a calm place. Get rid of all excess stimulation around you. Have a candlelit meal with nice soft music. Take a bubble bath, if that is what appeals to you. Do things that are just fun, and watch your blood pressure come down.

CHAPTER 6

PREVENTING OR FACING CANCER

Strategies for Protecting Ourselves

THE LONG DARK ROAD TO CANCER

In Chapters 2 and 3 you read how our toxic environment flooded with over one hundred thousand chemicals is affecting us and why we age. I know a lot of that information is shocking but I think you'll agree that it's much better to know what we're up against. Armed with that knowledge, you can take a stand. Armed with the information in this chapter, you can counter any notion from friends, family, or even your doctor that the causes of cancer are unknown. That's why this chapter is jam-packed with science and research to prove my point.

I've already mentioned many possible diseases that can result from the ongoing accumulation of toxins in the environment, but of all the diseases associated with aging, the most terrifying is cancer. We all hear the news about the escalating numbers of prostate and breast cancer cases in our aging population. Even though heart attacks and stroke are also associated with aging, in my experience, people are not as fearful of them. Perhaps there has been enough information linking heart disease with lifestyle, diet, and personality type that people have some idea of its origins. But most people have a hard time coming to grips with cancer; and even fewer people realize that we *can* do something about it. This is probably because, as a nation, we've been told that the causes of cancer are unknown. And that's what I want to address.

The darkness around cancer is understandable; medical experts say they don't really know what's causing the epidemic of cancer in our midst and we are told there is no cure. In 1970 President Nixon declared war on cancer, expecting to find a cure by 1990, but we seem to be no closer to a panacea than we were then. Cancer takes the lives of one in four people now. Soon the statistics will show that one in two people will develop it in their lifetime. Cancer in our grandchildren has increased several hundred percent in the last thirty years. After accidents, the leading cause of death in children is cancer. However, the greatest and most recent increase is in hormone-dependent cancers of the breast, prostate, and testicles in older adults.[1]

In 2002 the National Cancer Institute (NCI) in their annual report announced that double the present number of people will be diagnosed with cancer annually by 2050.[2] They used 1999 statistics in their calculations and found that in that year 1.3 million new cases of cancer were diagnosed; in fifty years there will be 2.6 million new cases diagnosed annually. These extraordinary statistics are said to be due to the aging population, which according to the NCI is the "cancer population." In fact, for the over-seventy-five age group the cancer rate will more than double. By 2050, more than 1.1 million people seventy-five and older will be diagnosed each year, up from about 400,000 today. In 1999 the NCI statisticians estimated 8.9 million people were living with cancer in the United States at the beginning of 1999. About 60 percent of those were sixty-five or older.

To us Power Agers, these should be fighting words. I certainly don't want to be a statistic lumped into a "cancer population" just because of my age. What I do want to share with you is why cancer seems to be epidemic and what we can do about it. In the mid-1970s I wrote a series of articles in *Penthouse* magazine about cancer. What I learned thirty years ago still applies today. I interviewed many cancer experts for that series, one of whom was Dr. Samuel Epstein, an occupational medicine expert who, in 1978, published a groundbreaking book called *The Politics of Cancer*. Even way back then, he and I shared grave concerns about the effects of DDT on our health, and we both worked to have that toxic chemical banned.

I believe Dr. Epstein is right when he states in *The Politics of Cancer* that there are four basic causes of cancer:

1. Cancer is caused mainly by exposure to chemical or physical agents in the environment.
2. The more of a carcinogen present in the human environment, hence the greater the exposure to it, the greater is the chance of developing cancer from it.
3. Although environmental carcinogens are the predominant causes of human cancer, the incidence of cancer in any population of animals or humans exposed to a carcinogen may be influenced by a variety of factors.
4. There is no known method for measuring or predicting a "safe" level of exposure to any carcinogen below which cancer will not result in an individual or population group.[3]

CANCER IS CAUSED BY CHEMICALS

Even though Dr. Epstein says cancer is mainly chemically induced, he does acknowledge that there are some genetic forms of cancer and that viruses may play a part in some cancers. These, however, count for only a small percentage of cancer cases. Dr. Epstein says that "Just as germs cause infections, so do certain chemical and physical agents, carcinogens, cause cancer."

And he may be right because a recent study shows that cancer does not occur in any greater numbers in twins than in the general population.[4] This certainly dampens the enthusiasm of some genetic researchers who insist that cancer is primarily genetic. Those who want to manipulate genes to "cure" us of cancer are very unhappy with the results of this study, but the rest of us can now simply take action and eliminate cancer-causing chemicals from our body and environment. Jeffrey Bland, Ph.D., a well-known nutritionist and health educator, says that it's not your genes so much as the environment your genes are floating in that controls your health.

The *New England Journal of Medicine* helps us understand what happens when chemicals attack the body. A 2000 article called "Roads Leading to Breast Cancer" said that, "Cancer results from the accumulation of mutations in genes that regulate cellular proliferation."[5] And it's chemicals that mutate these genes. Cells are created and operate under the direction of genes in our DNA. Our very existence is dependent on the precise genetic regulation of our cells. Healthy young cells have relatively perfect genes. Aging and environmental factors cause genes to mutate, resulting in damaged cells turning healthy cells into malignant cells. As gene mutations accumulate, and the body's immune system can't keep up with the necessary repairs, the risk of cancer sharply increases.

WHAT CAUSES GENES TO MUTATE?

Even the scientific literature on human studies shows that about 70 percent of gene mutation is environmental. Clearly, cancer is much more under our control than it would be were it a genetic disease that we were born with. Let me be very clear on this point. Genetics research is trying to prove that most cancers are inherent in our genes, and so in order to cure these cancers, gene therapy must alter our basic gene structure. But environmental gene mutation is not about a genetic code present at birth, but instead a disruption in the day-to-day work of our genes, as they make muscle or bone or send messages from one part of the body to the other. Our diet, lifestyle, and exposure to carcinogens, including chemicals and radiation, can control such environmental gene mutation.

Free Radicals

I talked a lot about free radicals in Chapters 2 and 3 but it's important to mention them here, because free radicals are an important cause of cancer. To review, free radicals are atoms with unpaired electrons that can cause damage in a normal metabolic process known as oxidation. We talked about oxidative stress in Chapter 3. Although the destructive effects of free radical activity have been heavily implicated in cancer, we don't usually hear about free radicals. We hear about carcinogens. Carcinogens are toxic substances that enter the body and cause free radical formation that in turn mutates normal cells into cancer cells. In earlier chapters we talked about a number of carcinogens and the importance of avoiding them: pesticides on our produce; nitrosamines in food; bromates in baked goods; food dyes and colorings; DEPC, a chemical that in a laboratory kills microbes but in our body combines with ammonia to harmful effect; and a list of chemicals used in food. These include glycerides, monosodium glutamate (MSG), propyl galate, sodium citrate, sulfiting agents, and disodium phosphate; DDT shows up in imported foods from countries that still use this deadly pesticide; and radioactive substances from nuclear plants and mining can be found in our water.

Diet and Cancer

In Chapter 3 you were probably surprised to hear that the food we eat every day could be harming us and causing chronic disease, inflammation, and cancer. We learned that "well-done" foods inflict massive damage to the genes. In particular, we looked at the University of Minnesota study that showed women who eat very well done hamburgers have a 50 percent greater risk of breast cancer than women who eat their burgers rare or medium. This famous Women's Health Study found that women who consistently eat well-done steak, hamburgers, and bacon have a 4.62-fold increased risk of breast cancer.[6] So, remember that cooking foods at high temperatures causes the formation of gene-mutating heterocyclic amines and can lead to many types of cancer. If you follow the Power Aging diet and drastically reduce or eliminate your meat intake, you will avoid this particular type of assault and substitute healthy, organic vegetables, grains, beans, nuts, and seeds.

For many health conscious people, avoiding hamburgers is already second nature. But the situation gets trickier when seemingly healthy foods can be carcinogenic by virtue of the way they are cooked. Grilled salmon, for example, contains a potent dose of gene-mutating heterocyclic amines. The carcinogenic dangers of heterocyclic amines have been thoroughly discussed in the scientific literature, yet the public is largely unaware of these dangers and continues to consume foods that inflict massive numbers of gene mutations. Recent studies indicate that heterocylic amines cause more cases of cancer than previously indicated. Heterocyclic amines, however, are not the only dietary culprit involved in gene mutation. As mentioned above, other mutagenic agents found in food are nitrosamine preservatives, aflatoxin molds, and pesticide–herbicide residues.

The bottom line is that we need to eat a certain number of calories and this inevitably exposes us to agents that mutate our genes. But we can also learn how to detoxify and get rid of these toxins from our body and take the right antioxidant nutrients to protect us. We'll talk more about how to protect ourselves from cancer at the end of this chapter, and in Chapter 9 we'll outline a detoxification process, and an eating plan that can help us get and stay healthy.

Not only does eating the wrong foods get us into trouble, *not* eating the right foods can also interfere with our health. A 2001 study involving thirty-four thousand postmenopausal women shows that bad diet choices can lead to breast cancer. Women who drink even half a glass of alcohol a day and eat few vegetables have low levels of the important cancer-protective B vitamin folic acid and a 60 percent increase in the likelihood of getting breast cancer.

Alcohol use has been linked in the past to a slight increase in the risk of breast cancer due to its breakdown into acetaldehyde, but it is particularly dangerous for people who do not eat vegetables. Folic acid is necessary to repair certain kinds of chemical-induced damage to genetic material. Until we get to our diet and treatment chapters, be reminded that you can get your folic acid from green leafy vegetables, dried beans, and peas.[7]

We hear a lot about drinking milk these days, the expensive "Got

Milk?" ads are everywhere, but dairy can be dangerous. An important editorial in the *British Medical Journal* by several experts from the University of Bristol in England warns about the growing body of evidence implicating insulin–like growth factor-1 (IGF-1) in cancer. This hormone is normally found in cows, but in humans it can trigger cancer cell production. The introduction of injectable, genetically engineered, synthetic bovine growth hormone, which drastically increases the amount of IGF-1 in milk, only adds to the cancer potential.[8] The authors say that, "The risk of cancer is higher among people with raised concentrations of insulin-like growth factor-1." They even agree that "The effects are sizeable and stronger than the effects seen in relation to most previously reported risk factors." The authors end by actually giving some advice and issue a warning, "Given the increasing evidence of the risk of cancer, caution should be exercised in the exogenous use of either insulin-like growth factor-1 or substances that increase concentrations of it." Of course, they should say *Stop drinking milk* instead of "exercising caution about these substances," but that's the decision you must make based on reading this material and doing your own research.

Sugar and Cancer

We talked about the dangers of sugar in great detail in Chapter 3, but did you know that indulging in our favorite vice can also set up an environment for cancer growth? Epidemiological studies consistently find that people who consume the most calories have significantly higher incidences of cancer. There are several mechanisms that explain why overeating causes cancer, but one reason is that more gene mutations occur in response to higher caloric intake. Moreover, we've known since 1931 that cancer cells crave sugar just as much as we seem to!

German Otto Warburg, Ph.D., was awarded a Nobel Prize in medicine for his discovery that cancer cells depend mainly on glucose as their food supply. They devour glucose without the aid of oxygen in what is called anaerobic metabolism and consequently produce a large amount of lactic acid. The build-up in lactic acid produces a more acidic pH in cancerous tissues and contributes to the overall physical fatigue experienced by cancer patients.[9] Numerous studies in peer reviewed journals show that sugar increases prostate, colon, and biliary tract cancers.[10] Yet we continue to eat it to the tune of $2 billion spent on Easter candy in 2003.

Why doesn't the average person know this valuable information? Why isn't it headline news? Why don't all the smiling news anchors drop this bombshell as we bite into our morning donut? Well, that donut probably *is* the reason why. The economy is partly propped up by the food industry, which depends on feeding you a lot of over-priced synthetic foods sweetened with sugar or loaded with fat. You may not know that low-fat junk food is high in sugar and low-carb junk food is usually high in fat! The economy is so tied into the marketing of food and shifts in consumer trends that if Oprah Winfrey stood up on her show and told everyone just how bad sugar really is, the sugar industry would not only have a heart attack, they'd suffer a huge loss in profits. That very thing happened when Oprah spoke out about the problems with eating meat; she had to suffer the consequences of angering a whole industry.

Here's another way sugar wraps us in a tight vicious circle. Excess sugar can cause increased weight gain and lead to obesity. We know that obese women have more estrogen in their tissues and we also know that toxic pesticides, many of which mimic estrogen, can become stored in fat cells. Because synthetic hormones and a lot of other chemicals are fat soluble, they migrate to fat tissue and dissolve right into them. There are dozens of studies showing the link between pesticides and cancer. Organochlorine (DDT and DDE) pesticides are especially dangerous. They are very common in agricultural and industrial products, and because of their weak estrogen-like effect they get trapped in the body's fat cells. Both play a role in the development of breast cancer.

Carcinogens in the Water

We talked about our water supply in Chapter 3. Let's talk about it now in relation to cancer. We naturally assume that our chlorinated water supply is safe from bacteria and dangerous contaminants, but it appears that the very substance used to kill organisms might be causing some ill effects. Two studies following 2,200 people in Iowa found that merely drinking chlorinated tap water can more than double the risk of bladder and rectal cancers in some individuals. Chlorine in the laboratory is different from chlorine put into the water supply. In the lab a drop of chlorine can annihilate bacteria introduced into a sterile medium. However, when chlorine is used in water-treatment plants, it can react with natural organic compounds in water and create certain by-products that are carcinogenic. It's the case of one plus one adding up to something other than two. In the lab, one plus one gives you two, but in the real world that extra factor of organic compounds creates something very toxic and dangerous.

Surveying a group of people who suffered from bladder, colon, or rectal cancers, researchers concluded that men who smoked and drank chlorinated tap water for more than forty years had twice the risk of bladder cancer than those who did not drink chlorinated tap water. In one study the rates for women smokers drinking chlorinated tap water were not significantly elevated. However, a second study had elevated rates for both men and women. Further results showed that people on low-fiber diets washed down with chlorinated water for over forty years more than doubled their risk for rectal cancer, compared with nonchlorinated-water drinkers. Looking at exercise showed the same pattern. Those who did not exercise had more cancer risk than those who exercised even once a week.[11]

Dioxin and Cancer

Dioxin is the deadly defoliant known as Agent Orange that American soldiers sprayed across the Vietnamese countryside during the Vietnam

War. It is still used in industry and enters the food chain through waste run off. Dioxin accumulates in the fatty tissue of animals and fish. And when humans eat those animals and fish we too accumulate dioxin. In the May 17, 2000, edition of the *Washington Post* there was an alarming headline: "Dioxin a Serious Cancer Threat." A report from the Environmental Protection Agency (EPA) disclosed that dioxin poses more of a cancer threat than previously believed. According to the EPA, which had placed the chance of getting cancer from dioxin at 1 in 1,000, the risk by 2000 was increased to 1 in 100. According to the *Washington Post* article, low levels of the toxic chemical have already been linked to diabetes and birth defects. Now the link to cancer is more defined.[12]

Let's get specific about pesticides that we may be silently ingesting in our diet. In 1998 a study published in the journal *The Lancet* showed that risk of breast cancer was twice as high in women with the highest concentrations of a pesticide called dieldrin (an organochlorine) in their blood compared with women who had the lowest concentrations.[13] A study in Spain published in *The Lancet* confirmed that pesticides may cause cancer. Patients with cancer of the pancreas were up to ten times more likely to show elevated levels of organochlorines in their blood than other, noncancer patients in a hospital setting.[14]

Pesticides and Lymphoma

An incredible body of research linking lymphoma (cancer of the lymphatic system) to pesticides is available from the Lymphoma Foundation of America.[15] The directors of this foundation recruited a scientific review panel of twelve doctors and scientists to help compile a report on the association between cancer and pesticides. Their paper "Do Pesticides Cause Lymphoma?" is extremely comprehensive. The report cites almost eighty scientific studies and almost forty editorials that highlight the pesticide–lymphoma connection. When defining the causes of cancer, the Lymphoma Foundation does not shrink from the task. Instead they give a very balanced answer:

. . . there are many things to consider: heredity, viruses, our exposure to chemicals, and toxic substances in our air, water, and food. These factors and exposures may vary, depending in part on our chosen occupations and where we live. Any or all of these may weaken a person's immune system. These are only some of the possible—even probable—"causes" of cancer. It appears that pesticides may be one piece of a larger lymphoma puzzle.

They urge us not to fall into the victim role and be blamed for our condition:

One of the most publicized stories about the "cause" of cancer is the ongoing drama of the cigarette companies and their attempts to show, in extended legal battles, that people develop lung cancer not from smoking, but from their own inherent problems and weaknesses.

The Politics of Cancer

The authors of "Do Pesticides Cause Lymphoma?" are quite aware that there is hidden bias in the reporting of the pesticide problem, which makes it very difficult to warn people about the hazards of these chemical contaminants. The primary researcher, who may be hired to do the study by the pesticide industry, may well be biased. After all, he or she wants to be paid. His or her team may come up with inconclusive results or say that further research must be done. Even the way a study is titled can deny its results. An abstract may be biased, and in many cases, it is not until a properly qualified expert reads a scientific study in its entirety that flaws are discovered. Or, as Lymphoma Foundation says, some researchers will maintain that they will never draw a conclusion, but keep asking for more studies and more research funding "unless everyone, or almost everyone, who is exposed to a substance later develops cancer." They say that some people still don't believe cigarette smoking causes cancer because not everyone gets it.

For the past thirty years, Dr. Janette Sherman, a practicing physician in Alexandria, Virginia, has been an advocate for patients' rights. In her book *Life's Delicate Balance: Causes and Prevention of Breast Cancer* she writes:

> There is a massing, in a few hands, of the control of production, distribution, and use of pharmaceutical drugs and appliances; control of the sale and use of medical and laboratory tests; the consolidation and control of hospitals, nursing homes, and home care providers. We are no longer people who become sick. We have become markets. Is it any wonder that prevention receives so little attention? Cancer is a big and successful business![16]

At a 1999 conference Helke Ferrie found evidence that some pharmaceutical companies enjoy profits from both cancer-causing and cancer-treating drugs. She said that "Zeneca's annual revenues from the cancer drug tamoxifen are at $470 million; the same company also makes over $300 million annually on the carcinogenic herbicide acetochlor and other chlorine products."[17]

Prescription Drugs and Cancer

Common sense tells us that chemicals like pesticides, herbicides, and fungicides are created specifically to kill things, so it's doesn't take a lot of imagination to realize that they may be also be toxic to humans. But when we look at prescription drugs we assume that they are beneficial or harmless. In the beginning chapters of *Power Aging* we talked about the overuse of drugs in our society. But we still can't imagine our friendly family doctor prescribing a drug with drastic side effects. Yet it happens all the time.

Antidepressants and Cancer. Researchers in Canada found that doses of three antihistamines—Claritin, Histamil, and Atarax—enhanced cancer growth in mice. Two years later the same group of researchers published a study on the antidepressant selective serotonin reuptake inhibitors (SSRIs) like Prozac. They found that SSRIs may be associated with an increased risk of breast cancer.[18] A 2000 study showed that breast cancer risk was seven times greater in women taking Paxil.[19] A follow-up study by the same investigators, following more than five thousand women, found a 70 percent increase, much lower than the previous study but still significant. In the first study women taking tricyclic antidepressants were found to have twice the risk of breast cancer compared to normal controls. Comments have been made that Paxil was only on the market for about three years before the breast cancer cases were diagnosed.[20]

Antihypertensives and Cancer. Power Agers should be alert to another study that indicates that women over age sixty-five who take certain blood pressure lowering medications have more than twice the risk of developing breast cancer. The class of blood pressure–lowering drugs tested are called calcium channel blockers, or CCBs. Common types of CCBs include verapamil, Diltiazem, and Nifedipine. A further warning should go to women who are taking hormone replacement therapy with estrogen in addition to calcium channel blockers. The women in the study taking both drugs appeared to have the most risk. Other previous studies on the calcium channel blockers have indicated that the risk for all cancers is higher among people taking high doses of these medications.[21]

Cholesterol-Lowering Drugs and Cancer. Since cholesterol is believed to be the "bad guy" in heart disease, most conventional medical doctors go after it tooth and nail. It turns out that teeth and nails might represent a safer approach. A review paper published in the *Journal of the American Medical Association* on all the available safety studies on cholesterol-lowering drugs (also known as lipid-lowering drugs) done on animals shows the danger. Investigators made sure they left no stone unturned in collecting their baseline data. Their sources were the 1992 and 1994 *Physicians' Desk Reference* (*PDR*), studies from the U.S. Food and Drug Administration (FDA), and all published articles identified by computer searching, bibliographies, and consultation with experts. Their findings were astounding. "All members of the two most popular classes of lipid-lowering drugs (the fibrates and the statins) cause cancer in rodents, in some cases at levels of animal exposure close to those prescribed to humans."[22]

It is through animal testing that scientists find out whether a drug is safe enough to investigate as a medication for humans. In spite of the fact that these lipid-lowering drugs were causing cancer in animals, they were tested and released to the public as if they were safe. The researchers waffled when they reported on the possibility that lipid-lowering drugs could cause cancer. They said that "evidence of carcinogenicity of lipid-lowering drugs from clinical trials in humans is inconclusive because of inconsistent results and insufficient duration of follow-up."

We might ask whose fault was it that there wasn't enough follow-up! Certainly not the public's.

Even though researchers are warning doctors that these drugs should be avoided except for short-term use, millions are taking these drugs for life! How disheartening. And you can be sure that "careful postmarketing surveillance" *over the next several decades* is just going to show us the rising "body count" and make us wonder why we didn't stop these drugs years earlier. It will also allow plenty of time for the drug companies to make as much money as possible from these deadly drugs. Especially since an aggressive pharmaceutical marketing campaign has targeted half the population with slick television ads that sing the praises of cholesterol-lowering drugs. Some doctors who try to avoid drugs complain that they spend half their clinic time trying to talk people out of the drugs that are promoted on TV.

By 2000, not only was there a general consensus that cholesterol-lowering drugs were associated with cancer but the mechanism for *how* they cause cancer was also uncovered. Apparently cholesterol-lowering drugs promote the growth of new blood vessels, which may have the potential to promote cancer. Tests were done in human cell samples and in live rabbits showing that the cholesterol-lowering drug simvastatin (Zocor) seems to activate a pathway through which cells communicate and act very similarly to a naturally occurring growth factor. Growth factor is not just a "factor," it's a hormone.

This study is saying that Zocor is a hormone-mimicking drug. To make matters even worse, simvastatin seemed to act on a different hormone called vascular endothelial growth factor (VEGF) that also stimulates new blood vessel growth. The researchers couldn't make themselves say it, but an accompanying editorial spoke some truth. Dr. Michael Simons, of Beth Israel Deaconess Medical Center in Boston, concedes that if statins do promote angiogenesis (the formation of new blood vessels), the effects may not always be helpful. This wishy-washy statement is followed by an admission that an example of those effects might be to increase the growth of blood vessels in cancerous tumors.[23]

A study published a month following the VEGF study found that VEGF is associated with the spread of colorectal cancer. It further found that survival time was diminished in patients whose cancerous tumors tested positive for VEGF.[24] Another team of researchers found that VEGF plays a role in diabetic retinopathy, a complication of diabetes that causes blindness.[25]

Breast Implants and Cancer

Breast implants, both saline and silicone, pose another threat to the body's immune system.[26] A thirteen-year study involving 13,500 women conducted by the National Cancer Institute revealed a link between implants and cancers of the lung and brain. It became clear that women in the breast implant group were three times more likely to die of diseases of the respiratory tract, primarily lung cancer, as the women in the plastic surgery control group, and twice as likely to die of brain cancer. But the Associated Press release about the announcement showed the side-stepping action on the part of the researchers.[27] Dr. Louise Brinton was careful to say that "the study demonstrated only a link between implants and the two types of cancer, not a cause-and-effect relationship." And she gave the all too familiar researcher's remark that we need more studies to really know what's going on. But I don't think scientists will ever get to the point of taking a stand on anything. Dr. Brinton went even further to discredit the findings by saying that "its significance is unclear."

What, we ask, could be more clear? We know that some scientists still refuse to say that cigarettes cause cancer, but can we afford to wait any longer before making dramatic changes in our chemical-filled lives? Dr. Brinton, for some reason, even tried to put a positive spin on the study. She said, "What the study showed is no difference for most of the cancer sites, which I think is good news. And for the few sites which we did find differences, we have no ready explanation. So I would not want to alarm women on the basis of one study."

There's a key word: alarm. We don't want to alarm the public, we don't want people to get upset and sue us or stop using our products. Fortunately there was another interview with Dr. Diana Zuckerman, director of the National Center for Policy Research for Women and Families, who served on the study's scientific advisory panel. Dr. Zuckerman was more forthcoming and realistic. She said, "I see this as a warning. I think this is very alarming." However, she also remarked that you can't draw any conclusions from one study. I suppose this protects her from being hauled up on the carpet for "alarming" people.

If an increasing array of prescription drugs might be triggering abnormal cancer cell production after only a few years of use, what will the results be after twenty years? This brings up the important point of the timing and impact of chemicals on our body. Dr. Sandra Steingraber, author of the book *Living Downstream: A Scientist's Personal Investigation of Cancer*, gave a keynote address at the Everyday Carcinogens conference in Canada. According to Dr. Steingraber,

> Each of us go through various what we call windows of vulnerability during our life span, during which time we are exquisitely sensitive to the effects of small amounts of chemicals that can set us up for future cancers, even though larger amounts at some other time when we're not so vulnerable might not have an effect. So in other words, we're not all one hundred fifty pound

white men, which is the basis on which we historically have regu-
lated a lot of toxic chemicals, and we are forced now by the new
science to revisit that kind of regulation.[28]

Hormones and Cancer

I talked about hormones in Chapters 3 and 4 but what do we know
about hormones and cancer? In *Rachel's Environment & Health News*
this important topic is met head on.[29] The author, Peter Montague,
says that breast cancer kills 46,000 women in the U.S. each year, cutting short women's lives by twenty years. The human and economic
costs are enormous. But Mr. Montague fears that a

> medical establishment dominated by male doctors pretends that
> the breast cancer epidemic will one day be reversed by some
> miracle cure, which we have now been promised for 50 years. Un-
> til that miracle arrives, we are told, there is nothing to be done ex-
> cept slice off women's breasts, pump their bodies full of toxic
> chemicals to kill cancer cells, burn them with radiation, and bury
> our dead.

It seems a very harsh statement but I've been saying the same
thing for countless years. And anyone who steps back and takes a
close look at the evidence will agree.

Mr. Montague continues,

> Meanwhile, the normal public health approach primary pre-
> vention languishes without mention and without funding. We
> know what causes the vast majority of cancers: exposure to car-
> cinogens. What would a normal public health approach entail?
> Reduce the burden of cancer by reducing our exposure to car-
> cinogens. One key idea has defined public health for more than
> 100 years: PREVENTION. But with cancer, everything is differ-
> ent. In the case of cancer, prevention has been banished from po-
> lite discussion.

The balance of this issue of *Rachel's News* is then taken up with a thorough review of a new book by medical doctor Janette Sherman, who challenges the cancer establishment with a hard-hitting book of irrefutable facts. Dr. Sherman says, "If cancers are not caused by chemicals, endocrine-disrupting chemicals, and ionizing radiation, what are the causes? How else can one explain the doubling, since 1940, of a woman's likelihood of developing breast cancer, increasing in tandem with prostate and childhood cancers?" She continues, "Actual prevention means eliminating factors that cause cancer in the first place."

Specifically addressing breast cancer, Dr. Sherman asks, "What is the message running through all of these 'risks'? Hormones, hormones, and hormones. Hormones of the wrong kind, hormones too soon in a girl's life, hormones for too many years in a woman's life, too many chemicals with hormonal action, and too great a total hormonal load." Peter Montague and Dr. Sherman agree that "there is something in the environment of the U.S. (and other western industrial countries) causing an epidemic of this hormone-related disease. The medical research establishment likes to call it 'lifestyle factors' but it's really environment. Air, food, water, and ionizing radiation."

Hormone Replacement Therapy (HRT) and Cancer

A 2000 study links hormone replacement therapy (HRT) with increased breast cancer risk in postmenopausal women. We found out in the 1980s that estrogen prescriptions used to treat menopausal symptoms caused uterine cancer. The pharmaceutical companies' answer to that problem was to use a synthetic progesterone along with estrogen to supposedly stop any side effects. And the effects of the combination had never been adequately tested, until now. This 2000 study found that the combination of progestin and estrogen causes even more breast cancer risk than estrogen therapy alone. A June 2003 study found that women on long-term hormone replacement therapy had an increase in breast cancer, strokes, and dementia. More than

3,500 women taking progestin and estrogen were followed for five years. The addition of progestin to estrogen therapy resulted in an increased risk of breast cancer by 24 percent, which was four times higher than estrogen therapy alone. This study provides the strongest evidence to date that progestins not only do not protect the breast from the (cancer-causing) effects of estrogen, but also increase substantially the estrogen-related increase in breast cancer.[30]

Tamoxifen and Cancer

To help deal with the epidemic of breast cancer, which in all likelihood is due to overuse of hormones, drugs, and chemicals in the first place, another synthetic hormone, amazingly enough, is being offered as a "cure." Tamoxifen is a synthetic estrogen that apparently blocks natural estrogen from binding to breast tissue receptor sites and is supposed to cut down on the occurrence of breast cancer. Yet, as I've said earlier, there is evidence it is a carcinogen. The FDA allowed it to be used as a preventive drug for long-term use in women at high risk for breast cancer. But in 1996 the World Health Organization designated tamoxifen as a "probable carcinogen." Even so, it is still offered to all premenopausal women with breast cancer who test positive for estrogen hormone receptors and in all postmenopausal women with breast cancer.

The manufacturers would like tamoxifen to be a preventive treatment for all women at risk for breast cancer. However, two long-term studies found a fivefold-increased risk of another type of cancer, uterine cancer. One study followed 1,372 patients on tamoxifen over nine years, and 23 of those women developed uterine cancer compared to only 4 women developing uterine cancer who were taking a placebo. A second study reported in the same paper, which followed a group of women over almost seven years, had the same findings.[31] How insidious that these cancer-causing drugs are knowingly put on the market and it is only in "post marketing surveillance" that the true nature of the drug is realized.

Let's look at the National Cancer Institute Web site. It is striking that the site contains no discussion of the causes of cancer—none at all. You may also be interested in what the NCI considers cancer "prevention." The following list is as it appears, and in the order it appears, on the NCI Web site as preventive measures for breast cancer.[32] Be aware that every twelve seconds a woman dies of breast cancer.

1. Tamoxifen for Prevention of Breast Cancer: Tamoxifen is a drug that blocks the effect of estrogen on breast cancer cells. A large study has shown that tamoxifen lowers the risk of getting breast cancer in women who are at elevated risk of getting breast cancer. However, tamoxifen may also increase the risk of getting some other serious diseases, including endometrial cancer, stroke, and blood clots in veins and in the lungs.

Often doctors tell their patients about the benefits of tamoxifen and neglect to mention that they may be trading breast cancer for endometrial cancer. Why a toxic medication is the first advice offered to women to prevent breast cancer is a mystery.

2. Hormonal Factors: Hormones produced by the ovaries appear to increase a woman's risk for developing breast cancer. The removal of one or both ovaries reduces the risk. The use of drugs that suppress the production of estrogen may inhibit tumor cell growth. The use of hormone replacement therapy, also called hormone therapy, may be associated with an increased risk of developing breast cancer, mostly in recent users. The use of oral contraceptives may also be associated with a slight increase in breast cancer risk.

Surgical removal of the ovaries seems a very extreme and even tragic approach to preventing breast cancer.

Beginning to menstruate at an older age and having a full-term pregnancy reduces breast cancer risk. Also, a woman who has her first child before the age of 20 experiences a greater decrease in breast cancer risk than a woman who has never had children or who has her first child after the age of 35. Beginning menopause at a later age increases a woman's risk of developing breast cancer.

3. Radiation: Studies have shown that reducing the number of chest x-rays, especially at a young age, decreases the risk of breast cancer. Radiation treatment for childhood Hodgkin's lymphoma may put women at a greater risk for breast cancer later in life. A small number of breast cancer cases can be linked to radiation exposure.

Limiting the number of chest X rays is good advice. The same can be said for mammogram X rays. Nothing about mammograms appears here because they are widely used to detect breast abnormalities; however, thermography is becoming a more accepted screening tool. It's less invasive, has no side effects, is not painful, and does not bruise breast tissue as mammograms do.

4. Diet and Lifestyle: Diet is being studied as a risk factor for breast cancer. Studies show that in populations that consume a high-fat diet, women are more likely to die of breast cancer than women in populations that consume a low-fat diet. It is not known if a diet low in fat will prevent breast cancer. Studies also show that certain vitamins may decrease a woman's risk of breast cancer, especially premenopausal women at high risk. Exercise, especially in young women, may decrease hormone levels and contribute to a decreased breast cancer risk. Breast feeding may also decrease a woman's risk of breast cancer. Studies suggest that the consumption of alcohol is associated with a slight increase in the risk of developing breast cancer. Postmenopausal weight gain, especially after natural menopause and/or after age 60, may increase breast cancer risk.

All of this is very important information that should be shouted from the rooftops. In fact, this material should have topped the list, not appeared halfway through. Not to mention that the wishy-washy way in which this section is written seems to imply that the NCI isn't convinced any of this information is reliable.

5. Prophylactic Mastectomy: Following cancer risk assessment and counseling, the removal of both breasts may reduce the risk of breast cancer in women with a family history of breast cancer.

This advice is the most shocking of all. Worse, it is being followed by terrified women who don't understand that the causes of cancer are known and cancer can be prevented.

6. Genetics: Women who inherit specific genes are at a greater risk for developing breast cancer. Research is underway to develop methods of identifying high-risk genes.

There has been a considerable amount of research focused on the genetic cause of all cancers, not just breast cancer. Certainly the participants in the conference "Everyday Carcinogens" do not believe that cancer is genetically inherited. Even if cancer is caused by faulty genes it is impossible to treat until we find out how to safely manipulate genes.

Fenretinide and raloxifene are 2 other drugs that are being studied for their usefulness as potential breast cancer prevention agents.

This is yet another proposed drug solution to a condition that many researchers are saying is due to the chemicals and toxins in our environment.

ARRESTING THE CANCER PROCESS

I've spent a lot of time telling you in Chapter 3 and in this chapter what causes cancer. Now let's find out ways of increasing our odds of staying healthy and preventing cancer. In her article "New Perspec-

tives in the War on Cancer," Helke Ferrie offers the following strategies gleaned from attending conferences, doing interviews with top
cancer researchers, and from material published by the World Health
Organization.

Avoid Known Cancer-Causing Sources

1. Do not smoke, or tolerate smoking, in your family's
   presence.
2. Avoid excessive exposure to sunlight and ultraviolet rays.
3. Do not consider breast implants.
4. Do not use dark hair dyes; check out safe alternatives.
5. Avoid perfumes, air-fresheners, and perfumed deodorizers
   and antiperspirants. If they contain benzene, aluminum,
   lemon-scented chemicals, or lack a full list of all
   ingredients to permit a checkup in a toxicology manual—
   do not use them.
6. Treat all cosmetic products with extreme suspicion until
   you have proof positive that they contain no known
   carcinogens; safe alternatives exist.
7. Avoid dry-cleaned clothes; find a non-chemical dry
   cleaner.
8. Avoid chlorinated water.
9. Do not drink fluoridated water or use fluoridated
   toothpaste.
10. Avoid electromagnetic fields (EMUs), especially with
    children. EMUs have been linked to childhood leukemia
    and brain cancers. Use appropriate protection on your
    computer screen, avoid using a microwave oven, avoid
    living near hydro towers.
11. Do not use hormone disrupting or mimicking substances
    such as chemical pesticides, herbicides, fertilizers,
    fungicides, and bug killers.
12. Do not use cleaning, polishing, renovation materials in
    your home that list unspecified "inert ingredients." If

they have toxic warning symbols; require calling a doctor; are "corrosive"; give special disposal instructions; or require "well-ventilated areas" for use—look for substitutes. If you cannot avoid some of these substances (e.g., oil paint, furniture stripper, car maintenance materials, etc.), wear the best charcoal-filtered mask available and minimize exposure, especially to skin and lungs.

13. Reduce consumption of salt-cured, smoked, and nitrate-cured foods.

14. Do not use the meat or dairy products from animals routinely treated with antibiotics and raised with hormones. Safe, certified organic milk and meat products are widely available in health food stores and some grocery stores. Better still, for you, the planet, and the animals, become a vegetarian.

15. Never heat shrink-wrapped foods or food in plastic containers. The plastic molecules migrate into the food when heated. They are xenobiotics.

16. Avoid food additives, especially Red Dye No. 3 found in most junk foods and many pop products. Avoid emulsifiers such as carrageenin; do not consume hydrogenated vegetable oils or margarine.

17. Limit sport fish consumption to the guidelines provided seasonally by the government.

18. Do not drink or eat foods that contain sugar substitutes such as NutraSweet, aspartame, etc., and avoid refined sugar, which usually contains silicon. Stevia, unpasteurized honey, maple syrup, and brown rice syrup are healthy substitutes easily available.

19. Avoid antibiotics unless your doctor has done the necessary test to identify the exact bacteria this antibiotic kills (except in extreme emergencies, e.g., meningitis); keep treatment period to a minimum.

20. Avoid prescription drugs unless your doctor also gives you a photocopy of the full drug information from the

annually updated *PDR* (*Physicians' Desk Reference*) and explains this information to you; if the drug requires regular liver function tests, insist on discussing alternatives or keep treatment to the minimum.

21. Avoid birth control pills, antihypertensives, antidepressants, hormone replacement therapy in pill form (toxic to the liver), and do not take tamoxifen preventively; get the full data on those drugs; check them out first on the Internet at www.preventcancer.com.

22. Do not invest your savings in known cancer source polluters.

Do Something Constructive About Cancer

1. Have your mercury amalgams removed by a dentist trained in the proper protocol.

2. If you are overweight, have your hormone levels checked and find out if you have food allergies. Overexposure to estrogen, lack of progesterone, thyroid problems brought on by pesticide exposure, or an adaptation to allergenic foods (often wheat products and refined sugar) are frequent causes of obesity, which promote cancer through excessive estrogen and pesticide storage.

3. Exercise regularly and moderately.

4. Eat cruciferous vegetables (cauliflower, brussels sprouts, broccoli, etc.), preferably organically grown; if that doesn't fit your budget, wash all your fruits and vegetables in VegiWash. This will remove pesticide surface residues.

5. Buy your foods in glass containers; avoid cans and plastic.

6. Take supplements, especially vitamins C and E, and minerals such as magnesium. Check out the literature and take charge of your health. If you need hormones, consider primarily natural ones and/or transdermally administered varieties in the smallest possible doses—they bypass the liver.

7. Join a health or cancer activist group.

8. Start a pesticide education group in your neighborhood; demand from your local representatives mandatory toxicology disclosure of all chemical ingredients being sold today; approach your local golf course manager and discuss alternative ways of maintenance; go to your city council and get them to explore alternatives to chlorine in public swimming pools and to put a stop to the use of chlorine and fluoride in the water supply.

9. Read the *Journal of Pesticide Reform* for basic information. Read Steingraber's *Living Downstream*, 2nd ed., 1999 (paperback). Read R. N. Proctor's *Cancer Wars*, 1995. Don't go shopping without Dr. Epstein's *Safe Shoppers Bible*, 2nd ed., 1999, or *Additive Alert*, 1999. If you have reason to be concerned about cancer, read Dr. Epstein's *The Breast Cancer Prevention Program*, 2nd ed., 1999, and give it to your daughters, women friends, and others.

10. If you have been recently diagnosed with cancer, search the Web and the literature for the latest alternative treatments. Your doctor is no doubt sincere, but possibly functions on automatic pilot, especially if he or she relies on drug representatives instead of the medical journals.

11. Thoughtfully consider, but carefully doubt all information (including this article) and start your own search. Only a determined consumer revolt and informed resistance will turn the cancer tide.[33]

COMPLEMENTARY THERAPIES FOR CANCER

We know now what we can do to prevent cancer, and how we may avoid sources of cancer: We must turn our backs on chemicals and detoxify our bodies. I'm not going to describe the dozens of anti-cancer modalities that are prescribed by complementary alternative medicine doctors or naturopathic doctors. That is best done on an individual basis. In this section I'll talk about some common, accessible anticancer nutrients.

First, however, we need to understand what happens when chemicals enter the body, so we can learn how to support the body's own ability to thwart them. We touched on this in Chapter 3, but it's worth a review because it helps you understand how you can support your body's ability to defend itself.

The long and slippery road to cancer begins when a toxin enters the body and is filtered through the liver. Detoxifying liver enzymes single out the toxin as a foreign entity and try to attach it to a neutral substance so that it can be ushered out of the body through the urine or feces. The water-soluble toxins are the easiest ones to deal with. But the fat-soluble ones, like pesticides that bind to fat cells, can form even more toxic chemicals when the liver tries to disarm them. These sinister chemicals are the ones that bind with our own cellular DNA, where they cause mutations and cancers. When mutations occur in tumor suppressor genes they can no longer stop cancer cells and they grow out of control. The growth of cancer cells is supported by their ability to form their own blood vessels. They also thrive on estrogen, which is everywhere in our environment in the form of xenoestrogens, or chemicals that mimic estrogen.

Preventing Gene Mutation

We learned in Chapter 3 and also earlier in this chapter that cancer is caused when gene mutation occurs. The first lines of defense against the many carcinogens in our diet are antioxidants that prevent gene mutation. As we know, antioxidants also act as free radical scavengers. Many antioxidants that prevent gene mutation have been identified in fruits and vegetables, the most potent being the indole-3-carbinols, the chlorophylls and chlorophyllin.[34] Chlorophyllin is the modified, water-soluble form of chlorophyll that has been tested as an anti-mutagenic agent for more than twenty years.

In one of the great ironies of natural-product science, it seems we now have a very large body of data concerning the anticancer, antimutagenic, antioxidant, and potentially life-extending benefits of chlorophyllin processed from chlorophyll, but much less information on the effects of natural chlorophyll itself. For example, chloro-phyllin can cross cell membranes, organelle membranes, and blood-brain barriers, while chlorophyll cannot. Chlorophyllin even enters into the mitochondria, the energy-producing organelles of the cell where 91 percent of oxygen reductions occur and where the majority of free radicals are produced.[35] Chlorophyllin neutralizes all the ma-jor reactive oxygen species, such as superoxide radical, hydrogen per-oxide, singlet oxygen, and even the most dangerously reactive hydroxyl radical at very low doses. It has been shown to be a potent mitochon-drial antioxidant that not only protects mitochondria from their own auto-oxidation (considered to be one of the major components of ag-ing),[36] but also protects mitochondria from external chemicals and ra-diation.[37] But I imagine that anything the processed chlorophyllin can do, the natural chlorophyll can do as well or even better! In Chapter 9 I'll talk about how you can get large amounts of chlorophyll in your diet by juicing and eating several servings of vegetables a day.

Antioxidant supplements have become popular because they re-duce gene damage inflicted by free radicals. You will also notice that each of these supplements strengthens the immune system. In essence, I'm not giving you a vitamin drug to prevent or treat cancer, I'm rec-ommending the proper nutrients that are necessary for your own amazing and vital immune system to be able to do its job. If you are deficient in even one of the nutrients you need, then your whole body suffers. Even so, it may take some time for that deficiency to give way to chronic disease or cancer, and you won't even know the reason why. But on the Power Aging program you will be filled with the nourishment of organic foods, plenty of freshly made vegetable juices and green drinks, and lots of oxygen from regular exercise, and will not experience these deficiencies. You can also add supplements to your program for extra insurance.

Let's look at the list of easy-to-find nutrients that can be used in our fight against cancer and to boost the immune system in its effort to stay healthy and cancer-free. Much of what you see here will be

elaborated on in further chapters. The dosages for cancer-prevention and health maintenance supplements are listed in Chapter 11. For cancer treatment dosages, which may be higher or lower depending on your condition, please consult your holistic health doctor.

Vitamins

Vitamin A. A fat-soluble vitamin that enhances immunity against tumor cells.[38] You will be getting lots of vitamin A and its precursor, beta-carotene, in your fresh vegetable juices and green drinks.

Folic Acid. A B vitamin that is abundant in green vegetables as well.

Vitamin B$_6$. A B complex vitamin, which is important for a strong immune system and nervous system. This B vitamin is necessary for RNA and DNA synthesis; making natural tryptophan in the body to elevate moods; making red blood cells; metabolizing fat and protein; and inhibiting tumor growth.[39]

Vitamin C. A water-soluble vitamin, which is also going to be high in your freshly made juices. Citrus fruits, broccoli, and most other fruits and vegetables contain high amounts of vitamin C. It's necessary for a strong immune system and protects against cancer. It's a powerful antioxidant and boosts certain enzymes in the body that destroy free radicals.[40] Linus Pauling was famous for proving that vitamin C cuts down symptoms of a cold but he also did important work on vitamin C's beneficial effect on colon polyps and colon cancer.

Vitamin E. A fat-soluble vitamin that protects cell membranes and is necessary for a strong immune system.

Minerals

Calcium. A mineral that's required in more than trace amounts. Studies show that people with colon cancer are calcium deficient. But

it must be taken in conjunction with magnesium in a 1:1 ratio for the best utilization of calcium. Both minerals are required for hundreds of functions in the body.

Iodine. A trace mineral that is very important in maintaining a healthy thyroid. The thyroid, in turn, is responsible for the metabolism that occurs in every cell in the body.

Manganese. A trace mineral that is part of the antioxidant system, superoxide dismutase, and as such is important as a cancer preventive.

Molybdenum. A trace mineral that is required in microgram amounts. It is essential in several enzyme systems in the body and assists the liver in detoxifying drugs and toxins.

Selenium. A trace mineral that works in association with vitamin E; together they could be called the "anti-cancer twins." Many studies have shown the benefit of selenium. Selenium is a necessary component of a major antioxidant system called glutathione peroxidase and is therefore necessary in liver detoxification pathways. Selenium works at the level of DNA synthesis and stabilizes the structure of the cell membrane. Unfortunately selenium deficiency is common in the population and even more so in cancer. Heavy metals like cadmium (from smoking), mercury (from dental amalgams and fish), and lead (from industrial and auto pollution) inactivate selenium.[41]

Zinc. A trace mineral that has gained a lot of attention because it is used in the form of throat lozenges for colds to help kill viruses in the throat. However, it should not be used alone; it needs to be balanced with copper. For every 20 mg of zinc you need from 1–2 mg of copper in your supplement program. Zinc is a cofactor in the superoxide dismutase antioxidant enzyme system. Low zinc levels means natural killer cells are less active and therefore less able to keep the body free of foreign bodies and precancerous cells.[42]

Essential Fats

Omega-3 Fatty Acids. Found in flaxseed oil and fish oils, omega-3 fatty acids can't be made in the body but must come from our food. The omega-3 fatty acids are necessary in the manufacture of our hormones, important for our heart, and necessary for the development of our brain. They also play a role in preventing cancer.

Herbs and Foods

Bromelain. An enzyme product usually derived from pineapple stems. It has been used to treat inflammation in all civilizations that grow pineapples and is used in many alternative medicine cancer protocols.

Chlorella. A freshwater single-celled green algae consisting of 60 percent protein, high levels of chlorophyll and vitamin A, and dozens of other nutrients. It's being researched as both an antiaging supplement and a cancer preventive.

Garlic. This herbal condiment has strong anti-infective properties. Hundreds of studies have been done over the years to show its beneficial effects.

Ginkgo Biloba. The leaves of the ginkgo tree have been used for centuries in Chinese medicine for lung problems, but research is exposing its effects against cancer and as an antioxidant.

Pau d'Arco. The pau d'arco tree does not support the growth of fungus on its bark. It grows in South America, where it is known to have antifungal and anticancer properties.

Sea Vegetables. Sea vegetables—the more acceptable name for seaweed—such as kelp contain an abundance of minerals, especially iodine.

Research on Diet for Cancer

We have the above list of supplements to guide us in cancer prevention. Now let's look at the science behind diet and supplements. Most of this research is going to sound very simple and obvious, and you're going to wonder why I've included all these studies on diet. But it is only because these studies have been presented in scientific journals that any credence is given to the type of Power Aging diet that I am advising. It's an unfortunate fact that even common sense has to be "scientifically proven" today. These are the types of facts you need to use when your friends and relatives ask you why you won't indulge in fried meat, white bread, cakes, cookies, and candies!

Simopoulos reviews the "Mediterranean diet" and its effects on aging and chronic disease. He found that there have been extensive studies on the pre-1960s traditional diet of Greece, which consisted of a high intake of fruits, vegetables (particularly wild plants), nuts, and cereals with more sourdough bread than pasta; olive oil and olives; cheese but less milk; more fish than meat; and moderate amounts of wine. Detailed study of the diet of Crete shows a number of protective substances, such as selenium, glutathione, a balanced ratio of (n–6):(n–3) essential fatty acids (EFA), high amounts of fiber, antioxidants (especially resveratrol from wine and polyphenols from olive oil), vitamins E and C. Simopoulos agrees that some of these nutrients have been shown to be associated with lower risk of the diseases of aging, including cancer.[43]

Fortes and a group from the Department of Epidemiology, Lazio Regional Health Authority, Rome, Italy, surveyed the diet of 162 independent residents in a home for the elderly. They found that high intake of ascorbic acid, riboflavin, and linoleic acid was associated with a 50–60 percent decrease in mortality risk. They concluded that high consumption of meat was associated with a higher risk of mortality among subjects with chronic diseases. And frequent consumption of citrus fruit, milk, and yogurt; low consumption of meat; and high intake of vitamin C, riboflavin, and linoleic acid are associated with longevity.[44]

A review study by Meydani found "further support for the consumption of fruit and vegetables, which contain several forms of phytochemicals with antioxidant activity, in order to reduce the risk of cardiovascular disease and cancer, the leading causes of morbidity and mortality among the elderly."[45]

Bonnefoy et al, in their article on antioxidants to slow aging, say that epidemiological data suggest that antioxidants may have a beneficial effect on many age-related diseases, including cancer. He and his colleagues comment that "the beneficial impact of antioxidants on various age-related degenerative diseases may forecast an improvement in life span and enhance quality of life . . . antioxidant-rich diets with fruit and vegetables should be recommended."[46]

Bouic from the Faculty of Health Sciences, University of Stellenbosch, South Africa, writes a review on the role of phytosterols and phytosterolins (derived from plant sources) in modulating the immune system. Bouic says that plant sterols were chemically described as far back as 1922, but until fifteen years ago their role in health had been under-researched and underestimated. Not only do they lower blood cholesterol, but the most recent research has shown that phytosterols decrease inflammation and stimulate the immune system in cancer patients. Bouic also found that since 1990, studies have shown the ability of phytosterols to modulate cancer is due to its effects on human lymphocytes.[47]

Salminen and a group of researchers at the Department of Radiotherapy and Oncology, University of Turku, Finland, researched the dietary attitudes of women who were diagnosed with breast cancer. Thirty percent of breast cancer patients changed their diets by reducing animal fat, sugar, and red meat and increased consumption of fruit and vegetables. The researchers reported that they expressed a concern that they could not get diets appropriate for their disease from their hospital treatment center.[48]

A research facility in France decided to study the relationship between diet and the risk of lung cancer in New Caledonia in the South Pacific. Between 1993 and 1995 they analyzed data from 134 patients with a new diagnosis of lung cancer. In the men, high consumption of dark-green, leafy vegetables was associated with decreased risk of lung cancer, particularly among Melanesians. A similar protective effect was also suggested for high consumption of poultry and fresh fish.[49]

Harnack and colleagues at the Division of Epidemiology, School of Public Health at the University of Minnesota wanted to study the adherence to sound nutrition in the Dietary Guidelines for Americans and its association with the development of cancer. They studied 34,708 postmenopausal women and found that for all cancers, including cancers of the colon, bronchials, lung, breast, and uterus, the women's relative risk of getting cancer lessened with a greater adherence to a healthy diet.[50]

Lahmann and colleagues from the Department of Medicine, Lund University, Malmo, Sweden, wanted to study the relationship of high Body Mass Index as a risk factor for postmenopausal breast cancer. They collected data from the Malmo Diet and Cancer Study that followed a group of 12,159 postmenopausal women since age twenty. They found weight gain and body fat can indeed be a predictor of breast cancer.[51]

Kasim-Karakas and a group from the Departments of Internal Medicine, Division of Endocrinology, Clinical Nutrition, and Vascular Medicine at the University of California at Davis observed that if there is more biologically inactive estrogen by-product released into the urine compared to a biologically active estrogen by-product, there is a lower risk of breast cancer. They also observed that a high fiber intake is associated with decreased cancer risk. Therefore they studied the effect of prunes with both soluble and insoluble fiber on the rate of estrogen by-product eliminate.[52]

Burdette and a large group of researchers from the Department of Medicinal Chemistry and Pharmacognosy and UIC/NIH Center for Botanical and Dietary Supplements Research, and College of Pharmacy, University of Illinois, investigated reports that the herb black cohosh treats menopausal symptoms and has an effect on breast can-

cer. The researchers concluded that their data suggests that black cohosh can protect against cellular DNA damage.[53]

Parcell reviews the importance of sulfur in human nutrition and
as applied to medicine and found, among other things, that sulfur
compounds such as SAMe, dimethylsulfoxide (DMSO), taurine, glucosamine or chondroitin sulfate, and reduced glutathione may be
used in the treatment of a number of disorders, including cancer. He
concluded that because there are very few, if any, side effects with
these sulfur compounds, and the potential for benefit is great, that
human clinical trials should continue.[54]

Alternative Medicine and Cancer

There are many survey studies that estimate the high frequency of
use of alternative and complementary medicine for treatment of various forms of cancer in spite of the fact that it's not "sanctioned" for
cancer treatment. In this section I'll present some of those studies
and then go into a handful of studies proving that various vitamins,
minerals, and herbs are helping to prevent and fight cancer. Again,
this is the type of information that you need to be armed with when
your doctor says, "You get all the vitamins you need in your diet."
I've done the research for you and it's only a drop in the bucket com
pared to what is available in the literature.

Lengacher and colleagues at the College of Nursing, University
of South Florida, questioned a series of 105 women with breast cancer and found that 64 percent regularly used vitamins and minerals
and 33 percent regularly used antioxidants, herbs, and health foods.
Of the 105 women, 49 percent prayed and received spiritual healing,
37 percent went to support groups, and 21 percent focused on humor
or laughter therapy. Massage was used by 27 percent of all participants at least once after diagnosis. Complementary alternative medicine (CAM) was used in participants who had undergone previous
chemotherapy treatment and those with more than a high school education. Being less than satisfied with their primary physician was

associated with patients' more frequent CAM use. The authors concluded that their studies found higher CAM use than in previous studies.[55]

Another frequency-of-use study was done in the University of California, San Francisco, obstetrics clinic. Interviewing 41 women with ovarian cancer, Powell et al found that 51 percent had taken herbs at some point since they were diagnosed with ovarian cancer. Most herbs were taken during chemotherapy. Only 12 percent saw or had their herbs prescribed by an herbalist or other health practitioner.[56]

Tough and his group in Alberta, Canada, examined the frequency of use of complementary alternative medicine (CAM) for patients with cancer of the colon and rectum. The results showed that 70 percent (871) of 1,240 participants completed the questionnaire, and 49 percent used CAM. CAM therapy usage in order of frequency were psychological and spiritual therapies (65 percent), vitamins and minerals (46 percent), and herbs (42 percent). Sixty-eight percent of CAM users informed their medical doctors, and 69 percent used CAM after conventional care.[57]

Herbs for Cancer

Many studies are being performed using herbs to treat cancer with excellent results. Zhao and a group at Shanghai University found that two Chinese herbal formulas, one called Chinese Jianpi herbs and one called SRRS, inhibit gastric cancer cell growth.[58] At the Cancer Research Institute at New York Medical College, Hsieh and his group studied the effects of an herbal formula called Equiguard on prostate cancer. Their results indicated that this formula was effective in killing prostate cancer cells and could be considered as a viable treatment for prostate cancer.[59]

Kapadia and his group at Howard University, School of Pharmacy, studied a number of herbal products in the lab and their activity against Epstein-Barr virus antigen, which serves as a model to test antitumor agents. In this experiment thirty-six extracts of thirty-two herbs belonging to twenty-seven families in use as herbal remedies were studied. They included ginkgo, black cohosh, echinacea, kava-kava, saw palmetto, turmeric, angelica, wild yam, cat's claw, passionflower, muira puama, feverfew, blueberry, chasteberry, licorice, nettle, goldenseal, pygeum, ginger, valerian, and hops. Turmeric showed the most potent anti–Epstein-Barr virus activity, which was ten times more than passionflower, next in the order of activity. Several of the herbal remedies tested inhibited the Epstein-Barr virus by more than 90 percent. The group also reported for the first time the activities of sixteen new medicinal plants as potential anticancer herbs.[60]

Many researchers like Abdullaev at the National Institute of Pediatrics in Mexico City make the comment that considering the prevalence of cancer and the fact that it is a leading cause of death, it is important to investigate readily available natural substances from plants, vegetables, herbs, and spices that might be useful in the prevention and treatment of cancer. Abdullaev focuses on saffron from the crocus plant, which is used as a spice, a food coloring, and a medical drug. This review paper shows that there is a growing body of research that has demonstrated saffron extracts possess anticancer and cancer preventive properties.[61]

Carnesecchi and a group of researchers in France studied the action of geraniol, a component of essential oils of fruits and herbs in human colon cancer cells. They found that geraniol caused a 70 percent inhibition of cell growth with no signs of toxicity.[62]

Surh and coworkers were interested in the effects of plant chemicals in turmeric and red pepper on various stages of cancer. They found that turmeric and red pepper exert antitumor effects by suppressing tumor promotion of RNA.[63]

Tatman and Mo at the Department of Nutrition and Food Sciences at Texas Woman's University concur with numerous researchers who report the beneficial association of fruits, vegetables, and plants in preventing cancer. Their research was focused on what part of the plant was the most active in this regard. They concluded that isoprenoids, a broad class of plant chemicals found everywhere in the plant kingdom, suppress the growth and spread of tumor cells and the growth of implanted tumors.[64]

Wargovich and his group acknowledge that herbs for medicinal purposes have been used by most every culture, both ancient and modern, throughout the world. They focus on the natural anti-inflammatory properties that are very common in herbs such as green tea, turmeric, rosemary, feverfew, and others. They conclude that because nonsteroidal anti-inflammatory drugs (NSAIDs) are associated with a reduced risk for several cancers, then natural plant anti-inflammatories should be investigated as possible anticancer agents.[65]

Sadava and colleagues at City of Hope Medical Center in California studied the pharmacology, cell biology, and molecular biology of a particular type of lung cancer called small-cell lung carcinoma by observing these cancer cells treated with four extracts of Chinese herbal medicines that are in common use in alternative cancer therapies. They found that Chinese herbal medicine extracts OLEN, SPES and PC-SPES kill lung cancer cells but not normal cells in a way that is similar to conventional chemotherapeutic drugs but without the side effects.[66]

Apparently some forms of PC-SPES have been either intentionally or unwittingly contaminated with certain medicinal drugs, therefore the FDA banned their use. This is especially tragic since, as the following studies demonstrate, this formula seems to have been having some remarkable results.

Pirani reviewed the effects of PC-SPES herbal formula on prostate cancer and found that the prostate cancer marker prostate-specific antigen was lowered and quality of life was improved. Pirani felt that clinical trials have proven that PC-SPES is a valid treatment for prostate cancer but further study needs to be done to discover how, precisely, it works.[67] Chenn at New York Medical College went on to do this, studying what doctors call the "mechanism of action" of PC-SPES, which contains seven herbs, and found that it is complex. It involves multiple metabolic pathways, with a crossover of action such that the whole extract is much more effective than any of its parts.[68]

Huerta and his group found that PC-SPES inhibits colon cancer growth. Mice given PC-SPES had a 58 percent reduction in tumor number and a 56 percent decrease in tumor load.[69] Schwarz and his colleagues studied the possible effects of the Chinese herb formulas SPES and PC-SPES for the hard-to-treat disease pancreatic cancer. They found that both formulas had the potential to treat pancreatic cancer and should undergo proper clinical trials.[70] Thomson and his group did a review of PC-SPES and its possible use in prostate cancer because they felt the present allopathic treatment of this disease was "woeful ineffective."[71] However, Hsieh and his group at New York Medical College are trying to find the most active ingredient in PC-SPES, synthesize that, and make it an anticancer treatment.[72]

Calcium

Researchers from Stockholm, Sweden, followed 61,463 women over 11 years and observed 572 incident cases of colorectal cancer. They found that high calcium intake may lower colorectal cancer risk.[73] Wu and a group at the Harvard School of Public Health also determined that higher calcium intake is associated with a reduced risk of distal colon cancer.[74]

Garlic

In *Aging Research Review*, Rahman finds that numerous studies on garlic indicate that it can help prevent arthritis along with cardiovascular disease, inhibit platelet aggregation, thrombus formation, prevent cancer, diseases associated with cerebral aging, cataract formation, and rejuvenate skin, improve blood circulation and energy levels. He feels that there is strong evidence that garlic's antioxidant properties may either prevent or delay chronic diseases associated with aging such as cancer.[75]

CONCLUSION

What have we learned from this in-depth look at cancer prevention and treatment? We've learned that you have a greater role to play in keeping yourself cancer-free than you ever believed. You've learned that there's no magic pill or magic treatment that's going to cure you once you're on the road to cancer. But you have learned about some of the studies that are the basis of the Power Aging diet. And now you can take a major detour toward health by putting the lifestyle and cancer-prevention techniques I've outlined into action. Join millions of other people who are on the Power Aging wavelength and spread the word.

CHAPTER 7

STAYING MENTALLY SHARP AS WE AGE

Strategies for Fighting Alzheimer's, Parkinson's, and Depression

Who hasn't heard about Alzheimer's disease? Famous people get it, our friends and family members get it; it's becoming almost commonplace. The same is true of Parkinson's. Sadly, the fact that they are ubiquitous doesn't make these conditions any less devastating. In this chapter I want to show you the problem that we are facing with the increase in "brain diseases" such as Alzheimer's and Parkinson's, and then show you the research that indicates that we can take action to prevent and treat them. We need not live in fear of mental decline.

First, however, I'll show you the reasons why our brains succumb to degeneration. You've heard about some of them already in previous chapters: bad diets, toxins, and chemicals in the environment and in our bodies. The evidence is all there, documented in scientific journals, but allopathic medicine and science is still determined to find a drug to "cure" these conditions. I don't believe that is going to happen. I don't believe it's even possible. Instead, I've seen these conditions reversed on Power Aging protocols, and I believe they represent the best approach. Here you'll find a general discussion of age-related brain dysfunction, and two specific programs—one for Parkinson's, one for Alzheimer's—as well as a discussion of depression.

As we age we suffer a progressive decline in our cognitive ability—basically, our ability to memorize and recognize. This decline often begins with short-term memory loss and the inability to learn new information. Simple memory deficits, if not addressed, can worsen over time. A group from the USDA-Neuroscience Laboratory, Research Center on Aging at Tufts University, warns that by the year 2050, about 30 percent of the population will be age sixty-five or older and at increased risk for neurodegenerative disorders such as Alzheimer's disease and Parkinson's disease.[1] What this means is that we need to act *now* to keep our minds sharp.

WHAT CAUSES THE BRAIN TO AGE PREMATURELY?

Neurological diseases such as senility, dementia, and Alzheimer's manifest most commonly in the elderly. The good news is that many of the underlying reasons why people suffer memory loss and other neurological disturbances can be corrected. First, let's look at the factors that can cause age-related cognitive dysfunction:

1. Chronic inflammation, which injures both cerebral blood vessels and neurons (brain cells)
2. A bad diet that leads to nutrient deficiencies (many older people become deficient in critical nutrients)
3. Hormonal imbalances and decreased levels of key hormones, especially DHEA, thyroid, and testosterone (see Chapter 4)
4. A decrease in oxygen to the brain cells because of impaired circulation due to disease (for example, atherosclerosis or heart disease)
5. A lifetime of poor health habits (for example, smoking, drinking, and stress)

6. Declining energy output of brain cells due to nutrient deficiencies

7. Essential fatty acid deficiencies (every brain cell requires EFAs in its cell membrane)

8. The damaging effects of chronic free radical exposure

9. Adverse side effects from prescription medications

FREE RADICALS AND ANTIOXIDANTS

I've talked about free radicals many times already, but they are such an important factor in aging that they bear additional mentioning in conjunction with neurological disease. Once again, we know that free radicals are atoms with unpaired electrons that can cause damage in the normal metabolic process known as oxidation. Brain cells are particularly vulnerable to oxidation because of their high-energy production; they are constantly firing messages back and forth. The more energy produced, the greater the number of damaging free radicals can occur. The destructive effects of free radical activity have been implicated in many disease processes, including Alzheimer's and Parkinson's disease.

Halliwell studied and reviewed the action of free radicals that are produced in the brain on a minute-by-minute basis. He says that some arise by normal "accidents of chemistry." He gives the example of "leakage of electrons" from the energy-producing mitochondrial electron transport. Other free radicals, he says, are generated for useful purposes, such as the role of nitric oxide in neurotransmission and the production of oxygen. But because the brain requires constant energy in the form of ATP (adenosine triphosphate) it consumes oxygen rapidly, and it thus produces these "accidents of chemistry" regularly. In order to deal with the constant production of free radicals, the brain contains a battery of antioxidant defenses. Two of the most important defenses are the mitochondrial superoxide dismutase (containing manganese) and glutathione. Halliwell reminds us that iron is a powerful promoter of free radical damage. Even though most iron in the brain is stored in ferritin, when the brain is damaged or injured, iron is released and causes more injury.

The importance of free radicals and the aging brain is being studied fervently in the hopes of finding a drug that will stop free radicals. There are increased levels of free radical damage to DNA, lipids, and proteins found in postmortem tissues from patients with Parkinson's disease, Alzheimer's disease, and amyotrophic lateral sclerosis. There is some speculation that at least some of these changes may occur early in disease progression. Halliwell says these findings account for the rush to develop antioxidants that can cross the blood-brain barrier and decrease oxidative damage. Unfortunately natural antioxidants such as vitamin E (tocopherol), carotenoids, and flavonoids do not easily cross the blood-brain barrier. So other antioxidants must be found.

Halliwell warned that little is known about the impact of dietary antioxidants upon the development and progression of degenerative brain diseases, especially Alzheimer's disease, and that is where the research should begin. He mentioned that several drugs are already in therapeutic use and might be exerting some of their effects by antioxidant action. They include selegiline (deprenyl), apomorphine and nitecapone.[2] However, we must all be very cautious about using chemical drugs that immediately place the burden of detoxification on our liver. That is why it is important to look for natural nutrients that have an impact on the brain and will not damage the liver.

In fact, there have been many studies, some of which I'll outline below, that show a healthy diet is beneficial to brain health. As you read them, remember these studies were not conducted on people eating organic diets, juicing, or taking powerful natural supplements. They were done on people who were simply adding more fruits and vegetables to their diets. And even so, researchers are finding significant improvement in brain health.

Drewnowski and Shultz reviewed the current government guidelines for a healthy diet, remarking that the exact same dietary recommendations were made to young adults, older adults, and the elderly. They questioned whether diets should be modified according to age, since different age groups require different nutrients and nutrient absorption lessens with age. They reminded us that despite the fact there is a growing population of elderly adults, few studies have been done on their specific nutrient requirements. Yet there is a growing list of problems associated with aging, including physiological, psychological, economic, and social changes that may adversely affect nutrition. Moreover, the elderly have, "a higher prevalence of chronic disease, take multiple medications and supplements, and tend to be sedentary." The authors acknowledge that simply living longer does not necessarily mean living healthier. Indeed, in our efforts to increase longevity, quality of life is something we must take into account.

Drewnowski and Shultz concluded that "optimal nutrition promotes both functional health status and mental well-being. Dietary diversity and variety promotes enjoyment and satisfaction with the diet. Regular physical activity promotes strength and endurance, helps to maintain appropriate body weight, and contributes to independent physical functioning. Improving health-related quality of life is a key element in promoting the health and well-being of older adults."[3]

A research team lead by Cantuti-Castelvetri reviewed the effects of antioxidants on behavioral and cellular changes in the aging brain and found numerous studies that show positive benefits of antioxidants in altering, reversing, or preventing symptoms associated with aging. They also found experiments that examined the effects of diets rich in fruits and vegetables or herbal extracts in reducing certain types of cancer and cardiovascular diseases. They said that evidence emerging from such experiments suggests that these kinds of dietary modifications can, indeed, be beneficial.[4]

Joseph and a group of researchers at the USDA Human Nutrition Research Center came to similar conclusions in another study on antioxidants. In this experiment, supplements of strawberry, blueberry, and spinach fed for eight weeks to a group of rats were found to be effective in reversing age-related neuronal and behavioral deficits.[5]

Galli and a team at Tufts University did a study on rats and found that increasing their dietary intake of fruits and vegetables high in antioxidant activity can retard and even reverse age-related declines in brain function.[6]

A study published in the *Journal of the American Geriatric Society* compared the link between antioxidant intake and memory performance in groups of older people. The study found that recall, recognition, and vocabulary were significantly related to vitamin C and beta-carotene levels. The levels of these antioxidants were found to be significant predictors of cognitive function even after adjusting for possible confounding variables.[7]

Casadesus and his colleagues at the Human Nutrition Research Center on Aging at Tufts University reviewed the literature surrounding two antiaging strategies, caloric restriction (more on this later) and antioxidant foods and supplementation. They concluded that both approaches are successful at protecting the brain from age-related oxidative damage.[8]

WHAT YOUR BRAIN NEEDS

Your brain requires a lot of energy to perform its myriad functions. However, with aging there is a decline in the ability of neurons to take up glucose (the primary fuel for the brain) from the blood and to produce energy. This decrease in energy production not only causes problems with memory but also slows down metabolism, which results in the accumulation of cellular debris that eventually kills brain cells. When enough brain cells have died from accumulated cellular debris, senility sets in.

Vitamins

There are many supplements and nutrients that we cover in Chapter 6 and Chapter 8 that have the cumulative effect of nourishing the brain as well as the body. Vitamins can protect and enhance our cognitive function, which means our reasoning, intuition, and perception. B vitamins in particular play an integral role in the functioning of the nervous system and help the brain synthesize chemicals that affect moods. A balanced complex of the B vitamins is also essential for energy and for proper production of hormones. One recent study determined not only that low folate (a B vitamin) levels are associated with cognitive deficits, but also that patients treated with folic acid for sixty days showed a significant improvement in both memory and attention.[9]

In a six-year study to determine the relationship between nutritional status and cognitive performance, 137 elderly people were studied and several significant associations were observed between cognition and vitamin status. Higher intake of vitamins A, C, E, and B complex, both past and present was significantly related to better performance on abstraction and visuospatial tests.[10]

In addition to a direct effect, we are also learning that vitamins indirectly impact mental function by altering the levels of harmful or beneficial substances in the body. For instance, elevated homocysteine levels have been linked to heart disease and poorer cognitive function. Studies show that vitamin B_6 and folate taken at higher than recommended dosages reduced blood levels of homocysteine. One study revealed that less-than-optimal levels of vitamin B_6, vitamin B_{12}, and folic acid can also lead to a deficiency of S-adenosylmethionine (SAMe). SAMe deficiency can cause depression, dementia, or demyelinating myelopathy (a degeneration of the nerves).[11] In fact, we are finding out that we just can't function properly without a wide array of vitamins and minerals that act as necessary cofactors in all the metabolic processes in the body.

And unfortunately the typical American diet does not provide us with enough essential vitamins. Because vitamin C and the B complex vitamins are water soluble and rapidly excreted from the body, they must be replenished daily. Older people are at greater risk for vitamin deficiency because they tend to eat less of a variety of foods, although their requirements for certain vitamins such as B_6 are actually higher. Older people may also have problems with efficient nutrient absorption from food. Even healthy older people often exhibit deficiencies in vitamin B_6, vitamin B_{12}, and folate, as well as zinc.

And I found more studies that show the absolute need for nutrients. An article published in the journal *Psychopharmacology* described a study of seventy-six elderly males given vitamin B_6 versus placebo in relation to memory function. The authors conclude that vitamin B_6 improves the storage and retrieval of information in the elderly patient.[12] And an article published in the *Archives of Internal Medicine* concludes that both memory problems and neuropathy have been improved with vitamin B_{12} injections or supplementation.[13] Furthermore, an article published in the *New England Journal of Medicine* concludes that many common difficulties, such as memory loss and muscle weakness, might well be a product of vitamin B_{12} deficiency without the normal clinical indicators.[14] Methylcobalamin is a coenzyme form of vitamin B_{12} that has been identified as a nutrient that is useful in treating neurological disease associated with aging. Most sources of B_{12} come from meat products, not vegetarian sources. So, if you are following a vegetarian diet, you may need to take B_{12} supplements.

Martin and his colleagues reviewed the many human trials using dietary sources of vitamins E and C and found that these nutrients may improve immunity, vascular function, and brain performance. They say that an optimal intake of these nutrients has been associated with decreased risk of developing cognitive impairments associated with aging and should be studied further.[15]

Villeponteau and colleagues discuss the use of nutraceuticals in the treatment of age-related diseases, including Alzheimer's and Parkinson's disease. They reported on two human clinical trials using antioxidant supplements, and concluded that based on the available data, human life expectancy can be significantly increased by optimizing diet and using nutritional supplements.[16]

Vatassery and a group from the Research Service at the VA Medical Center in Minneapolis, Minnesota, researched the use of high doses of vitamin E in the treatment of central nervous system (CND) disorders of the aged. They found that one study showed that the use of 2,000 IU of alpha-tocopheryl acetate (vitamin E) was beneficial in the treatment of Alzheimer's disease, and that two large clinical trials using 2,000 IU of vitamin E per day for two years suggest that vitamin E is relatively safe at this level. However, they call for more clinical trials on the use of vitamin E in treatment of disorders of the CNS in the aged.[17]

I find it unfortunate that even when studies show the importance of vitamin supplementation, there is no call to implement its use. Researchers never conclude that they must take action, but only that they need to conduct further studies. In doing so, they keep the grant money that pays their salaries flowing. It seems they care very little for the health of the people afflicted with the conditions they study. I can only assume they believe the job of implementing their results belongs to an appropriate government body. And unfortunately these government bodies are often swayed by lobby groups hired by pharmaceutical companies to downplay the importance of nutrients and promote the use of drugs. I hope you can see my point here that we can no longer wait for the government to tell us what to do, or what to take, for our health. It's up to you to read, research, and find out for yourself what makes you feel better. I've tried to lay the groundwork with these literature searches for the studies that prove diet and nutrients are the key to better physical, mental, and emotional health.

These studies are also being conducted outside the United States. In Hamburg, Germany, Kontush and colleagues in the Clinic of Internal Medicine, University Hospital Eppendorf, investigated the influence of vitamins E and C on fat oxidation in Alzheimer's patients. They acknowledged that increased oxidation is a feature of Alzheimer's disease and that low concentrations of the antioxidant vitamins E and C are found in cerebrospinal fluid (CSF) of Alzheimer's patients. They theorized that giving these supplements might delay development of Alzheimer's disease. Twenty patients were divided into two groups. One group was given 400 IU vitamin E and 1,000 mg vitamin C; the other group 400 IU vitamin E alone for one month. Supplementation with vitamins E and C significantly increased the concentrations of both vitamins in plasma and CSF, which meant that susceptibility of CSF and plasma lipoproteins to in vitro oxidation was significantly decreased. However the supplementation with vitamin E alone, although it substantially increased its levels in CSF and plasma, did not decrease the lipoprotein oxidizability. The researchers concluded that there was a superiority of a combined vitamin E plus C supplementation over a vitamin E supplementation alone in Alzheimer's disease, and a biochemical basis for its use.[18]

I feel this last study emphasizes a very important point. Science usually studies one thing at a time, one vitamin at a time, to the exclusion of all else. But the body doesn't work that way; it works synergistically as thousands of factors come into play. So we must remember that we are never going to find a single "magic pill" that will do it all. We have to eat a varied diet and take a complex of nutrients in order to meet all our body's many requirements.

Bourdel-Marchasson and colleagues in France studied the blood of elderly Alzheimer's patients for antioxidant defenses and oxidative stress markers. The subjects in this study were twenty normally nourished patients with Alzheimer's disease and twenty-three healthy elderly control subjects. They found lower plasma concentrations of vitamin E and vitamin A in the Alzheimer's group than the normal healthy elderly controls. They concluded that these antioxidant vitamins had been consumed as a result of excessive production of free radicals in Alzheimer's patients.[19]

Desnuelle and a group of researchers from the Physical Medicine and Rehabilitation Service in Nice, France, say that there is evidence that oxidative stress may be involved in the pathogenesis of ALS (amyotrophic lateral sclerosis, also known as Lou Gehrig's disease). They say that past research shows that the antioxidant vitamin E slows the onset and progression of paralysis in mice. Their study using 500 mg twice daily of alpha-tocopherol (vitamin E) was designed to determine its effects on ALS. The study recruited 289 patients with ALS for less than five years. They were on an ALS drug called riluzole. They received either vitamin E or placebo for one year. The results were that patients receiving riluzole vitamin E remained longer in the milder states of ALS, and at three months there were changes in biochemical markers of oxidative stress. The researchers urge further studies.[20]

Acetyl-L-carnatine and Lipoic Acid

Researchers in the Division of Biochemistry and Molecular Biology, University of California, Berkeley, studied the oxidative damage to various structures and building blocks in the brain. They wanted to see the effects of oxidation on mitochondria, protein, and nucleic acid in terms of neuronal and cognitive dysfunction. A group of elderly rats were fed two substances that the mitochondria require for their metabolism: acetyl-L-carnitine and alpha-lipoic acid. In testing memory they found that both nutrients improved memory but the combination of both was the most effective. They analyzed the oxidative damage to nucleic acids and found that the damage did increase with age in the brain's hippocampus region, which is important for memory. The greater oxidative damage to nucleic acids occurred predominantly in RNA and not DNA. But even in this regard giving acetyl-L-carnitine and alpha-lipoic acid significantly reduced the extent of damaged RNA; again the combination of both nutrients was the most effective. At the cellular level they were able to show with electron microscopic studies of the hippocampus that the two nutrients reversed mitochondrial structural decay that was related to aging. The researchers concluded that their results suggest that feeding acetyl-L-carnitine and alpha-lipoic acid to old rats improves performance on memory tasks by lowering oxidative damage and improving mitochondrial function. Unfortunately they made no recommendations as to how aging humans could benefit from this research.[21]

A Word about Mitochondria

It's no accident that acetyl-L-carnitine was chosen for the above study; it's an amino acid closely involved in the transport of fatty acids into the cell's mitochondria as a building block in the production of energy. More and more studies are indicating that acetyl-L-carnitine can slow neurological aging.

But what about mitochondria themselves? I've mentioned these powerhouses several times already but they are so important in the functioning of a healthy brain that they deserve another look. Mitochondria are long, oval-shaped specialized structures located inside cells that pull in nutrients from the cellular fluids and convert them into energy. They are unique in that they have their own DNA separate from the cell's DNA. They are thought to have originated from one-celled animals millions of years ago.

Believe it or not but these pint-sized powerhouses utilize more than 80 percent of the oxygen that we breathe and put it to good use in making about 95 percent of all the energy that cells need to function. Mitochondria have many other unique aspects that make them powerful energy workhorses; they have a double membrane surrounding them. The outer membrane is smooth and the inner one is arranged in deep folds called cristae. The inner membrane is where all the action happens between oxygen uptake and electron release to the rest of the body. In the study of mitochondria, researchers have come to realize that one of the most important substances involved in the electron transport chain is a small molecule, coenzyme Q10, also called ubiquinone, which acts as an electron carrier.

When mitochondria diminish in numbers or in their ability to function, we are in trouble. That means when we don't have enough coenzyme Q10 as a building block for the production of energy, then our energy is diminished. It's no wonder that many diseases of aging are now being called "mitochondrial disorders." Brain cells require a high level of cellular energy to properly function and coenzyme Q10 gives them that energy.

Coenzyme Q10

Let's take a closer look at this amazing molecule. Coenzyme Q10 was first identified in 1957 as a natural component of the body. Coenzyme is a name that is given to a lot of molecules that support metabolic functions in the body. As its name suggests, it promotes the activity of an enzyme and helps it to work. Coenzyme Q10 functions as an energy transporter in the mitochondria and also as an antioxidant. One of the most important things that scientific research has found out about coenzyme Q10 is that it is destroyed by cholesterol lowering drugs and other medications. This is very important information for Power Agers who are still on medications!

Coenzyme Q10 is made in the body but when it is given orally, it is incorporated into the mitochondria of cells throughout the body where it facilitates and regulates the breakdown of fats and sugars into energy. Scientists have been researching the effects of coQ10 and have come up with some pretty exciting results.

Here are the highlights from a study published in the Proceedings of the National Academy of Sciences.[22] When coenzyme Q10 was administered to middle-aged and old rats, the level of coQ10 increased by 10 percent to 40 percent in the cerebral cortex region of the brain. This increase was sufficient to restore levels of coQ10 to those seen in young animals. After only two months of coQ10 supplementation, mitochondrial energy expenditure in the brain increased by 29 percent compared to the group not getting coQ10. The human equivalent dose of coQ10 to achieve these results is 100–200 mg a day.

When a neurotoxin was administered to the above group of rats, coQ10 helped protect against damage to the region of the brain where dopamine is produced. When coQ10 was administered to rats genetically bred to develop ALS (Lou Gehrig's disease), a significant increase in survival time was observed. The conclusion by the scientists was that coQ10 can exert neuroprotective effects and could be useful in the treatment of neurodegenerative diseases.

This National Academy of Sciences study showed that short-term supplementation with moderate amounts of coQ10 produced profound antiaging effects in the brain. Previous studies have shown that coQ10 may protect the brain via several mechanisms including reduction in free radical generation. This study documented that orally supplemented coQ10 specifically enhances metabolic energy levels of brain cells. Based on the types of brain cell injury that coQ10 protects against, the scientists suggested that coQ10 might be useful in the prevention or treatment of Huntington's disease and ALS (Lou Gehrig's disease).

It was noted that while vitamin E delays the onset of Lou Gehrig's disease in mice, it does not increase survival time. Thus, coQ10, which studies show may increase survival time, was suggested as a more effective treatment strategy. In my opinion, the answer would be to use both nutrients together.

CoQ10 might also be effective in the prevention and treatment of Parkinson's disease. One study showed that the brain cells of Parkinson's patients have a specific impairment that causes the disruption of healthy mitochondrial function. It is known that "mitochondrial disorder" causes certain cells in the brain to malfunction and die, thus creating a shortage of dopamine.[23] An interesting finding was that coQ10 levels in Parkinson's patients were 35 percent lower in a control group of the same age. This deficit of coQ10 caused a significant reduction in the activity of enzyme complexes that are critical to the mitochondrial function of the brain cells affected by Parkinson's disease.

Another impressive study showed that high-dose coQ10 supplementation slows the progression of Parkinson's disease by 44 percent.[24] The ramifications of this study are significant. Parkinson's disease is becoming more prevalent as the human life span increases. This new study confirms previous studies that Parkinson's disease may be related to coQ10 deficiency. The scientists concluded that, "The causes of Parkinson's disease are unknown. Evidence suggests that mitochondrial dysfunction and oxygen free radicals may be involved in its pathogenesis. The dual function of coQ10 as a constituent of the mitochondrial electron transport chain and a potent antioxidant suggest that it has the potential to slow the progression of Parkinson's disease."

We do know however that Parkinson's is being associated with mercury poisoning, aluminum overload, and exposure to pesticides. These three very toxic metals and chemicals may be the underlying cause of damage to the mitochondria and significant factors that we must eliminate both from the external environment and our internal body environment.

A multicentered study by the Parkinson Study Group researched the effects of coenzyme Q10 in early Parkinson's disease. They acknowledged that Parkinson's disease is a degenerative neurological disorder for which there is no known treatment that even slows its progression. Eighty patients with early disease were randomly given coenzyme Q10 at dosages of 300, 600, or 1,200 mg per day, or placebo and followed for sixteen months. They found that coenzyme Q10 is safe and had no side effects up to 1,200 mg per day. Coenzyme Q10 subjects showed less disability than those taking placebo. The higher the dosage the more benefit with coenzyme Q10. They concluded that coenzyme Q10 appears to slow the functional deterioration in Parkinson's disease.[25]

Another important fact in the story of coQ10 and aging is that levels seem to naturally decrease with age. Depletion is caused by reduced production of coQ10 in the body along with increased use of coQ10 in the mitochondria. A coQ10 deficit results in the inactivation of enzymes needed for mitochondrial energy production, whereas supplementation with coQ10 preserves mitochondrial function. It appears that aging humans have only 50 percent of the coQ10 compared to young adults, thus making coQ10 an important nutrient for Power Agers to put in their supplement regime.

Choline and Lecithin

Various forms of choline and lecithin, the most commonly used memory-enhancing nutrients, are precursors to the neurotransmitter acetylcholine. Because acetylcholine helps brain cells communicate with each other, it plays an important role in learning and memory, especially short-term memory. When you can't remember where you left something, it may be because of a deficiency of acetylcholine.

In a 2001 issue of *Mechanisms of Ageing and Development*, an extensive review was published about the multiple effects of one type of choline known as glyceryl-phosphorylcholine (GPC).[26] The review analyzed thirteen published clinical trials examining a total of 4,054 patients with various forms of brain disorders, including adult-onset cognitive dysfunction, Alzheimer's disease, stroke, and transient ischemic attack. The overall consistent finding was that "administration of GPC significantly improved patient clinical condition." The researchers stated that the effects of GPC were superior to the results observed in the placebo groups, especially with regard to cognitive disorders relating to memory loss and attention deficit. They noted that the therapeutic benefits of GPC were superior to those of acetylcholine precursors used in the past such as choline and lecithin. What most impressed the researchers was data indicating that GPC helps facilitate the functional recovery of patients who have suffered a stroke.

Brain aging is partially indicated by neurotransmitter deficiency, along with structural deterioration to neurons and their connective transmission lines (axons and dentrites). A significant body of research indicates that GPC may be of benefit in helping to prevent this deterioration. It may thus be possible to both protect against underlying causes of brain aging while partially restoring cognitive function. GPC is also available in the United States as a dietary supplement, even though it is sold as a prescription "drug" in European countries.

Essential Fatty Acids

The basic building blocks of your brain cells are essential fatty acids such as EPA (eicosapentaenoic acid) and DHA (docosahexaenoic acid) from fish oil. These fatty acids are also used as fuel for brain metabolism and they help control chronic inflammatory processes involved in degenerative brain disorders. When it comes to protecting brain health, DHA may be the more important fatty acid. One study found that DHA supplementation significantly decreased the number of reference memory errors and working memory errors in aged male rats and in young rats.[27] Fish has long been referred to as "brain food," and newly published scientific studies reveal that the oil of cold-water fish (high in omega-3 fatty acids such as DHA) functions via a variety of mechanisms to protect against common neurological impairments.

Vinpocetin

We know that normal aging results in a reduction of blood flow to the brain and a decrease in the metabolic activity of brain cells. Fortunately, however, there are dietary supplements that specifically enhance circulation to the brain. An extract from the periwinkle plant called "vinpocetin" was introduced twenty-two years ago in Europe for the treatment of cerebrovascular disorders and symptoms related to senility. Since then, it has been used increasingly throughout the world in the treatment of cognitive deficits related to normal aging.

The biological actions of vinpocetin initially showed that it enhances circulation and increases oxygen utilization in the brain, increases tolerance of the brain toward diminished blood flow, and inhibits abnormal platelet aggregation that can interfere with circulation or can cause a stroke. Vinpocetin relaxes cerebral vessels and increases cerebral blood flow. The effect of vinpocetin on memory functions was studied in fifty patients with disturbances of cerebral circulation. Improvement of cerebral circulation was observed after administration of vinpocetin. Blood flow was most markedly increased in the gray matter of the brain. Improvement of memorizing capacity evaluated by psychological tests was recorded after one month of vinpocetin treatment. Longer-term use of vinpocetin was associated with alleviation or complete disappearance of symptoms of neurological deficit. No side effects attributable to the drug were observed. The authors of this paper stated that vinpocetin is indicated in the treatment of ischemic disorders of the cerebral circulation, particularly in chronic vascular insufficiency.[28]

Ginkgo Biloba

Extracts from ginkgo biloba have been shown to thin the blood, improve blood flow to the brain, and protect against free radicals. Ginkgo is approved in Germany for the treatment of dementia. There are over 1,200 published studies in the scientific literature on ginkgo biloba extract.[29] An article published in the journal *Physiology and Behavior* showed that treating rats with ginkgo biloba extract not only improved their learning and memory, but also significantly extended their life span. Those rats fed ginkgo biloba took fewer training sessions to reach the performance criteria as well as fewer errors in a complex maze.[30] A study done on old rats showed that treatment with ginkgo extract can also partially prevent certain harmful, age-related structural changes as well as free radical damage to the mitochondria.[31]

Phosphatidylserine (PS)

New methods of extracting phospholipids from soy can give us a more concentrated source of nutrients that protect brain cell membranes. One of these phospholipids, phosphatidylserine (PS), plays an important role in maintaining the integrity of brain cell membranes. The breakdown of these membranes prevents glucose and other nutrients from entering the cell. By protecting the integrity of cell membranes, PS facilitates the efficient transport of energy-producing nutrients into cells, enhancing brain cell energy metabolism.

Abnormalities in the composition of PS have been found in patients with Alzheimer's disease,[32] and European studies show enhancement in cognitive function when PS is administered to those in various stages of dementia. PS is sold as a dietary supplement in the United States, but is approved as a drug to treat senility in Europe.

In his e-Alert newsletter in March 2003, Dr. William Campbell Douglass broke the news that PS manufacturers are now allowed to make certain claims for PS.[33] They can say that phosphatidylserine may reduce the risk of cognitive dysfunction and dementia in the elderly. Dr. Douglass says that nutritionist Dr. Kyl Smith petitioned the FDA to allow the health claims. Accompanying his petition were over two dozen studies demonstrating that PS may help improve memory impairment associated with aging.

Dr. Douglass wrote in his newsletter that PS is required for optimal function. It acts as a potent antioxidant, and it helps to open brain cells to receive nutrients. PS also is in charge of instantaneous bursts of information and the reaction to those bursts. Moreover, it can help increase the number of neurotransmitter sites in the brain.

As we age, the production of PS diminishes, and therefore it makes sense to supplement PS, especially if you are already having age-related memory problems. Unfortunately, you cannot get ample PS simply through foods, as there are only trace amounts in our diet. Now, however, with this new technology to extract PS from soybeans, we have a reliable source of the nutrient. The dosage of PS in studies showing improved mental function in subjects is 300 mg per day. PS seems to be safe, with no side effects associated with its use.

Garlic

We know garlic is good for the heart, fights infections, and is absolutely delicious, but it's also good for the brain. Borek at Tufts University School of Medicine in his study on garlic concluded that "compelling evidence supports the beneficial health effects attributed to aged garlic extract (AGE), i.e., reducing the risk of . . . the oxidant-mediated brain cell damage that is implicated in Alzheimer's disease."[34]

Melatonin

Reiter and his colleagues defined the role of melatonin in antiaging as a multifaceted free radical scavenger and antioxidant. It detoxifies a variety of free radicals including the hydroxyl radical, peroxynitrite anion, singlet oxygen, and nitric oxide. Additionally, it stimulates several antioxidative enzymes including glutathione peroxidase, glutathione reductase, glucose-6-phosphate dehydrogenase, and superoxide dismutase. On the other hand it inhibits a pro-oxidative enzyme, nitric oxide synthase. Melatonin also crosses the blood-brain barrier and the placenta, and distributes throughout the cell increasing its efficacy as an antioxidant. Melatonin protects both membrane lipids and nuclear DNA from oxidative damage. The authors conclude that in every experimental model in which melatonin has been tested, it has been found to resist the damage and the associated dysfunction commonly found with free radicals.[35]

Reiter continued his investigations and review of melatonin and found that in the past ten years, since it was discovered in 1990 to be a direct free radical scavenger, a considerable amount of research has been undertaken. He found that along with melatonin's ability to directly neutralize a number of types of free radicals, it also stimulates several antioxidative enzymes. This activity greatly increases its efficiency as an antioxidant. In addition many antioxidative enzymes are enhanced in their activity by melatonin: superoxide dismutase, glutathione peroxidase, and glutathione reductase. The authors conclude that melatonin is a protective agent against a wide variety of processes and agents that damage tissues via free radical mechanisms. It's use as antiaging molecule is becoming more widely researched.[36]

Abbott and a group of researchers in the Division of Biostatistics and Epidemiology, University of Virginia School of Medicine, found evidence in the literature that the area of the brain damaged in Parkinson's disease is associated with obesity. They analyzed fat measurements that were done from 1965 to 1968 in 7,990 men in the Honolulu Heart Program. These men were aged forty-five to sixty-eight years and without Parkinson's disease. The follow-up period was thirty years during which time 137 men developed Parkinson's disease. Data allowed them to conclude that increased triceps skin-fold thickness measured in midlife is associated with an elevated risk of future Parkinson's disease. [37]

TARGET: PARKINSON'S DISEASE

Parkinson's disease is a degenerative disorder of the brain in which patients develop tremor, slowness of movement, and stiffness of muscles. It affects approximately one percent of Americans over the age of sixty-five. Although certain drugs, such as levodopa, can reduce the symptoms of Parkinson's disease, no treatment has been shown to

slow the progressive deterioration in function. However, in a health support group that I conducted, I saw some individuals who showed astounding improvement from Parkinson's disease simply by putting a general wellness concept into practice. At the time I was not even aware they had Parkinson's but they knew all too well that they had progressive symptoms, which were resolved on a wellness protocol.

The main elements of the wellness concept that they followed included slow methodical detoxification of the body and environment, exercise, and training in stress management. People learned to see the stumbling blocks put in front of them, and by learning how to overcome them, they developed stronger, more resilient, and spiritual characters, and brought joy back into their lives.

Astonishingly enough, at the final meeting of the group, a seventy-year-old African American engineer revealed that for the past twelve years he had had Parkinson's disease. His symptoms had been so debilitating that he could not continue working because he could not hold a drafting pen, he could not feed himself because his hands shook terribly, and he suffered from severe brain depression, brain fog, and an inability to remember names or numbers. Prior to joining the group he had tried taking some nutrients and two neurologists prescribed medications, but he did not want to continue on that path.

This gentleman entered the group with a "what the heck" attitude and a willingness to try the protocol even though a specific protocol for Parkinson's was not offered. This man made all the changes recommended in the protocol and adopted it diligently. Here's what he did. First, he changed what and how he ate. He got rid of all the processed foods in his house, eliminated fried foods, dairy products, and mucous-producing foods. He substituted all organic food in a vegetarian diet that included all the essential fatty acids and large quantities of vegetable juices. He ate more frequent meals. By the end of the program he was drinking up to thirteen glasses of juice a day. It was his opinion that juicing was primarily responsible for the improvements he experienced. He ate more frequent meals and included many fiber-rich foods. He supplemented his diet with basic antioxidants like vitamin C, vitamin A, and beta-carotene to trap free

radicals, which we learned about in previous chapters, that attack the brain.

He also began exercising on a daily basis. He dealt with his emotional stress by working on anger, frustration, and resentment issues that he realized he was holding on to. He also cleaned his living environment because his entire concept of cleanliness and hygiene was transformed. He threw out everything in his home that was made of particleboard, which is usually steeped in formaldehyde and other harmful chemicals. He got rid of his wall-to-wall carpet, which traps mold and dust and infectious organisms. To impove his air quality he started using an air filter and bought a few common household plants that remove toxins from, and release oxygen to, the air. He had his central air and heating system thoroughly cleaned to remove the dust, fungus, and bacteria that can lead to a depressed immune system.

In our seminars I taught his group simple hygiene principles such as keeping the toilet seat closed when flushing. I explained, rather graphically, that flushing with the lid open has an effect similar to a giant sneeze, propelling bacteria from your feces into the air, on to your soap and toothbrushes, and thereafter, into your mouth. Initially, this gentleman and most of the group thought I was crazy when I said our culture doesn't practice proper hygiene; he equated a "neat" house with a clean house. Then, at my behest, he wiped all the handles and surfaces that he normally touched in his house with paper towels soaked in hydrogen peroxide and was amazed to see that paper had turned shades of black. As part of his hygienic routine, he now cleans surface areas including telephones, doorknobs, and the refrigerator in his home three to four times a day.

Everyone in his household takes off their shoes before entering so that heavy metals, animal waste, and toxins in dust don't get tracked throughout the home. His family changes the bed linens frequently and uses nonchlorine bleach. Full spectrum lighting was added and the microwave oven and electric blankets were given away. He also makes sure to keep his head at least six feet away from digital clocks, and when he watches TV, to be at least eight feet away.

This gentleman's newly activated hygienic awareness naturally

began extending beyond his home. He told the wellness group that he observed a man sneezing into his hand and saw the mucus spray everywhere. When this man approached him to shake hands, he did not want to shake a bacteria/virus-covered hand. Instead, he followed a recommendation from our group and grasped the man's forearm just above the hand to avoid infection.

Three weeks after he began the wellness protocol, he felt his energy soar as if he were rising from the dead. He felt so energetic, it was easy for him to follow the protocol and make a gallon of juice in the morning to last through the day. He added three to four tablespoons of the powerful antioxidant vitamin C to the juice. He also had one or two drinks of high quality vegetable-based protein, which included a mixture of antioxidants, and alpha-lipoid acid. By making conscious choices, not only did he feel good but his tremors were completely gone, the brain fog lifted, and his mental clarity sharpened. He reported that every neurological and physical symptom was gone simply by eliminating processed and unhealthy foods, eating live, healing foods (including nuts, seeds, vegetables, tubers, and fruits), drinking juices, allowing only positive thoughts, reorganizing his day, exercising, cleaning the environment, and cleaning his colon. Without any medical treatment his condition was reversed. He was not the only person in the group to show tremendous improvement; another woman with Parkinson's disease reported an improvement of about 90 percent by adhering to the protocol.

Nutrients for Treating Parkinson's Disease

If I were designing a program specifically to meet the needs of a Parkinson's patient, I would extend the general wellness protocol (see Chapter 11) to repair the body even further. The nutrients I would recommend include some or all of the following, and would be taken in divided doses throughout the day.

DHEA: 15 mg
Lycopene: 25 mg

Lutein: 25 mg

Vitamin C: 2,000–10,000 mg

Aloe vera: 10–12 oz per day

Green tea: 400 mg

Green juices: up to 13 glasses a day

Conjugated linoleic acid: 1,000 mg

Melatonin: 1–5 mg

Acetyl-L-carnitine: 2,000 mg

Phosphatitylserine: 2,000 mg

Alpha-lipoic acid: 1,000 mg

Coenzyme Q10: 100–1,500 mg

Ginkgo biloba: 300 mg

Siberian ginseng: 200 mg

Pine bark extract: 500 mg

Under medical supervision, IV chelation therapy consisting of certain safe chemicals to pull out heavy metals, excess calcium plaques, and toxins and IV therapy introducing 5 mg of hydergine and 1,500 mg of intravenous glutatione can also be used as part of a Parkinson's program. Unfortunately, these treatments are not being administered, even though conventional treatments are problematic, and even though, as you will read further in this chapter, there are many scientific studies that clearly point to both the cause and the treatment of Parkinson's. Allopathic medicine relies on strong medications to try to correct an imbalance in brain chemistry, but these medications have unpleasant side effects and don't often work. In order to relieve Parkinson's tremors, treatments are administered that actually destroy parts of the brain: nerves may be cut or alcohol may be injected into certain areas. Clearly, the natural approach is much healthier and safer.

I believe this approach could help Muhammad Ali, Janet Reno, and Michael J. Fox, well-known people with Parkinson's disease. If they were willing to try this approach, others might follow their lead. Well intentioned as they are, efforts to start foundations and fundraising to support research into drug therapy miss the mark, because traditional methods have not yielded the beneficial results that our nutritional programs have.

I believe there are numerous causes of Parkinson's disease. The accumulation of viruses, all forms of heavy metal poisoning, and exposure to carbon monoxide can destroy parts of the brain. I encourage all Parkinson's disease patients to remember that living foods and antioxidants are crucial to help protect the brain.

The Alexander Technique

Although the Alexander Technique can be helpful for a variety of conditions, I want to discuss it here because of the possibility it holds out to Parkinson's patients. The Alexander Technique is a way of learning how you can get rid of harmful tension in your body by improving the way you move your body in your day-to-day activities. Stallibrass, Sissons, and Chalmera at the School of Integrated Medicine, University of Westminster, London, set out to investigate whether the Alexander Technique would benefit Parkinson's disease patients. Ninety-three patients were placed in three groups: an Alexander Technique group received twenty-four lessons in the Alexander Technique; a massage group received twenty-four sessions of massage; a third group received no intervention. The Alexander group had less depression and on self-scoring were improved over the other two groups. The researchers concluded that the Alexander Technique may offer sustained benefit to Parkinson's disease patients.[38]

Exercise and Parkinson's Disease

Miyai and a group of researchers from the Neurorehabilitation Research Institute, Bobath Memorial Hospital, Osaka, Japan, set out to determine whether body weight–supported treadmill training had a long-term benefit in Parkinson's disease patients. They concluded that there was lasting benefit in this type of exercise particularly in their short-gait stride.[39]

TARGET: ALZHEIMER'S DISEASE

Presently, Alzheimer's disease affects millions of Americans. We have seen its effects on people both well-known and people whom we love. A diagnosis of Alzheimer's is a terrible blow to the patient and to his or her family. Alzheimer's is a debilitating, degenerative brain disease that affects the hippocampus and cerebral cortex of the brain, where memory, language and cognition are located. People can no longer remember, speak, or even know where there are or who they are with. One finding common to everyone with Alzheimer's is deposits of a waxy plaque called beta-amyloid in certain regions of the brain, particularly the hippocampus. When beta-amyloid plaque builds up, degeneration of nerve tissue occurs. Although scientists say they are still trying to determine exactly what causes the build-up, many are pointing to chemicals and heavy metals that accumulate in our bodies as we age.

In Chapter 3, I touched on the role that oxidative stress and inflammation from chemicals play in causing Alzheimer's disease. When the neurons located in the front of the brain are destroyed, acetylcholine production is interrupted. Acetylcholine is the most important neurotransmitter in the brain. It facilitates our quick reactions to stimuli, as well as muscle activity. When production of acetylcholine is diminished, we experience all sorts of problems with motor skills, concentration, and memory.

What can we do about Alzheimer's? We want to stop the amyloidal plaque formation in the brain. We also want to turn off the inflammatory process and turn on the healing process. To accomplish this, I recommend the Power Aging diet and supplements. For advanced cases, I would recommend intravenous chelation therapy, because this disease is promoted by heavy metals like aluminum, mercury, and lead playing havoc with the mitochondria. As we know, when they are destroyed, extreme fatigue and neurological damage can occur.

Nutrients for Treating Alzheimer's Disease

Acetylcholine: 1,000–3,000 mg

Coenzyme Q10: 400–1,000 mg

Boron: 3 mg

DL phenylalanine: 500 mg

Glutamine: 1,000–3,000 mg

L-taurine: 500 mg

L-glutathione: 1,000–10,000 mg

Acetyl-L-carnitine: 1,000 mg

Phosphatitylserine: 1,000 mg

Caprilic acid: 25 mg

Essential fatty acids: 2,000 mg

Melatonin: 2–5 mg

Alpha lipoic acid: 1,000 mg

B complex: 100 mg

Vitamin C: 5,000–15,000 mg

Vitamin E: 400–800 IU

Ginkgo biloba: 125 mg three times a day

5-hydroxy tryptophane as a precursor to tryptophan is also
recommended

There are even some "smart" drugs, given under medical supervision, that may be important for some. They have few or no side effects and enhance the flow of oxygen to the brain. Among these are Deprenyl and Hydergine. Deprenyl protects the neurons and the substantia nigra of the brain, which is commonly affected by Parkinson's disease. However, this drug may also help with Alzheimer's. Piracetam, a drug similar to Hydergine, slows down the destruction of brain cells.

As I've mentioned before, I think it's important to show you what researchers are finding out about the natural treatments for neurological diseases. It is empowering to know that science is proving that we do have recourse when it comes to coping with chronic conditions such as cancer and neurological diseases. Even so, the general public seems to believe that these conditions are a death sentence. They haven't developed the Power Aging attitude that compels you to shout from the rooftops, "I can be as healthy and happy as I wish to be!" Often the best way to combat critics who seek to discourage you from maintaining a healthy lifestyle is simply to say, "There are studies that prove this works."

Mattson at the Laboratory of Neurosciences National Institute of Aging insists that Alzheimer's is preventable. He says the risk of several other prominent age-related disorders, including cardiovascular disease, cancer, and diabetes, is known to be influenced by the level of food intake—high food intake increases risk, and low food intake reduces risk. An overwhelming body of data from studies of rodents and monkeys has documented the profound beneficial effects of dietary restriction (DR) in "extending life span and reducing the incidence of age-related diseases."[40] Dietary restriction is just what it sounds like—eating fewer calories per day.

Fillit and Hill, from the Institute for the Study of Aging in New York, did a strange study. They wanted to determine the costs to Medicare of vascular dementia in comparison with Alzheimer's disease. Vascular dementia is a term for dementia associated with problems in the circulation of blood to the brain. It is the second most common type of dementia after Alzheimer's.

The results showed that vascular dementia costs Medicare more than Alzheimer's because people with vascular dementia often have coexisting heart and circulatory complications.[41] I mention this study because it is emblematic of the way disease is viewed in this country—in terms of its cost to the economy. This study made no mention of how to prevent these conditions, and its conclusion, like many studies of this sort, was simply that more research needs to be done into drugs to treat these conditions because they are so costly.

Otsuka at the Department of Neurology, Jichi Medical School, Omiya Medical Center in Japan, wanted to determine the role diet has to play in the development of Alzheimer's disease. Sixty-four Alzheimer's disease patients and eighty controls were studied. The researchers found that Alzheimer's disease patients ate more meat and avoided fish and green-yellow vegetables compared to controls, and thus ate less beta-carotene, vitamin C, and polyunsaturated fatty acids. The author suggested that the findings imply that Alzheimer's disease might be a lifestyle-related disease such as coronary heart disease, a western style diet-associated cancer, and a hyperallergy. In a second phase of the study the patients were given a supplement of the essential oil EPA, at a dose of 900 mg/day, which improved signs of dementia. The author concluded that the present study showed that nutritional intervention could be useful both for the prevention of Alzheimer's disease and for the treatment of dementia.[42]

Capurso and a group of researchers in Bari, Italy, studied the causes of age-related cognitive decline (ARCD). They said that the causes of ARCD are unknown, but they found some studies that suggested it may be prevented. These studies indicated that protection from ARCD comes from a variety of factors: avoidance of cardiovascular and other chronic diseases, high level of education, and good vision and hearing. Conversely, risk factors for ARCD included hypertension, effects of altered metabolism of steroid hormones, smoking, low-complexity occupation, higher density of persons/bedroom in home, and low level of physical activity. They also commented on a recent study done on an elderly population of southern Italy: they ate a typical Mediterranean diet high in monounsaturated fatty acids, and seemed to show a high protection against cognitive decline. The researchers concluded that dietary antioxidants, specific macronutrients, estrogens, and anti-inflammatory drugs may act synergistically with other protective factors, opening new therapeutic interventions for cognitive decline.[43]

Years ago scientists used to say that once a brain cell dies it's gone forever; unlike most other cells in the body, neurons, or brain cells, don't constantly replace themselves. But now some research findings are showing that even the brain's neurons can regenerate. Other studies show that the neurological impairment caused by normal aging, or by damage to the brain, such as stroke, can be reversed.

DEPRESSION

In my book *7 Steps to Overcoming Depression and Anxiety* I speak about the fact that too often, doctors and the public in general have the mistaken idea that it is normal for the elderly to feel depressed. Based on the work I've done with older people over the past thirty years, I say that's just not true. I believe that most older people feel satisfied with their lives. Sometimes, however, even they may dismiss their moods as a normal part of aging. But I want to assure you Power Agers that you don't have to be depressed.

With alarming frequency, it seems that when an older person goes to a doctor, symptoms that can't be traced to a physical cause are deemed "psychological." Or if you're an older patient with a few nonspecific symptoms such as fatigue, insomnia, and apathy, doctors jump to the conclusion that you're suffering from depression, instead of a lack of vitamins and minerals or a bad diet. If you admit to having stress in your life (and who doesn't?) then the doctor is further convinced that you're depressed. You may be told that you should learn to relax and slow down but, for a doctor, the easiest and most common treatment of depression is medication.

In my book on depression I list the following conditions that are often misdiagnosed as depression.

1. Sugar intolerance causes symptoms of hypoglycemia and prediabetes that go undiagnosed.
2. Gluten allergy from rye, oats, wheat, and barley causes particular chemicals to affect the brain.
3. Allergy to dairy products and the resulting intestinal flora imbalance leads to brain allergy symptoms.
4. Mold allergy from various foods including peanuts and two-day-old leftovers, mold allergy from tobacco, and mold allergy from mildew in your home can all cause mental and emotional symptoms that some people misinterpret as depression. Allergy to fermented foods and beverages including alcohol can cause emotional symptoms as can

sensitivity to the hundreds of additives, dyes, colorings, and preservatives in our food and beverages.

A word of caution: If you are on any form of medication, check out *The Physicians' Desk Reference* in your local library or at your drug store. This book lists hundreds of prescription drugs and their side effects, including emotional instability and depression. But depression is most common in the face of vitamin, mineral, amino acid, and essential fatty acid deficiencies. I remind you that none of these deficiencies are studied carefully in hospital settings where doctors can develop an appreciation of how important nutrients are to mental health. Even simple hormonal deficiencies such as adrenal insufficiency, thyroid hormone deficiency, and DHEA deficiency, along with the more common estrogen, progesterone, and testosterone deficiencies, are mostly overlooked by busy doctors who still view the mind and body as separate. I take up the fascinating subject of hormonal imbalance in Chapter 4.

If your doctor diagnoses depression, which could be a side effect of your medications, the most common treatment is *more* medication. The better solution would be to wean off medication, and, under a doctor's supervision, apply the Power Aging approach. Recent research also suggests that brief psychotherapy or talk therapy is effective in reducing symptoms in short-term depression in older persons.[44] I also make the point in my book that politicians are very concerned that the elderly can't afford their drugs. But I say that instead of arguing to make drugs less expensive and have them covered under Medicare, we need to implement Power Aging with proper diet, supplements, and lifestyle choices to keep ourselves healthy so we don't feel we need drugs.

CHAPTER 8

THE ANTIAGING ARSENAL

What's New, What's Tried and True

I deally, we'd be getting many of the nutrients we need from a varied, organically derived diet. Realistically, though, our diet sometimes falls short. Sometimes we're too busy to take the time to shop for food, cook, or even eat regular meals. Sometimes we have trouble utilizing the nutrients in regular foods. Or maybe organic food is just not available. If these factors affect you—and particularly if you're actively working to maintain health and vitality as you age—supplements are in order. They provide a way for you to optimize your nutritional intake, tailoring it precisely to your individual needs.

It's important that you supplement under the guidance of a holistic physician, as opposed to just starting to take things at random. Before you talk to your health professional, I offer you this survey of the best nutrition boosters to help maintain a Power Aging lifestyle. Let's start with today's "hottest," most touted weapons in the antiaging arsenal.

CUTTING-EDGE SUPPLEMENTS

Coenzyme Q10. Coenzyme Q10, also known as ubiquinone, is beneficial for heart function, for brain function, and for the gums. It is known to lower blood pressure. The heart is often adversely affected by a coQ10 deficiency, but an increasing body of evidence indicates that the brain is also likely to suffer from an inadequate supply of this substance.[1]

As we grow older, our natural production of coenzyme Q10 declines. Since cells need coQ10 for energy production and to counter mitochondrial free radical activity, the results of a coQ10 deficiency can be seen in a greater incidence of many degenerative diseases associated with aging.

About 95 percent of cellular energy is produced from structures in the cell called mitochondria, the cells' "energy powerhouses," and the diseases of aging have been referred to as mitochondrial disorders. A growing body of scientific research links a deficiency of coQ10 to a host of brain diseases related to mitochondrial disorders.[2] (See also Brain Boosters, page 189.)

When coQ10 is taken orally, it is incorporated into the mitochondria of cells throughout the body, where it facilitates and regulates the oxidation of fats and sugars into energy. Aging humans produce only 50 percent of the coQ10 that young adults do, which makes coQ10 one of the most important nutrients for people over thirty to take. CoQ10 is a fat-soluble nutrient. Taking this supplement in an oil-based capsule enables the coQ10 to be absorbed through the lymphatic canals for better distribution throughout the body. There is also evidence that coQ10 is an anticancer nutrient.

The recommended dose of coQ10 is 30 to 300 mg a day with meals.

Vitamin E. The vast majority of people who take vitamin E take only one form of it, alpha tocopherol, because that is the only tocopherol contained in most vitamin E products. But there is a growing body of scientific evidence that gamma tocopherol plays a critical role in preventing diseases, and that the combination of all the tocopherols is more potent than alpha tocopherol alone. The evidence is especially strong that gamma tocopherol is the most potent form of vitamin E.

Further evidence indicates that compounds called tocotrienols, in alpha, delta, and gamma forms, can synergistically work with vitamin E to help protect us against lipid peroxidation and other damaging processes. Tocotrienols have also been shown to lower the levels of LDL, the dangerous form of cholesterol that is a risk factor for heart attack and stroke. One study demonstrates that intake of tocotrienols can clear atherosclerotic blockage in the carotid arteries, a condition that can lead to stroke.

Symptoms of hearing loss improved when forty middle-aged to elderly patients were treated with vitamins A and E for twenty-eight to forty-eight days, but, again, this sort of treatment plan must be supervised by your alternative care physician.

Vitamin E may alleviate women's hot flashes and lessen vaginal thinning and dryness. Postmenopausal women may wish to increase gradually to 600 IU of vitamin E, although some may require up to 800 IU to reduce these symptoms.

Vitamin E is found in green leafy vegetables, eggs, and various oils.

The recommended dose of alpha tocopherol vitamin E is 200 to 600 IU per day, along with at least 200 mg of gamma tocopherol, plus 65 mg of palm-oil-derived tocotrienols. Do not take synthetic vitamin E (dl-alpha-tocopherol). (See also Brain Boosters, page 189.) Avoid higher doses of vitamin E if you have high blood pressure, ischemic heart disease, or rheumatic heart disease.

TMG (Trimethylglycine). TMG is the most effective facilitator of youthful methylation metabolism. This is important because research has shown that defective methylation is related to a variety of diseases, including cardiovascular disease, cancer, liver disease, and neurological disorders.

Enhancing methylation with TMG and other nutrients, such as vitamin B_6 and folic acid, improves health and slows premature and, perhaps, normal aging. The research shows three specific benefits:

1. Methylation lowers dangerous homocysteine levels, thus reducing the risk of heart disease and stroke.

2. Methylation produces SAMe (S-adenosylmethionine), which may have potent antiaging effects and has been shown to alleviate depression, remyelinate nerve cells, improve the condition of patients with Parkinson's disease, help arthritis patients, and protect against alcohol-induced liver injury.
3. Methylation protects the integrity of DNA, which lowers the risk of cancer and may slow cellular aging.

TMG should be taken with cofactors vitamin B_{12} and folic acid. The recommended dosage is 1 to 8 tablets a day with meals, depending upon what's needed to keep homocysteine levels below 7 micro mol per liter of blood.

BRAIN BOOSTERS FOR MEMORY AND INTELLIGENCE

Brain aging is a leading cause of disease, disability, and death in the elderly. The quest to slow brain aging, seen as a decline in the ability to learn, remember, and reason, is a major concern for millions of people. To help slow or reverse brain aging, the Life Extension Foundation offers a supplement called Cognitex, which contains compounds such as pregnenolone, phosphatidylserine, and several different forms of choline, the building block of acetylcholine, which regulates learning and memory.

Cognitex also contains a periwinkle extract called vinpocetin, which functions via several mechanisms to correct multiple causes of brain aging. It has been well established that normal aging results in a reduction of blood flow to the brain and a decrease in the metabolic activity of brain cells. The biological actions of vinpocetin show that it enhances circulation and oxygen usage in the brain, increases the brain's tolerance of diminished blood flow, and inhibits abnormal platelet aggregation that can interfere with circulation, which can lead to a stroke.[3]

Ginkgo is an ancient remedy available in standardized liquid, softgels, and capsules. An extract of the Ginkgo biloba plant is approved in Europe for the treatment of dementia, including the most common form, Alzheimer's disease. It improves circulation by reducing blood platelet formation. Ginkgo is a flavonoid that strengthens capillaries to improve blood flow to the brain and to counteract free radical activity.

Consult your physician before taking ginkgo if you are taking a blood-thinning medication or an MAO inhibitor, or if you are pregnant or nursing.

We've already discussed vitamin E, but we should mention it again as being very important in maintaining brain function. Vitamin E (not synthetic) slows memory loss at 400 to 800 mg a day. Other nutrients to take note of here are vitamin B_6, which improves memory—20 mg per day for 3 months (no longer); and, again, coenzyme Q10, which energizes brain cells—200 mg a day.

Aging's most dramatic effects are reserved for the brain. The only two antioxidants in the brain are glutathione and melatonin. Glutathione is three amino acids protecting brain cells—300 mg a day; melatonin, the pineal gland hormone best known for promoting sleep, is also cytoprotective, and is a free-radical scavenger—3 to 10 mg at night.

Phosphatidylserine from soybeans is excellent for reversing memory loss; it's generally recommended at 500 mg a day for up to twelve weeks. Research shows that when people over fifty receive supplemental phosphatidylserine, available at your health food store, all measurable brain functions improve, including memory.

As we age, the body produces less DHEA, an adrenal gland hormone that's been called the fountain-of-youth hormone. We've discussed this supplement in Chapter 4, on hormonal keys to health, but let's say here that DHEA may lead to significant improvement in middle-aged people with memory impairment. Before taking DHEA, be tested to see if you are deficient, because if you are not deficient, this should not be used. It becomes more important after age forty-five, and even then it should be used sparingly. A daily dose of 5 to 25 mg should be sufficient to restore your mind's alertness. Refrain from using DHEA if you have breast cancer, prostate cancer, or benign prostatic hypertrophy.

Acetyl-L-carnitine is a powerful antiaging nutrient that is beneficial for mild mental impairment; practitioners recommend 1,000 to 2,000 mg a day for up to ninety days.

Up to 42 percent of seniors are deficient in vitamin B_{12}, the absence of which impairs mental function. Take B_{12} lozenges—1,000 mcg per day. Zinc, at 15 mg daily, is another common deficiency involved with memory, because there are many zinc-containing enzymes that take part in the cell repair process.

Balance is a key to sound mental functioning; there's no need to take a million supplements. A high-potency multivitamin/mineral supplement and sound diet cover many of the above supplemental needs, but not all.

It's important to be patient with yourself and others if a forgetful moment occurs. It's an opportunity, really. In the midst of a desperate world, let that refreshing silence be filled with peace.

Carnosine. The amino acid L-carnosine, also known as carnosine, is widely accepted as an antiaging antioxidant that stabilizes and protects cell membranes.

As you age, pathological alterations occur in which sugar molecules bind to protein molecules to form nonfunctioning structures in your body. As we first explained in Chapter 3, this degenerative process of glycosylation, with massive accumulation of these altered structures, contributes to many age-related diseases. There is strong evidence that the proper dose of carnosine is the safest and most effective method of inhibiting glycosylation, which may help to prevent age-related conditions such as muscle atrophy, eye problems, and neurological degeneration.

The recommended dose of carnosine is 500 mg two to three times a day.

Acetyl-L-carnitine. A nutrient with a name similar to the last can provide help for the brain and heart, as well as in fighting cancer. This recently popular supplement is acetyl-L-carnitine. Elderly patients receiving acetyl-L-carnitine at doses of 1,000 to 2,000 mg a day for up to ninety days found relief from mild mental impairments such as slow memory. Acetyl-L-carnitine has also improved walking difficulties in the elderly. Numerous animal studies support the direct antiaging effects of this nutrient.

Acetyl-L-carnitine has proven helpful toward restoring short-term memory in Alzheimer's disease, as we discussed in the previous chapter. This supplement is also effective against dementia in non-Alzheimer's patients.

A common problem associated with aging is neurological damage. Administration of acetyl-L-carnitine at either 1 or 2 grams per day for seven days improves symptoms of Parkinson's disease. Patients with some types of facial paralysis receiving doses of 3 grams a day of acetyl-L-carnitine, along with 50 mg of methylprednisolone for two weeks, experienced significant recovery of nerve function.

There is evidence to suggest that acetyl-L-carnitine may be effective in cases of heart disease and stroke. Supplemental acetyl-L-carnitine administered to stroke patients brought improvements in memory, cognition, and task performance. Acetyl-L-carnitine at 1,500 mg intravenously per day brought increased cerebral blood flow to patients who had suffered a stroke at least six months before treatment.

Anticancer activity has been documented for acetyl-L-carnitine. Several animal studies also indicate that acetyl-L-carnitine may be useful in the treatment of diabetes. Acetyl-L-carnitine is also showing promise in cases of depression, AIDS, chronic fatigue syndrome, and alcohol-associated cognitive dysfunction.

Studies on depression in the elderly show this nutrient to be of benefit. Examples include one in which the administration of 3 grams per day of acetyl-L-carnitine for thirty-six days was shown to significantly reduce severe symptoms of depression in elderly senile patients. In another, depressed patients in their seventies improved significantly when they received a daily dose of 1,500 mg of the supplement. In yet another, elderly patients hospitalized for depression improved significantly, relative to controls, when they received acetyl-L-carnitine.

One thousand to 2,000 mg per day is the suggested dosage of acetyl-L-carnitine.

Alpha-lipoic Acid. Alpha-lipoic acid is a vital antioxidant that boosts the power of other antioxidants, including glutathione and vitamin E. Many studies document the benefits of alpha-lipoic acid in treating diabetes. One study shows that diabetic neuropathy can improve after oral ingestion of alpha-lipoic acid at doses of either 50 or 100 mg twice a day.

Other studies suggest that alpha-lipoic acid may be helpful for stroke and cardiac patients. Prevention of cataracts, memory improvement, and help in cancer prevention are all possible, according to studies on this supplement. Patients with stages I and II open-angle glaucoma receiving doses of 150 mg per day of alpha-lipoic acid for one month improved.

Alpha-lipoic acid is a sulfurous fatty acid that might be classified as a vitamin except that it is synthesized within the human body. The effects of this nutrient include normalizing blood sugar levels, improving nerve blood flow, reducing oxidative stress, alleviating diabetic neuropathy, and protecting membranes. Alpha-lipoic acid is a free radical scavenger, inhibits the damaging effects of the cross-linking of proteins, and is used to treat liver ailments and to protect the liver from the toxic effects of many pharmaceutical drugs. Alpha-lipoic acid also increases intracellular glutathione levels that slow the biological aging process.

A dietary note: Starchy vegetables and tubers, such as russet potatoes, sweet potatoes, and yams, are not fattening and actually contain alpha-lipoic acid to help your heart.

The daily dose of alpha-lipoic acid is 200 to 300 mg per day.

Essential Fatty Acids. Most people don't get enough essential fatty acids from foods. That's why dietary supplements such as borage, flax, and fish oils have become so popular among health-conscious people.

Fatty acids serve as building blocks for nerve cells and cell membranes. When levels of essential fatty acids are inadequate, dangerous saturated fats replace the essential fatty acids within cell membranes. This results in reduced membrane fluidity, and then inefficiency, which promotes premature aging and disease. You can maximize the production of beneficial prostaglandins, and minimize the production of harmful ones (such as prostaglandin E2) by taking the right proportions of essential fatty acids.

Deficiencies in essential fatty acids are linked to:

• Chronic inflammatory conditions (such as arthritis)
• Hypertension (high blood pressure)
• Memory loss
• Elevated triglycerides
• Dementia
• Cardiovascular disease
• Insulin resistance (leading to type II diabetes)

You need the right amounts of GLA (gamma linolenic acid), DHA (docosahexaenoic acid), and EPA (eicosapentaenoic acid) to ensure optimal fatty acid intake. Omega-6 fatty acids are good for your complexion and for proper joint flexibility. Extra dry skin and stiff, painful joints are symptoms of omega fatty acid deficiency.

Fatty fish, such as salmon, mackerel, cod, grouper, tuna, sole, and sardines, are all good-quality proteins, and they are also outstanding sources of omega-3 fatty acids that help turn off the inflammatory process, relieving fibromyalgia, asthma, emphysema, and digestive disorders.

Conjugated linoleic acid (CLA) is a group of isomers of the omega-6 essential fatty acid linoleic acid. Isomer cis-9 trans-11 CLA has been shown to appear to inhibit cancer formation, and to enhance muscle growth. The trans-10 cis-12 CLA isomer has been shown to eliminate lipogenesis, or the creation of fat cells, and to stop existing fat cells from increasing in size. CLA's ability to increase muscle mass and reduce fat mass, creating a leaner physique, without altering hormone levels, makes it effective for use by both men and women.

Flaxseed oil or ground flaxseeds are vegetarian sources of omega-3 and omega-6 essential fatty acids.

Note that omega-3 fatty acids must be balanced with omega-6 fatty acids. Here is a commonly recommended daily combination:

4,000 mg of borage oil, yielding 920 mg of GLA (omega-6)
2,000 mg of fish oil extract, yielding 1,000 mg of DHA (omega-3)
400 mg of EPA (omega-3)
1,000 mg of conjugated linoleic acid (CLA)

PROVEN AGE-BUSTERS

The rate at which your body ages is largely determined by a number of biological processes, which we discussed in Chapter 3. The following agents have been widely accepted as being effective in slowing the aging process and warding off disease. I'm going to group them into five categories: antioxidants; Chrono-Forte, an antiaging formula; bone-enhancing nutrients, which will be of particular interest to women, although men can benefit from these too; natural prostate-helpers for men; and herbal aids to health. As we discuss supplements in various sections of this book, there is going to be some overlap, with certain supplements popping up time and again. That's because many of them perform a variety of functions and can help in multiple ways. That's part of the wonder of natural substances!

THE ANTIOXIDANT ARMY (VITAMINS, MINERALS, AMINO ACIDS) AND MAJOR SUPPORTIVE NUTRIENTS

Antioxidants guard against many chronic diseases by removing chemicals that may damage your body. Many common chronic diseases such as cancer, cardiovascular disease, and arthritis arise from the same insidious source: mutations, caused mainly by free radicals. Your cells are protected against free radicals and lipid peroxidation when you are in peak health.

The antioxidant army is a complex system of human defense in which vitamins, minerals, amino acids, and certain enzymes guard your health. Antioxidants are substances that react chemically with free radicals to disarm them. Antioxidants break the vicious cycle of the decomposition of proteins and fatty aids, which would otherwise create new free radicals, leading to premature aging and cell death. Known antioxidants include:

- Vitamin C
- Vitamin E
- Some B vitamins, beta-carotene (use mixed carotenoids)
- Alpha-lipoic acid
- Manganese
- Selenium
- Zinc
- Some amino acids, such as L-carnosine, N-acetyl cysteine (NAC), and L-taurine, reduced L-glutathione
- Coenzyme Q10 (coQ10)
- Some hormones, such as melatonin
- Some enzymes, such as superoxide dismutase (SOD)

The Antioxidant Army may be compared to the pieces of a chess set. The antiaging superstars might then be King Vitamin C and Queen CoQ10, Sir Selenium, Bishop Vitamin E, and Castle Carnosine; but if, in your quest for rejuvenation, you were to welcome *only* these flashy antioxidant supplements, you would be missing vital support from other nutrients, such as Pawn Potassium.

A main message of this book is that balance is essential to health; that is why you will find several supporting supplements in this section. Just as an army cannot win victory without its humble foot soldiers, the Royal Family of Antioxidants cannot rule without help from its support staff. Copper, for example, is a handmaiden to vitamin C, assisting in making C bioavailable. Copper is also a component of the antioxidant enzyme superoxide dismutase (SOD). The Antioxidant Army that defends you is truly a team.

Beta-carotene and Mixed Carotenoids.

Beta-carotene is a precursor of vitamin A. The carotenoids are powerful antioxidants that are deeply involved in the aging process. Research indicates that beta-carotene alone and in combination with selenium enhances natural killer cell activity in the elderly.

Beta-carotene supplements of 30 mg a day or more for two months significantly enhanced immunity in elderly subjects. Low levels of beta-carotene are linked to the risk of cataract development. Beta-carotene is the best-known vitamin for the eyes, and it protects against macular degeneration as well as cataracts.

Research done at Johns Hopkins University shows that there were approximately 50 percent fewer cases of heart disease among study participants who had the highest blood levels of beta-carotene, compared with the group with lowest levels.

At Harvard University, scientists found that of two groups with prior evidence of heart disease, the group given a beta-carotene supplement had 40 percent fewer heart attacks than the group given a placebo.

Carrots, parsley, and collard greens are rich sources of beta-carotene. Peaches, apricots, cantaloupes, yams, beets, spinach, and romaine lettuce are also rich sources.

When you're taking this supplement, 10,000 IU of beta-carotene per day is the recommended dose. Remember, use of mixed carotenoids (not just beta) is most effective.

B Vitamins and Folic Acid (Vitamin B Complex).

B vitamins perform a whole array of functions, and they work best together. Depression and other emotional difficulties are favorably affected by B vitamins, including B_{12}. As you age, your stomach secretes less hydrochloric acid than before. This decreased secretion is known as atrophic gastritis. Reduced hydrochloric acid has an enormous impact on your ability to absorb several B vitamins. As a result, we find lower levels of vitamin B_{12} and folic acid in the blood of older people, and subsequently there is a greater need on their part for these nutrients.

Research at the University of Alabama in Birmingham and at Tufts University finds that folic acid aids in the prevention of stroke, as well as heart disease. People who consume the most folate (within usual dosages) are 50 percent less likely to have narrowing of the carotid artery leading to the brain.

Holding Homocysteine at Bay. Increased levels of homocysteine are very common in older Americans who don't consume enough B vitamins in their diet. Studies show that elevated levels of homocysteine are a contributing factor in the development of cardiovascular disease and stroke. By increasing their level of B vitamins, either through diet or supplements, older people can lower their risk of acquiring these conditions.

Dietary folic acid and vitamins B_6 and B_{12} have the strongest effects on helping to rid the human body of homocysteine, according to the American Heart Association. Several studies find that higher blood concentrations of B vitamins contribute to lower concentrations of homocysteine. The AHA also notes that other evidence ties low blood levels of folic acid to a higher risk of fatal cardiac disease and stroke. Clinical research is expanding on several continents to determine whether the lowering of homocysteine by vitamin B and folic acid leads to a decrease in cardiovascular disease over time.

Vegetables (especially cabbage, raw spinach, endive, and asparagus), whole grains, citrus fruit, papaya, and tomatoes are rich sources of folic acid.

Bananas, pears, and brown rice offer vitamin B_6, which is a superb antioxidant in its own right, and is even known as a painkiller. But it cannot be taken alone in high doses for too long.

Vitamin B_{12} is found in fermented tofu, tempeh, and in B_{12} lozenges of 500 to 1,000 mcg a day.

Avoid dietary intake of substances that deplete the B vitamin family, such as caffeine and prolonged alcohol consumption.

Vitamin B complex may be taken at daily doses of 50 mg per day; folic acid may be taken at 400 mcg per day.

Vitamin C and Bioflavonoids. Researchers have found that a high intake of glucose, or eating a high-fat, high-calorie, fast-food meal causes an increase in the blood's inflammatory components. This reaction inflames the lining of the arteries for up to four hours and increases the risk of atherosclerosis. Research shows that the antioxidant vitamins C and E can stop this inflammatory response.

High plasma vitamin C is also shown to be associated with high plasma HDL (good) and HDL2 (better) cholesterol, which may reduce atherogenic risk.

Bioflavonoids are antioxidant pigments from plants and fruits that protect us against free radical damage:

Pycnogenol. Pycnogenol is the bioflavanoid proanthocyanidin extracted from pine bark and grape seeds. It is a powerful antioxidant and free radical scavenger, known to exhibit anticancer activity.

Pycnogenol protects the brain by fortifying the blood vessel walls. It's protective against stroke and dementia. Pycnogenol keeps collagen elastic, and softens blood platelets for more efficient movement through the vessels.

Take a minimum of 400 mg of pycnogenol per day.

Grape Seed Extract, Grape Skin Extract, Red Wine Concentrate. These ultrapowerful anti-inflammatory bioflavonoids are available in one formula. Choose a naturally extracted product without chemical or solvent residues. A recent study shows that resveratrol, a polyphenol in grape skins, inhibits blood platelet aggregation, protecting your heart. It is scientifically documented to improve varicose veins, and reduce leg swelling and bruising. This complex increases peripheral circulation, improving vision. There is less aging of your skin, particularly with regard to maintaining skin elasticity. Fewer allergies and reduced inflammation are reported. This bioflavonoid complex also helps to heal ulcers by reducing histamine secretion and by binding to and protecting connective tissue in mucous membranes.

Dentists and their patients report that this bioflavonoid complex provides healing and preventive benefits for the teeth and gums, evidently through its anti-inflammatory effects, free radical deactivation, and connective tissue protection.

These potent antioxidant bioflavonoids help to protect cellular DNA from oxidative damage and from cell mutations that can lead to cancer.

This is one of the few antioxidants that is able to protect neural tissue by crossing the blood-brain barrier. Purchase products that state on their label that the contents are standardized (i.e., certified by analytical procedures). The standard concentration for grape seed extracts is 95 percent PCOs (oligomeric procyanidolic complexes).

These bioflavonoids are found in many types of foods, but usually only in tiny amounts. Some of the best sources are in seasonal fruits such as grapes, blueberries, cherries, and plums. The proanthocyanidins are found mainly in the peels, skins, or seeds. Food processing and storage will reduce bioavailability.

PCO selectively binds to the connective tissue of joints, preventing swelling, helping heal damaged tissue, and lessening pain.

PCO has also been shown to prevent the stickiness of blood platelets that can lead to blood clots and strokes. Patients taking PCO of grape seed extract have reported reduced blood pressure and cholesterol levels.

The American Heart Association showed that six glasses of grape juice were as effective as two glasses of wine in preventing heart disease.[4] This study offers convincing evidence that PCO from grapes, rather than the alcohol, provide wine's protective benefits to the circulatory system.

Health professionals monitoring the effects of PCO have reported that it also has helped in the prevention and treatment of glaucoma.

PCO strengthens skin connective tissue and fat chambers. People taking PCO of grape seed extract have noticed that it helps tone their skin and reduce cellulite, stretch marks, and old scars. There is speculation that cellulite may be a sign of bioflavanoid deficiency.

Some physicians report that patients with multiple sclerosis have improved while taking PCO. The ability of PCO to reduce the progressive symptoms of multiple sclerosis may be due to its potent antioxidant and anti-allergenic qualities. In addition, the ability of PCO to cross the blood-brain barrier, where it may protect the brain's nervous tissue from oxidation, may explain why patients taking PCO often report improved mental clarity.

PCO of grape seed extract has also been found to reduce the coughing, wheezing, weakness, mucus, and recurring respiratory infections usually associated with emphysema. PCO apparently reduces the inflammation and damage to the air sacs of emphysema patients.

A recent symposium in Europe gave a general guideline for taking 1 mg of PCO per day for every pound of body weight for the first week, enough to saturate the body tissues. Then the amount may be reduced to as little as one half of that amount. This reduced dosage would be for general protection, not for specific health problems, which may require higher doses.

Effective dosage varies with the severity of the condition. It is always wise to consult a knowledgeable practitioner on dosage for specific conditions. Allergies, for example, may require 100 to 200 mg two to three times per day for several days until the body builds up a sufficient amount to stabilize the condition. As an adjunct to cancer therapy, 150 to 200 mg, four times per day, might be taken to enhance immune response. Dosages far greater than these have been shown to have no toxic effects.

Quercetin. The bioflavonoid quercetin shows anticancer properties in the lab. Animal trials provide evidence of cardioprotective and antidiabetic activity, as well as inhibition of gastric ulcers.

Rutin. Animal studies show that the bioflavonoid rutin can inhibit tumors associated with colon cancer, and slow hypercholesterolemia and peroxidation. Rutin is an in vitro antioxidant and free radical scavenger, and it offers protection against gastric injury in rats. Rutin enhances vitamin C absorption, promotes circulation, and is a popular remedy for bruises, high cholesterol, muscular pain, cirrhosis, cataracts, stress, hemorrhoids, and constipation. Natural dietary sources of rutin include the pith of citrus fruits, the white core of green peppers, prunes, rose hips, apricots, cherries, rhubarb, mint, buckwheat, and chamomile.

Dietary sources of vitamin C include citrus fruits; cruciferous vegetables; raw or cooked green or red sweet peppers; raw or cooked snow peas; cooked kohlrabi; baked or boiled sweet potato; boiled green or ripe plantain; cantaloupe; honeydew melon; frozen, unsweetened peaches; cooked asparagus; raw or frozen unsweetened strawberries; and papaya.

Take bioflavonoids with vitamin C because bioflavonoids enhance the benefits of vitamin C to fortify your immune system. Bioflavonoids promote capillary health.

A commonly recommended dosage for vitamin C is 2,000 to 10,000 mg per day orally, preferably from ascorbyl palmitate, with 500 to 1,000 mg per day of bioflavonoids such as pycnogenol, grape seed extract complex with grape skin extract and red wine concentrate, quercetin, and rutin.

Take a little vitamin C after a meal to speed digestion and protect against heart disease. Vitamin C also protects against diabetes and cancer. A little vitamin C taken at bedtime will launch system repairs while you sleep.

Calcium. Calcium may lower blood pressure, and lower total cholesterol while inhibiting platelet aggregation. It helps prevent osteoporosis, taken with cofactors (see Bone-Enhancing Nutrients for Women, page 209).

Green leafy vegetables, especially collard greens, contain calcium. Avoid dairy sources, which are not well absorbed anyway.

Take 1,500 to 1,800 mg per day of calcium citrate, which is more easily absorbed than other forms, and is especially better for people over age sixty. Always take digestive enzymes with calcium to assist assimilation.

Vitamin E. (See Cutting Edge Supplements, page 186.)

Coenzyme Q10. (See Cutting Edge Supplements, page 186.)

Copper. Trace amounts of copper are present in all human tissues, but copper is most concentrated in your liver, kidneys, brain, bones, and muscles, and it is essential in blood. Copper is a component of the antioxidant enzyme superoxide dismutase (SOD).

Copper increases iron assimilation. Copper and iron form hemoglobin and red blood cells. In fact, anemia can be a symptom of a copper deficiency. Various enzyme reactions require copper. Copper influences overall healing and protein metabolism, improves oxidation of vitamin C, and is required for RNA formation. Low or high copper levels can be found in those with mental and emotional problems. Also, copper may help rid the body of parasites.

Symptoms of copper deficiency are diverse, and include allergies, parasites, Parkinson's disease, reduced glucose tolerance, aneurisms, arthritis, dry brittle hair, hernias, high blood cholesterol, hyper- and hypothyroidism, hair loss, liver cirrhosis, heart disease, edema, osteoporosis, breathing difficulties, ruptured disc, skin eruptions or sores, white or gray hair, varicose veins, and wrinkled skin.

Whole grain cereals, almonds, and green leafy vegetables are natural sources of copper.

For a daily copper supplement, one would use copper, as gluconate, at 2 mg. Liquid forms may be more bioavailable.

Magnesium. Magnesium calms the nerves. As this mineral mediates digestive processes, a lack is associated with many eating-related problems, including vomiting, indigestion, cramps, flatulence, abdominal pain, and constipation.

When under stress, we use up much magnesium. Chocolate cravings may be a sign of magnesium deficiency, because chocolate is high in magnesium.

Magnesium deficiency has been implicated in depression, diabetes, heart disease, migraines, and menopausal symptoms.

Natural sources of magnesium include dark, leafy vegetables, sea vegetables, and whole grains.

The daily recommended dose of magnesium is 1,200 mg.

Manganese. Manganese is an important antioxidant that is an essential trace mineral. Manganese activates many enzymes, including those that help to maintain blood sugar levels, metabolism for energy, and healthy thyroid function. The enzymes activated by manganese are necessary for proper use of biotin, choline, thiamine, and ascorbic acid. Manganese helps to control insulin reactions.

As an antioxidant, manganese plays a role in the function of superoxide dismutase (SOD). Supplemental manganese increases SOD activity, which stimulates increased antioxidant activity.

Manganese is involved in the metabolism of cholesterol, fatty acids, and mucopolysaccharides. Functions of manganese include normal skeletal development, a healthy immune system, healthy brain and nerves, and sex hormone production.

Manganese is found in green and sea vegetables.

Excessive dietary intake of manganese might interfere with iron absorption. High calcium and phosphorus intake increases the need for manganese.

The recommended daily dose of manganese is 10 mg.

Potassium. Epidemiological and clinical studies demonstrate that potassium has an important effect on blood pressure regulation. Increasing potassium levels and lowering sodium intake has the overall effect of lowering blood pressure. By increasing the level of potassium in the blood, we can reduce the risk of a variety of heart problems. This mineral also has potential benefits for diabetics.

Potassium aids iodine in creating thyroid hormones to increase metabolism and regulate metabolism of glucose. Muscles, brain cells, and nerves all rely on potassium.

The best way to increase potassium intake is to eat fresh fruit, such as bananas. If you wish to avoid starchy fruit, you may take a 300 mg potassium supplement daily.

Selenium. Selenium, an essential trace mineral and vital antioxidant, works synergistically with vitamin E. One study concludes that supplemental beta-carotene and selenium enhanced immune function in a healthy elderly group. Dozens of animal and in vitro studies point to selenium in the prevention and treatment of cancer. A review article cites many epidemiological studies showing a significant inverse relationship between selenium intake and human cancer risk. Most recently, research has proven a role for selenium in the prevention of colon cancer.

Selenium may also help to prevent diabetes and heart disease. Selenium and vitamin E given together to rabbits protected their heart muscle from changes associated with a diet high in fat. And this mineral may enhance the body's capacity to fight infectious diseases.

Selenium appears to be involved in thyroid hormone metabolism.

Immune function can be strengthened by selenium. Kidney damage, lupus, ulcers, dental caries, and poor mood are other conditions that respond positively to selenium supplementation.

Cooked sockeye salmon and raw mushrooms contain this nutrient. The recommended daily dose of selenium is 200 mcg.

Zinc. Zinc is an essential trace element involved in many human biological functions including cell division and differentiation, gene transcription, apoptosis (programmed cell death), biomembrane function, and many enzymatic actions. Zinc is central to the process of aging well. This antioxidant protects against macular degeneration, which is an age-related vision impairment. Arthritis responds to zinc supplementation. In one study, 220 mg of zinc sulfate was given three times a day for twelve weeks to rheumatoid arthritis patients. They reported feeling significant improvement in the areas of joint swelling, walking time, and morning stiffness.

Cancer patients taking 250 mg a day of oral zinc gluconate for three weeks showed enhanced immune function. Animal studies suggest that zinc may protect against stroke and mitigate the negative effects of chronic stress in mice.

Zinc shows promise in treatment of male infertility. Many studies point to zinc in treatment of skin disorders such as eczema, herpes, and acne. Many older people have anorexic symptoms because they do not have normal diets. Zinc doses in the range of 40 to 90 mg a day help anorexic patients to gain weight. Zinc affects improvement in patients with sickle cell anemia, cerebral palsy, and inflammatory bowel disease.

Lutein. Lutein is a yellow-pigment carotenoid found in vegetables and fruits. It acts as an antioxidant, protecting cells against the damaging effects of free radicals. Since it's not made in the body, lutein must be obtained from food or vitamin supplements.

This substance is important to all of us because it helps maintain eye health. Research shows that people with diets rich in lutein and zeaxanthin are at a lower risk for degeneration of the macula, which is a part of the retina. Macular degeneration is the leading cause of blindness in older adults.

Leafy green kale is a fine source of lutein. Other sources include spinach, broccoli, romaine lettuce, tomatoes, oranges and orange juice, carrots, and celery.

Lycopene. The carotenoid lycopene is a powerful antioxidant that is stronger than beta-carotene. The human body does not produce lycopene, so it must be obtained from dietary sources. Look for foods that have red pigment when you're thinking about this nutrient—e.g., tomatoes, a great source, as well as watermelon, beets, guava, and even pink grapefruit.

Recent studies cite lycopene for maintaining heart health, and for cancer prevention. Lycopene exhibits anticancer properties in animal studies, in vitro, and in human beings. A large human case-control study found that increased consumption of lycopene-containing foods, especially tomatoes and tomato products, may lead to reduced myocardial infarction risk. Lycopene prevents LDL (bad) cholesterol from oxidizing and building deposits on walls of arteries; it thus curbs development of atherosclerosis. The role of lycopene in prevention of prostate cancer is documented.

Reduced L-Glutathione. Alpha-lipoic acid may aid in absorption of the tripeptide glutathione. The reduced form is more assimilable.

This is a master antioxidant with a major role in cancer prevention and treatment. The highest concentration of glutathione is in your liver for cellular detoxification. Glutathione reconstitutes vitamins C and E after they have been oxidized, and therefore glutathione plays a role in the function of these vitamins.

Low glutathione levels are linked to compromised immunity, leading to a host of neuro-degenerative diseases, such as multiple sclerosis, ALS, Alzheimer's, and Parkinsonism; also, atherosclerosis, cataracts, and pharmacological drug damage have been associated with low levels.

Take two 75 mg capsules of reduced L-glutathione daily, preferably with an alpha-lipoic acid supplement. Do not exceed 200 mg per day.

L-Taurine. L-taurine is a major antioxidant that prevents hardening of the arteries and strengthens heart contractions, increasing blood flow to prevent heart failure.

The recommended daily dose is 500 mg of taurine taken twice a day.

NAC (N-acetyl Cysteine). NAC, a potent antioxidant, is an altered form of the amino acid cysteine that the body synthesizes; it is also commonly found in food.

NAC inhibits oxidation of LDL cholesterol and inhibits carcinogens in tobacco smoke; it counteracts excessive generation of free radicals during exercise, and it protects lungs from free radical damage and lung ailments.

A dosage of 1,200 mg of NAC per day helps to prevent the flu, relieves symptoms of existing flu infection, and reduces the duration of the disease, especially in the elderly and in those who are chronically ill.

This antioxidant administered at 1,800 mg per day is currently being tested as an immune system enhancer in people with AIDS. NAC has been suggested as a viable alternative to other protease inhibitors for AIDS treatment because NAC itself is an effective pro-tease inhibitor.

NAC inhibits proliferation of *Streptococcus pneumoniae*, especially in bronchial tissue of smokers with chronic bronchitis. It also facili-tates the excretion of arsenic from the body; victims of arsenic poi-soning are saved from death when NAC is administered upon arrival at the hospital.

It has even more benefits. NAC helps to remove (chelate) toxic mercury from the body. It reduces the toxic side effects of cyclophos-phamide, a cancer drug. And it prevents the liver damage that leads to death after Paracetamol overdose.

It's important to know that NAC helps to prevent various types of cancer by exerting antimutagenic effects against a wide variety of toxic chemicals. Also, NAC enhances the effectiveness of interferon alpha in the treatment of hepatitis C, primarily by counteracting the depletion of the antioxidant glutathione.

The recommended daily dosage of NAC is 1,000 mg.

Superoxide Dismutase (SOD). Superoxide dismutase (SOD) is an antioxidant enzyme that counters free radical damage at the cellu-lar level. It shows benefits for osteoarthritis. Also, in many animal tri-als, SOD protects against lung damage.

Topical application of SOD helps to heal burns. TMJ patients who do not respond to traditional therapy may find that intra-articular injection of SOD is effective. Many animal studies support SOD to prevent and treat heart disease.

CHRONO-FORTE: THE ANTIAGING FORMULA

Chrono-Forte is a compound supplement that combines the benefits of several well-known antiaging nutrients, such as carnosine and oth-ers, described earlier.

Tumor necrosis factor-alpha (TNF-a) is a dangerous chemical that stimulates the immune system to attack healthy tissues. Elevated

TNF-a causes a systemic inflammatory cascade that may result in painful arthritis along with lethal neurological or vascular complications. Increases in TNF-a play a role in catabolic wasting seen in cancer and advanced aging. Nettle leaf extract has been shown to inhibit TNF-a at 1,000 mg.[5]

Many scientific studies show that acetyl-L-carnitine and alpha-lipoic acid promote youthful cellular levels of glutathione, sustain mitochondrial energy production, and protect against immune dysfunction.[6] Acetyl-L-carnitine and alpha-lipoic acid work with coenzyme Q10 to maintain healthy energy levels. Chrono-Forte combines these nutrients for a synergistic advantage, as follows:

Acetyl-L-carnitine HCL 2,000 mg
Alpha-lipoic acid 300 mg
Carnosine 1,000 mg
Nettle leaf extract 1,000 mg
Zinc 15 mg
Quercetin (water-soluble) 100 mg
Biotin 3,000 mg

BONE-ENHANCING NUTRIENTS FOR WOMEN

Osteoporosis is a common consequence of aging that can cause disabling fractures (most commonly hip fractures), or even death. Since osteoporosis has no symptoms in its early stages, prevention with mineral supplementation is critical. Living bone is never at rest metabolically. Its "walls" or matrix and mineral stores are being remodeled constantly, and minerals such as calcium play crucial metabolic and structural roles in bone.

For this reason, calcium supplements are often prescribed for women. However, osteoporosis is associated with deficiencies of a wide range of nutrients, including magnesium, vitamin D_3, manganese, and zinc.[7] In order for calcium to prevent bone loss, adequate amounts of vitamin D_3 and certain trace minerals must be available so that calcium, magnesium, and phosphorus will be incorporated into the bone matrix.[8] The following formula, compounded in absorbable capsule form as Bone Assure by the Life Extension Foundation, is designed to prevent bone loss:

Elemental calcium (as bis–glycinate) (equals 1,800 mg of elemental calcium citrate)	1,000 mg
Magnesium (oxide)	320 mg
Zinc (citrate)	12 mg
Manganese (citrate)	3 mg
Boron (amino acid chelate)	2 mg
Copper (sulfate)	1.5 mg
Oat straw (10:1) (silica source)	40 mg
Vitamin D_3	400 IU
Folic acid	200 mcg
TMG	100 mg
Vitamin B_6	15 mg

NATURAL PROSTATE HELPERS FOR MEN

Benign prostatic hypertrophy (BPH), or prostate enlargement, is a consequence of aging for most men. An extract from the saw palmetto berry may prevent BPH, and possibly reduce the risk of prostate cancer. Saw palmetto is derived from the berries of a small bushy tree found in the southeast United States. It inhibits the binding of DHT (dihydrotestosterone) to prostate cell receptor sites and also acts as an alpha–adrenergic receptor inhibitor, reducing urinary urgency and inflammatory action in the prostate gland. Saw palmetto has been used for decades to treat urogenital disorders. European researchers document its effectiveness in alleviating symptoms of benign prostatic hyperplasia.[9]

Nettle root extract (*Urtica dioica*) helps suppress the effects of estrogen and sex-hormone-binding globulins by stopping them from binding to the prostate.[10]

Pygeum, which has anti-inflammatory properties, has been shown to alleviate symptoms associated with benign prostate enlargement.[11]

The Life Extension Foundation offers a therapy called Natural Prostate Formula. Each capsule of this formula contains the identical herb extracts used in Europe to alleviate symptoms of benign prostate disease by 86 percent after three months of use. This formula contains:

Saw palmetto super critical extract	160 mg
Pygeum extract	50 mg
Urtica dioica (nettle root) extract	120 mg
Lycopene extract	5 mg

HERBAL AIDS

Herbal Brain Boosters. Diaphoretics are the class of herbs that increase sweating to eliminate waste; many will cause dilation of surface capillaries, helping poor circulation, and memory. Cayenne, garlic, and ginger are diaphoretics that can be simply prepared.

Ginger has been used in traditional Chinese medicine for over 2,500 years. In India, it's called the universal medicine. Like garlic and cayenne, ginger has circulatory benefits that protect the vessels in the brain. Enjoy bracing cups of fresh ginger tea with raw honey; or simply add cayenne powder to green tea (coat the tea leaves with cayenne to taste, then steep) for a surprisingly pleasing spice treat that restores concentration immediately; or bake a head of garlic (cloves intact) in parchment paper for one hour at 325°F for an aromatic garlic pâté. All of these can help strengthen your memory, with many attendant benefits. Take herbs such as gotu kola (see page 214) capsules for clarity by day, and for better sleep at night (quality sleep enhances concentration).

Herbal Infection-Fighters. Postmenopausal women tend to contract cystitis frequently; herbs used to treat this condition fall into the antiseptic, demulcent, and diuretic categories. Antiseptic herbs for bladder infections include uva-ursi, buchu, goldenseal, juniper berries, and garlic. Demulcents soothe inflamed mucous membranes inside the urethra and bladder, and these include corn silk, juniper berry, and marshmallow root. Diuretic herbs stimulate urine production and excretion, which helps to wash out bacteria. Parsley and goldenrod are common diuretics.

Antiaging Herbs. The following herbs may be taken as powders, capsules, tinctures, or teas.

Angelica (*Guardian Angel*). Tea made from this herb is useful in fighting infections, including colds and flu. Angelica is sometimes recommended for long-term use to prevent wintertime illnesses. Angelica also helps digestion, but note—it is not for use by diabetics because it may increase blood sugar levels.

Arnica. Given at times to ease pain, arnica is available in topical products for relief of bruises, sprains, and sore muscles.

Bach Flower Remedies. These remedies may offer relief from emotional pain and difficulties (so you can retain a more youthful positive outlook; irritability and fear will age you fast). "Rescue Remedy" is the best known of these, and it is recommended and used by many professional nurses and herbalists. These are available at health food and vitamin stores. They help pets, too. These go beyond aromatherapy.

Bilberry. Bilberry is even higher in antioxidants than blueberry.

Black Cohosh. Tincture of black cohosh can be part of an effective treatment for depression. This herb has proven benefits for women suffering from symptoms of menopause.

Burdock Root. Burdock is a diuretic and diaphoretic herb. It is one of the best blood purifiers, and a skin disease remedy.

Calendula. This one helps with varicose veins.

Capsicum. Capsicum stimulates circulation and elimination. It is a mild diuretic that helps to cleanse the kidneys.

Cayenne (*Red Pepper*). Cayenne lowers cholesterol to help lower blood pressure, and prevents hardening of the arteries (atherosclerosis) by preventing blood from clotting in your arteries.

Chasteberry (Vitex). This is noted for relieving hot flashes and other menopausal symptoms.

Chisandra. This is another antioxidant.

Comfrey. This is used particularly to help with varicose veins.

Damiana. A diuretic that also acts directly to tone and stimulate reproductive organ function, this herb is said to be an aphrodisiac.

Dong Quai. This herb increases circulation in the pelvic area.

Fo-Ti. Devotees say that this is an excellent digestive tonic that rejuvenates the endocrine system.

Garlic. Nutritionists have been singing the praises of garlic for a long time, and with good reason. This herb is antiviral, antibacterial, and antifungal. It also boosts energy. Garlic stimulates detoxification of the liver and colon, and it may have anticancer properties.

The power of garlic to "clear the arteries" was recorded as early as the first century A.D. Today we know that standardized garlic ingestion at 900 mg per day reduces serum total cholesterol and LDL-cholesterol. The mechanism responsible for this effect seems to center around various components of the bulb, mainly allicin, ajoene, and diallyldisulfide. These compounds affect how cholesterol is made in the liver; they fine-tune the regulation of this pathway. The reaction between garlic-derived organosulfur compounds and intracellular signaling pathways leads to reduction of total serum cholesterol. These features demonstrate that garlic is a natural and relatively safe therapeutic tool for treatment of mild cases of hypercholesterolemia, or high cholesterol. What's more, allicin-standardized dried garlic powder also significantly lowers triglycerides.

Garlic lowers blood pressure slightly; it helps to thin the blood by reducing platelet aggregation (blood coagulation). A 900 mg a day garlic regimen has been shown to help reverse arterial plaque build-up, reducing the risk of cardiovascular disease.[12]

Warning: Taking garlic with prescription blood-thinning drugs is generally contraindicated. If you take Coumadin (warfarin), aspirin, heparin, or Trental (pentoxifylline), which are all blood-thinning drugs, do not use garlic unless you are following medical advice to do so. As a rule, do not use garlic with any blood thinners.

Garlic with vitamin or herbal blood thinners: Taking garlic with high doses of vitamin E or with ginkgo may cause bleeding.

Ginger. Ginger is a heart tonic. It lowers cholesterol, and makes blood platelets less sticky, and thus less likely to form obstructive clots. It's fun to use this herb creatively in cooking, which can be a process as simple as just sprinkling it on a salad. Or you can brew fresh ginger tea using one or two teaspoons of grated ginger root per cup of boiling water. Do not use crystallized ginger.

Ginkgo Biloba. Ginkgo improves circulation to microcapillaries to carry vital nutrients and oxygen to all tissues of the brain and heart. It works to prevent strokes, and is also prescribed for stroke survivors. It's yet another free-radical fighter.

Ginseng. A Chinese symbol of longevity, ginseng is considered a rejuvenation herb. Research shows that ginseng is an antioxidant that slows the free radical damage of aging. It promotes better focus under stress, and boosts energy levels.

Gotu Kola. Gotu kola, another herb associated with longevity, increases vitality and stamina, and reinforces memory. Elephants graze on gotu kola and live to be seventy in the wild, where they usually die of starvation, not illness. This herb may lower blood pressure.

Green Tea. Chinese green tea, in particular, has well-documented cancer-fighting properties in animals and humans. Regular consumption of green tea appears to counteract the negative effects of mutagens and carcinogens released in meat cooked at high temperatures. Green tea extract inhibits malignant gastrointestinal tumors in humans. Plus there's even more good news about this widely available substance: Green tea exhibits antibacterial action, and Chinese green tea polyphenols are effective preventive agents against dental cavities.

Green tea is an antioxidant for the health of heart cells. It may be a powerful free-radical scavenger protecting against peroxidation of lipids, a cause of atherosclerosis. It may also help prevent strokes as well. Use a standardized extract with at least 50 percent catechins and

90 percent total polyphenols. A regimen of 100 mg three to six times a day is therapeutic. The tea form is not standardized, but drinking the tea is recommended as well.

Hawthorn. Hawthorn may be helpful in the management of mild forms of arteriosclerosis, angina, and arrhythmia. It may also lower cholesterol and blood pressure. Standardized hawthorn products, such as tinctures, capsules, extracts, and teas from dried hawthorn are available. They contain flavonoids and procyanidins.

You may need to take hawthorn for at least six weeks, three times a day, for angina or heart failure. Follow recommended dosages. If pain or exhaustion increase, discontinue use. If your condition does not improve in six weeks, consult your health care provider.

Contraindications: If you are taking Lanoxin (digoxin), the medicine prescribed more than any other for heart ailments, or digitalis, do not use hawthorn, as hawthorn may adversely increase the effects of these drugs. Never take hawthorn with digoxin because the combination could lower your heart rate too much, cause pooling of blood, and bring on possible heart failure.

Hops. Hops may improve your appetite. It is a sedative as well, and it promotes sleep. A warm hops pillow can relieve earache and toothache, and it often calms nervous irritation.

Lavender. Stress is a significant factor in cardiovascular disease. Essential oil of lavender in the bath water relieves tension.

Licorice. Low doses of licorice extract (150 mg a day) have been proven effective against hyperkalemia (excess potassium in the blood) in diabetic patients. Licorice has antiviral properties in vitro, including inhibition of herpes virus growth. It's used to treat chronic hepatitis and cirrhosis of the liver, as well as ulcers.

Milk Thistle. Milk thistle can play an important role in rejuvenation because it enhances liver function, thus aiding in the removal of toxins from the body.

Motherwort. Angina, palpitations, and other heart conditions, as well as menstrual disorders including PMS, have all been treated with this herb.

Mugwort. This has often been recommended by herbalists for vaginal yeast infections and skin infections.

Muira puama. This one is used as an aphrodisiac.

Raspberry Leaf. As an astringent, raspberry leaf is useful in a wide range of cases, including diarrhea, leucorrhoea, and other loose conditions, often a result of the difficulty in proper food digestion associated with aging. It's also used for relief from oral problems, such as mouth ulcers, bleeding gums, and inflammations. As a gargle it will help sore throats.

Rosemary. This popular herb is known for the soothing properties of its oil on the nervous and digestive systems. Rosemary is also commonly used to treat headache, depression, muscle pain, gum disease, anxiety, flatulence, warts, hair loss, and high blood pressure. Rosemary exhibits anticancer activity in many animal studies. Rosemary oil is traditionally used to restore alertness and concentration.

Skullcap. This herb relieves nervous tension.

Theonine. Taken at a dose of 100 mg two to three times a day, this herb can stop a migraine headache, and calm you. Theonine is an active component of green tea.

Turmeric. Circumin is a compound in turmeric that helps prevent blood clots. Turmeric is also associated with anticancer activity. Curry dishes contain this valuable herb.

Valerian. Valerian root is currently the most widely used sedative and sleep aid in Europe, and it's interesting to note that it has been used for thousands of years for this purpose. Sometimes the ancients had it right! Valerian is taken as a tea, tincture, or in capsule form, and its benefits include relief of anxiety, digestive disorders, muscle spasms, fever, and high blood pressure. Research shows that extracts of valerian root can relieve depression in mice, and promote sound sleep.

Vervain. Vervain is another yet another calming herb with a long history. It has been used for hundreds of years as an emotion soother.

Wild Yam. Wild yam relieves hot flashes, depression, insomnia, irritability, and other menopausal symptoms. Wild yam supports the adrenal production of DHEA, which is a building block for estrogen, progesterone, testosterone, and cortisols, which decline with age. Wild yam is an adaptogen that balances the body's hormonal functions. It ameliorates many chronic conditions including heart disease, cancer, arthritis, and autoimmune diseases.

PART III

PUTTING IT ALL TOGETHER — FOR YOU!

CHAPTER 9

GARY'S NON-DIET DIET, NO-EXERCISE EXERCISE PROGRAM

Creating the Plan That's Right for You

DETOX FIRST

I've talked a lot about how our present-day body has to cope with many invaders and polluters: alcohol, sugar, caffeine, dairy products, meat, poultry, pesticides, herbicides; toxins that are in our home and work environment, equally polluting our air, food, and water. In fact, I've mentioned these obstacles to our health in many chapters of *Power Aging* but now we want to tell you how to eliminate them from your body. Even though many of these toxins are said to be present in "tiny amounts," we must realize that for a toxin like mercury, there is no safe level. And chemicals like organophosphate pesticides that disrupt the hormonal system and immune system are toxic at the nanogram and microgram levels. Unfortunately, no longer can we assume that every American has a strong and fully functioning immune system that can neutralize, detoxify, and heal from environmental assaults. The fact is that most Americans are sick with multiple illnesses in multiple stages. As we age and our immune systems become less capable of defending us, and our cells are under siege—bioelectrically, chemically, and hormonally—our first step must be to strengthen our overall immune system with a comprehensive detoxification program.

But, at the same time, I want you to remember what I said in

Chapter 1, under the heading "New Millennium, New Mind-set." I'm convinced that we can develop a healthy mind-set and change the way we look at the human life span. For every toxin or problem that we are encountering I'm convinced there is a nutrient or method of detoxification to get rid of it. For every obstacle in our path we can find the solution. So, let's discard those stereotypes of aging and dive into the modern era of scientifically supported life-enhancement, antiaging protocols. I'll show you how it's already been done by hundreds, if not thousands, of people. They set the example for you to follow; they've broken down the barriers to aging and raised the bar for what we can achieve as we age. In Chapter 11 I'll reinforce the wellness concept and give you more information on taking care of specific illness, but here I want to give you a formula for detoxification that anyone can use.

LIFE-ENHANCEMENT PROTOCOLS

In 1990 I began a number of well-designed, comprehensive, life-enhancement protocols that are still ongoing. Let me tell you about some of the first groups I ran. I think that once you know that thousands of other people have succeeded at changing their lifestyle and revitalizing their health you'll be raring to go.

Upon entering these study/support groups participants were given identical protocols. To enroll, first this group of individuals had to give a detailed medical history, including a current blood chemistry hormonal panel, weight impedance, and blood pressure measurements. Then we met once a week for three months, followed by meetings every other week for eighteen months. The size of the groups ranged from one hundred to eight hundred participants. The total number in all the groups now totals more than thirteen thousand people.

During each two-hour meeting I guided people in what were really very simple and basic lifestyle changes. At no time did we talk about their illnesses. I wasn't there to reinforce illness or negative thinking about health, I was there to help people shift their attitude to one of health and longevity. At no time, in all these years, did I even talk about the treatment of a disease. At no time did I give specific or individual protocols. If a person had arthritis, dementia, or urinary tract infections, I did not give specific nutrients or therapies that are known to help these conditions. Instead it was my belief that by providing people with sound, comprehensive, and inclusive lifestyle recommendations, that individuals would be able to naturally rebuild their immune systems and no longer feed the inflammatory process and the abnormal biochemical and hormonal processes that were causing disease. It was a very simple premise and it bore fruit.

LIFE-ENHANCEMENT RESULTS

At the end of eighteen months people were re-examined and had new blood work done, and their results were statistically charted. Without exception every single person in every single health support group had statistically significant improvement. In the group focused on reversing hair loss, the participants had to have balding, thinning, and graying hair for seven years prior to joining that support group. We did "before" and "after" photos of people and reviewed their journals. For those who kept to the protocols there was significant hair regrowth and recolorization back to their natural pigment and color and cessation of thinning. Since most of these people had male pattern baldness, which is genetic, in effect we had reversed the genetic process.

It was incredible to see these fantastic improvements in people's health with basic lifestyle changes. Isn't this what genetic engineering and allopathic medicine are trying to do? But they are failing. These groups, following basic lifestyle changes, are doing it naturally! More important, when people compare their initial symptoms to the final statistical analysis, they are amazed to find that if they had symptoms of arthritis, their symptoms are gone, their weight and blood pressure are down, and their vision has improved. Their whole body begins to rejuvenate. We see what had been missing in the American lifestyle: a healthy formula for living!

Let me give you some specific statistics on one group. In January 1997, 300 people participated in a "Reversing the Aging Process Study" that ran for eighteen months. Sixty-five completed the study, and the remaining 235 became controls. We then made many important observations on the blood chemistry, weight, physical measurements, physical appearance, memory, energy levels, sleep patterns, bowel movements, nighttime urination, muscle strength, digestion, olfactory senses, visual senses, tactile sense, skin texture, and stress levels of the people in these two groups.

Here are the results:

- 52 percent of participants had lower cholesterol and triglyceride levels
- 68 percent had increased DHEA levels
- 78 percent had a significant improvement in their fat to muscle ratio
- 90 percent had an increase in bowel movements
- 92 percent had a decreased need for sleep
- 95 percent had increased energy levels
- 97 percent had decreased stress levels

From this data and from diaries kept by participants we were able to conclude that my antiaging protocol, which has now become the Power Aging protocol, can benefit the vast majority of people over sixty-five. Even people in nursing homes and hospices can enjoy increased energy and vigor if they are able to follow my approach. Wouldn't it be wonderful to enlist the support of a nursing home, change their diet to organic, whole foods and just watch the amazing results? In my book, *The Ultimate Anti-Aging Program: How to Live Forever,* I talk about Harry Biele, who followed our antiaging protocol. Now here's an example for all of us to follow!

At age eighty Harry had chronic sinusitis, asthma, arthritis, an enlarged prostate, a precancerous condition in his lower bowel, and a blockage of his main coronary artery. Ten years later he's a marathon runner and looks and acts more like seventy than ninety. His cardiologist took him off his heart medication and his family doctor took him off his asthma inhalers. But I want to stress that Harry is not the exception—he's an example of someone who has taken this program and made it work for him.

DON'T BE A STATISTIC

We know that there are too many fad diets. Too many of us shuttle between two extremes, the high protein diet on one hand, and the high carbohydrate/low fat diet on the other. Although in some instances they may help you lose weight, they also tax the body's immune system, cause chemical imbalances that lead to high levels of inflammatory products, and cause hormonal imbalances as well as a variety of diseases. You might be thinner but now you're sicker.

We also see that a strictly medical approach is not working either. Instead of using diet, allopathic medicine has chosen to treat pain and inflammation with drugs. In the case of arthritis, nonsteroidal, analgesic, anti-inflammatory drugs caused the death of 16,400 Americans in 2000. To me, this is just unacceptable. But it doesn't seem to bother the medical community and there are no headlines and no media even talking about it. For the medical community these deaths seem to be non-events—just statistics. I began to wonder what would happen if hamburgers killed sixteen thousand people. What if it was shown that drinking coffee killed sixteen thousand people? Would there be an outcry? Then I realized they do kill people: fried meat from diseased cows causes heart disease, and infections and the stimulants in coffee spark heart arrhythmias. And there is no outcry!

YOU ARE WHAT YOU EAT

Most Americans have been conditioned not to fear what they eat, drink, and, for the most part, smoke, providing they do these things in moderation. I believe that over the past fifty years this conditioning process has been implemented by special interest groups that promote unhealthy products. At this stage, how can they now tell you that they were wrong; that what they've been saying about your basic four food groups is actually causing disease: that coffee, the "best part of waking up," could be promoting heart disease; that alcohol, which allows you to feel good and socialize, is leading to liver disease? Now we're caught between a rock and a hard place.

These special interest groups have been so successful and effective in exploiting people's ignorance, laziness, or indifference about their health that now we have a whole nation without the tools to change its lifestyle. To offer a sick person a proven way to change his whole life is completely ineffective when he is of the mind-set that all he needs is a pill. For many people, the idea that an aggressive and well-reasoned cleansing and rebuilding program could change their lives is just not on their radar screen of possibilities.

GIVE THE BODY THE RIGHT BUILDING BLOCKS

When the people in our study groups began to redress all the factors that could cause illness—cellular imbalance, inflammatory processes, hormonal imbalances, nutrient deficiencies—and when they eliminated these problems with our program, all their conditions improved. Then, by including various nutrients and healthy fruits and juices, they saw even greater improvement. In fact, they overcame all forms of illnesses. And this healing process began even without special supplementation and without individualized protocols. The programs are all based on cleansing and rebalancing through elimination, inclusion, and rejuvenation.

THE POWER AGING APPROACH

The studies discussed above are the reason I can offer you the Power Aging approach. It's based on our very successful, original protocols. It's a gradual process that may take between one to two years to produce maximum benefits, but day by day you will be able to see improvements. No two people have the same level of cell damage, pro-

grammed cell death, body toxicity, or heavy metal pollution. But I believe we can substantially expand our life spans, improve our quality
of life and eliminate a lot of illnesses because we're changing the mi-
lieu within which these illnesses manifest. Remember, many others
have done this program before you—indeed, you can read their stories in Chapter 13—and proven that it's possible to become a new
person!

GETTING THE GIST OF ORGANIC JUICING

In the Power Aging program you will begin by cleansing and detoxifying. I make the assumption that most people don't know what's
toxic and have never really experienced a real cleanse. So you begin
with the idea that you must eliminate everything from your system that
harbors pollutants. That's why I spent so much time telling you about
the chemicals and toxins in the environment, so you could understand what you have to avoid and why. And that's why we begin with
juicing. Fresh, organic juices are pure and unadulterated. They give
the body readily absorbable, easily digested nutrients, which become
the building blocks and cofactors for all the metabolic processes in the
body. We also know that juices contain hundreds of phytochemicals
(plant-based chemicals) that have an antiviral, antibacterial, and im-
mune-boosting impact. They carry a full spectrum of nutrients that
gradually heal on very subtle levels. And, the more variety of vegetables and fruits you use in juicing the better results you will have.

Imbibing the Juice

In the first four to eight weeks of your new detoxification and cleansing program I suggest that you drink one 10 oz glass of juice a day,
preferably diluted green juices. By diluted I mean that you should
have about 4 oz of dark or light green vegetables in 6 or 8 oz of water,
or one tablespoon of a green concentrate powder in 12 oz of water.
Also add 1 oz of aloe vera concentrate to help digest the mixture. In

this way your body begins to slowly acclimate to concentrated juice intake.

I remember the first time I took a 1 oz glass of wheat grass juice, I had a spinning sensation in my head. So the next time I tried it I put the 1 oz of wheat grass in 12 oz of water, drank it slowly, and had no problem as it gave my body a nice chlorophyll and phytonutrient boost. Eventually I was able to take a straight 1 oz glass of wheat grass juice. But it's a gradual process; normal American impatience can be a danger. So let me warn you. Do not jump ahead of the protocol. You can do yourself harm. Be patient. It has taken you decades to get as sick and toxic as you are, so, allow yourself some time to detoxify. The program I'm suggesting is designed to enhance your well-being and to make sure you don't suffer in the initial stages of the process.

You should try to get a juice extractor to make your juices fresh. If that is not possible, then visit a health food store that has a juice bar and get them to make your juice drinks. In six months you will be drinking almost a gallon of juice per day. As you can see the juices are a crucial part of the Power Aging protocol. At first you need to take the juices in small quantities by sipping gradually over a period of perhaps an hour. For some people juices are an acquired taste because they are not used to the taste of real concentrated vegetables. So you may have to take your time and add in vegetables slowly, or put a little apple in your juices to improve the taste.

The more chlorophyll you can get into your body over a period of time, the better, because it slowly chelates toxic heavy metals out of the body; it has strong antiviral and antibacterial activity; gives good-quality oxygenation to the cell; and is a great blood cleanser and rejuvenator. But you must start slowly and gradually and steadily increase the amount you drink.

For people who are not hypoglycemic or diabetic, or who know that their blood sugar is normal, you could also add some red and blue fruits. The best ones to begin with are the berries—raspberries, cherries, strawberries, blueberries, and blackberries. Berries are rich in the types of phytochemicals that help rebalance your lipid profile and your hormone levels. They also have a rejuvenating effect as they help repair damage to our DNA and enhance enzyme activity. The powerful living energy of these fruits, which are low in calories, is extremely beneficial to the body.

It is my experience that a high-quality juicing program with a great variety of vegetables and fruits, taken gradually from smaller to larger amounts over a period of time, is the best single thing we can do to cleanse and rejuvenate. These juices are cleansing the system, cleansing the blood, lowering the viral and bacterial levels, energizing the cells, naturally chelating toxins out, and purifying the blood. In effect, they are one of the best natural, single tonics available. I've had more positive feedback from individuals who've said they've been helped and felt much better when they added juices to their program and did nothing else—no extra vitamins, minerals, or herbs. Just doing the juices has made a tremendous difference.

How to Begin

I realize not everyone has the fortitude or the desire to make radical changes all at once. Instead I want you to realize that you are under going a gradual process. You should say to yourself: "Over the next twelve months of my life I will go from having no fresh organic juices in my diet to having up to six glasses per day." Accordingly, you will start with one glass per day for the first two months, then two glasses per day for the next two months, three glasses per day for the following two months, and then four glasses up to six. By the end of the year you'll be having six glasses a day. It is also possible to supplement your juices with power-foods that you add to your juice. The most important ones are garlic, sesame seeds, cayenne pepper, ginger, lemon, lime, grapefruit skin and seed, and flax seeds and flaxseed oil. Garlic is the single most important cleansing, detoxifying, and blood-purifying herb that we have. A pinch of cayenne pepper in your juice can help soothe the stomach and prevent ulcers and ginger can help upset stomachs.

HOW TO EAT RIGHT WITHOUT DIETING

You will never have to "diet" again once you learn about the Power Aging diet. As you develop these good eating habits you'll learn what to substitute, what to avoid, and what to add to your diet to make every meal healthy and energizing. The Power Aging diet will stay with you for a lifetime because it's not so much a diet as a way of life. The first rule is to be sure to *read labels* so that you can avoid dyes, additives, partially hydrogenated oils, hidden sugars, binders, fillers, preservatives and a host of chemicals that do nothing to keep your body healthy but just maintain shelf life for packed and processed food.

What to Substitute

Rather than red meats, consume fish. Instead of hamburgers and hot dogs, have soy-based alternatives. Instead of egg substitutes, there is Tofu Scrambler, a flavored tofu mixture, which is much better for you than Eggbeaters. Instead of high fat dairy products, consume low fat or nonfat dairy products or switch to soy, rice, or almond milk and cheese substitutes. Rather than butter and lard and other saturated fats, use various types of vegetable oils. Instead of ice cream, cakes, pies, cookies, use fruit. Instead of refined cereals and processed carbohydrates, use whole grains and millet bread, spelt bread, or rice bread. Instead of fried foods and fatty snack foods laced with chemicals, have fresh salads and vegetables and other types of healthy snacks that are readily available in any health food store. Instead of salt and salty foods, use low sodium or no sodium foods and/or use spices to flavor foods. Instead of coffee and soft drinks, have herbal teas and diluted fresh fruit and vegetable juices. If you need to remind yourself why you are giving up these dangerous, artificial foods, reread Chapter 2 where I talk about the harmful effects of chemical additives, food irradiation, and genetically engineered food.

Substitutes for Animal Protein

We avoid animal protein including beef, poultry, and shellfish because they are loaded with artificial hormones, antibiotics, and toxic pollution at the bottom of coastal waters. Replace these toxic protein sources with cold-water fish, such as salmon, trout, mackerel, sardines, cod, and sea bass, four to six times a week. Avoid farm-raised fish, which are grown in crowded conditions with chemicals and antibiotics to control their growth and with dyes to render their flesh "salmon-colored." Add nuts and seeds, which are vegetarian sources of protein. They include almonds, walnuts, sunflower seeds, pumpkin seeds, chia seeds, and sesame seeds. Nut butters are also highly concentrated protein sources. Don't forget soybeans and soy products, and little-known grains like quinoa, amaranth, spelt, and teff. Beans are also an excellent source of protein: There are over seventy varieties of bean commonly available, including black-eyed peas, navy beans, adzuki beans, lentils, split peas, lima beans, and turtle beans.

Substitutes for Dairy

Avoid dairy, including milk, yogurt, cheese, butter, ice cream, and cream sauces. Replace these products with rice milk, soy milk, almond milk, or oat milk. Eat nothing with casein (a protein found in the milk of all mammals) in the ingredients.

Substitutes for Caffeine and Alcohol

Do not take caffeine products or drink alcohol in any amount, including chocolate, coffee, tea, wines, hard liquor, etc. Replace them with decaffeinated herbal teas, grain beverages such as Postum, Caffix, Raj's lemon water, or green tea (which has small amounts of caffeine but it also has threonine, which neutralizes caffeine and has a very beneficial calming effect).

Substitutes for Sugars and Artificial Sweeteners

Avoid all sugars or artificial sweeteners. Replace them with stevia leaf, raw unfiltered honey, molasses, brown rice syrup, or natural food sweeteners.

Substitutes for Carbonated Beverages

On this protocol I don't allow carbonated beverages, including sodas or seltzer. Replace them with spring water, distilled water, filtered water, or fresh-squeezed organic juices.

Substitutes for Wheat

Stay away from processed bread or wheat products. Replace them with spelt bread, millet bread, kamut bread, sprouted whole grain breads, rice bread, or Essene bread.

What to Avoid

1. Avoid all nonorganic produce. Replace with certified organic produce. And this applies to all vegetables, fruits, beans, grains, legumes, nuts, seeds, and potatoes.
2. Avoid deep-fried or processed foods. Replace with sautéed, steamed, stir-fried, or broiled meals cooked at lower temperatures. The oils for cooking are coconut, macadamia, and safflower oils; for baking, hazelnut and macadamia; for salads, walnut, flaxseed, and extra virgin cold-pressed olive oil. (If cooking with olive oil, use it at the end of the cooking process, not at the beginning.)
3. Avoid all food additives, preservatives, coloring agents, flavorings, and MSG.
4. Avoid margarine and other foods containing trans-fatty acids, particularly partially hydrogenated oils. They

interfere with very important nutrients in the diet, the most important of which are the essential fatty acids.

Fiber Is Detoxifying

When you go on a Power Aging protocol, healthy fibers are gradually introduced into the diet in the form of whole grains, legumes, and the fruit fibers in berries. These are excellent for stimulating intestinal peristalsis, a wavelike rhythmic movement, to get food to go through your system faster, which will facilitate better and more complete digestion and elimination.

Basic Rules for Eating

1. Eat primarily during the day.
2. Try to have your largest meal between one and three in the afternoon; eat a very light breakfast and a light dinner.
3. Make sure to drink enough fluids throughout the day.

The right amount of fluid intake is very important for the body. Otherwise, we upset our electrolyte balance, our lymphatic balance, and our ability to cleanse and eliminate. Most people should drink a minimum of a gallon of water per day including purified water or juices, plus one or two cups of green tea, lemon juice to help alkalize the body, and digestive enzymes to help with the tea. But if you're sweating profusely or exercising vigorously, you may need more fluids.

More about Meat

If what I said about of meat contamination in Chapter 3 hasn't yet turned you away from flesh food, let me give you some facts about animal protein diet versus a vegetarian diet. Most people are under the impression that you must eat animal protein in order to sustain life. This is a myth perpetrated by the meat industry. In point of fact, my own original work with Dr. Hillard Fitsky at the Institute of Applied Biology and Dr. Victor Berman in 1984 showed that virtually all foods contain all eight essential amino acids. However, we have been led to believe that only animal foods contain these amino acids. As a result, we have relegated vegetables, grains, nuts, seeds, fruits, and herbs to an insignificant accompaniment, or garnish, to a meat-based or animal protein-based diet. We owe this misconception about animal protein to good propaganda and beautiful marketing on the part of the meat industry.

You must, however, be sure that you are getting high-quality amino acids from high-quality sources. You need 9/10 gram of protein per kilogram of body weight, which is approximately 60 grams per day for women and 80 grams per day for men. During pregnancy, lactation, recovery from various illnesses, surgery, and infection, you will require more. You need 40 to 50 grams of high-quality fiber per day from a variety of grains, legumes, nuts, seeds, millet, buckwheat, brown rice, spelt, rye, quinoa, oats, vegetables and fruits including yams, potatoes, sweet potatoes, gourds, squashes, and preferably five servings of cruciferous vegetables per day such as broccoli, cabbage, cauliflower, onions, asparagus, and mustard sprouts. During times that require extra protein you can add fatty deepwater fish, cod, tuna, sole, mackerel, grouper, salmon, or sardines.

Break Out of Your Breakfast Rut

When did bagels and coffee become the unofficial American breakfast? In Chapter 10, Chef Marcus Guiliano will guide you in an eating plan and give you wonderful and delicious options to start your day. Whether it's a smoothie, or a green drink, or a plate of scrambled eggs or scrambled tofu and spinach, breakfast should be fun and should be different every day of the week.

Let's Do Lunch—the Right Way!

Lunch should be the biggest meal of the day. Then you have the rest of the day to digest and utilize the energy from your meal. Otherwise unused calories will be stored in fat cells. If you eat fish, this is the time to do it. See Chapter 10 for recipes that are easy to prepare and incredibly tasty.

Your Diminishing Dinner

Dinner should be lighter than lunch. It should definitely be a vegetarian meal because vegetables and grains are digested much faster than fish or animal protein. Eat no later than 7 P.M. If you eat a heavy meal late at night, your body is focused on digestion rather than repair and regeneration. You'll find you'll sleep better if you eat early too. Again, in Chapter 9 you'll learn how to get the best out of your grains and vegetable meal using spices and herbs galore.

Snack Power

Snacks are foods that have become increasingly unhealthy. For the most part they are synthetic foods that have no nutritional value whatsoever. They are in fact very detrimental. They are loaded with trans-fatty acids, saturated fats, sugar, and dozens of food additives, dyes, preservatives, and chemicals to tempt and maybe addict us to their taste! It's a nutritional disaster. You can find and make plenty of snacks to keep you away from these horrific temptations.

Chapter 10 gives you a variety of snack choices and recipes made from fresh vegetables, fresh fruits, dried fruits, nuts, and seeds. It's good to keep healthy snacks on hand and in your bag so you don't get tempted with something unhealthy when you're away from home.

Low Calorie Diets

What we've been talking about in our Non-Diet Diet adds up to a lot less calories but without the bother of weighing every bite you eat. A mostly organic, vegetarian diet that avoids processed carbohydrates will very often be naturally low in calories. And that's exactly what you need as you age—fewer calories. A teenager or a pregnant woman needs a lot more calories that an older adult, and if you continue to eat like a teenager, then that extra food is going to show up as bulges and excess weight that is detrimental to your health. Let's look at the science behind low calorie diets.

It only took four weeks to find some answers about the low calorie approach in a group of aging mice. The genes of these elderly mice were showing the effects of aging, which was reversed in four weeks on a low calorie diet. In the *Washington Post* Dr. Stephen Spindler, who ran the study and is a professor of biochemistry at the University of California at Riverside, says "My work shows that calorie restriction not only prevents [age-related] changes in gene activity, but very quickly reverses the majority of the changes that take place with age."[1] The study made use of new technology that allows a "vast number of genes to be looked at" simultaneously.

To date, the only treatment that extends the life of mammals is "severe" caloric restriction, but there are really no studies to show effectiveness in humans. Of great interest to Power Agers is that Dr. Spindler's group were able to identify twenty genes that seemed to become more active with age. Further scrutiny showed that several of these genes were associated with inflammation, which itself is related to chronic pain syndromes, heart disease, autoimmune diseases, and chronic illness. In almost three quarters of the genes, calorie restriction completely or partially prevented the age-related changes. Another twenty-six genes had their activity curtailed over time and another large group of genes was responsible for detoxifying the body against drugs and chemicals. Long-term calorie restriction partially reversed the age-related changes in about half of these genes. Even though Dr. Spindler was very clear in his interview with the *Washing-*

ton Post that it would take years to create drug therapies to target these genes, we have the proof we need right now to decrease our caloric intake and receive healthy benefits. And we also know that drugs or genetic manipulation is not the answer.

Lane and colleagues at the National Institute on Aging studied caloric restriction and aging first in non-primates. Their extensive review of the literature showed seventy years of research proving that a 30 percent to 40 percent reduction in caloric intake leads to a significant life extension in a variety of short-lived species. They also said that since the late 1980s studies in longer-lived species, such as rhesus and squirrel monkeys, have been undertaken, which suggest that the effect of caloric restriction on aging is universal across species. Results in other caloric restriction studies indicate prevention or delay of onset of age-related diseases such as cardiovascular disease, diabetes, and perhaps cancer.[2]

THE IMPORTANCE OF EXERCISE

Remember Harry Biele, the ninety-year-old marathon runner? When he began the antiaging protocol he also began to exercise regularly. He took to it like a fish to water and became an incredible example for the older generation. Now, you certainly don't have to become a marathon runner in order to stay young. We all know that as a society we are not exercising nearly enough. Most people say they just don't have time for it. But we can show you studies that say even a few minutes of exercise a day can improve your health. So, that's where you begin, with a few minutes of exercise a day.

It's something that seems so basic but we constantly have to be reminded that sitting on a couch in front of your TV or sitting in front of your computer is not exercise! Astronauts in weightless flight develop osteoporosis and muscle wasting. These surprising findings made us realize that we depend on gravity pulling on our bones to keep them strong. Add a little regular exercise and you can prevent protein wasting away from your muscles and you can stop osteoporosis in its tracks.

A series of studies on exercise in a very ill population proved the benefits of physical activity. A group of researchers in a 2003 paper found from reviewing prior studies that both aerobic exercise training and resistance exercise (weight training) will increase protein mass. They concluded that "in general, patients with wasting conditions who can and will comply with a proper exercise program gain muscle protein mass, strength and endurance, and, in some cases, are more capable of performing the activities of daily living."[3] This is great news for people who imagine that it's too late to try exercise.

Let's look at chronic obstructive pulmonary disease (COPD). It's said to be incurable but, in fact, with the help of exercise, researchers are finding out that patients can suffer from far fewer symptoms. Schols wrote in the *International Journal of Cardiology* that while studying weight loss in COPD he was surprised to find that dietary intervention, oral nutritional supplements, and exercise resulted in less morbidity and mortality.[4] This is no surprise to people who understand the power of good nutrition. For us Power Agers, this study just reinforces what is possible.

Reviewing the following series of studies on COPD and exercise, I noticed that researchers spent a lot of effort trying to decide what is the best exercise for improving lung function. To my mind the money would be better spent actually setting up exercise programs, enrolling people in walking clubs, having simple stretching exercise programs on TV, even at prime time! The possibilities are endless. If only allopathic medicine would get into the business of health and not the business of disease, they could use the tremendous amount of research that has been done on aging and exercise, diet, and supplementation and take action!

Sadly, that was not the case: hundreds of thousands of dollars went into the next group of studies trying to define exactly what exercise people should do! Chavannes and colleagues spent their funding reviewing the effects of physical activity in mild to moderate COPD. They found that physical exercise can improve a patient's fitness.[5] Wright and colleagues tried to determine the best form of exercise for patients with chronic obstructive pulmonary disease. They found that short-term high-intensity strength training may improve pulmonary function in COPD and may be the preferred method.[6] Vogiatzis and a group of researchers suggested interval training as an alternative to continuous exercise in COPD patients. They concluded that interval training does produce substantial training effects that are similar in magnitude to those produced by continuous training at half the exercise intensity but double the exercise time.[7] Another team of researchers found that both resistance training (weight training) and endurance training have similar effects on "peripheral muscle force, exercise capacity and health-related quality of life in chronic obstructive pulmonary disease patients with peripheral muscle weakness."[8] And on it goes, the research juggernaut with no correlation to the real world and no thought of implementing on a grander scale what their research finds.

How Long Should I Exercise?

As for the amount of time you need to exercise to start getting benefits, a report in the March 2001 *Journal of the American Medical Association* effectively counters people's argument that they don't have time to exercise. The report says a nine-minute-a-day walk cuts women's heart disease risk by half. The study done by Harvard epidemiologists followed forty thousand women for five years. They found that minimal exercise had an impact on health; even walking one hour a week reduced the risk of heart disease. Even women who smoked, were obese, and had high cholesterol benefited from this low level of exercise. And it wasn't the speed of the walking that mattered, it was just the time doing it. So you can start out slowly, gradually build up your endurance, and then work up to thirty to sixty minutes of exercise every day. Just think what the gain in health benefits would be if you quadrupled the study's exercise time.[9] In Chapter 11 I talk about the Wellness Model and I advise people to strive for forty-five minutes of exercise every day as the optimum amount for improving metabolism, keeping limber, and keeping muscles toned.

CONCLUSION

It's up to you now. I recommend that you study the Non-Diet Diet, No-Exercise Exercise Program, set your goal for a year or two down the road to be healthy and happy, and slowly implement the program. Take one small step today toward health. You won't regret it, because the health benefits begin almost immediately.

RECIPES FOR POWER AGING

Jump-start Your Detox

To help you put the dietary advice of the previous chapter into practice and to jump-start your detox, Chef Marcus Guiliano and I offer the following seven-day plan. These recipes are founded on good, simple, clean, and fresh food. Some recipes are more involved than others, so start out at your own level. Whatever recipe you are trying, read and re-read it. Visualizing the procedures makes the process easier.

All of these recipes have been formulated without refined sugars, refined flours, processed foods, or dairy products. They include a wide variety of ingredients that one could obtain from a good-quality health food store. Always choose organic ingredients over conventional ones when that is an option. Try to buy produce that is in season and grown locally. A great way to do this is shop at your local farmers' market. When choosing seafood, make sure there is no odor and buy from a reputable seller.

Although we've given you seven days' worth of food, you need not follow the recipes in the precise order they appear. So long as you use the guidelines laid out in Chapter 9, you can make your own substitutions. You'll see that we've included only one juice recipe per day:

this is appropriate for people just embarking on the Power Aging plan, but if you're already well on your way, you can feel free to add juices as recommended. On some days you will notice that I don't include a breakfast suggestion. In those cases, you may choose to simply have a breakfast juice with protein powder.

Finally, some of the ingredients and flavors in these dishes may be new to you, which I hope will add to the adventure of cooking and mealtimes. Most important, we've selected these with delicious taste in mind—so enjoy!

SEVEN-DAY JUMP-START YOUR DETOX PLAN

Day One

Breakfast Juice: Pecan Shake
1 scoop of protein powder (optional)
Breakfast: Sprout Toast with Spirulina and Sunflower Honey
Lunch: Trout with Almonds and Parsley
Tropical Fruit Gazpacho
Dinner: Zucchini with Mint and Cumin
Mango Jello
After Dinner Juice: Apple Grape Sprout Juice

Day Two

Breakfast Juice: Peanut Butter Banana Shake
1 scoop of protein powder (optional)
Breakfast: Soy and Sunflower Pancakes
Lunch: Braised Red Cabbage with Tofu and Dried Bing Cherries
Alaskan Halibut with Black-Eyed-Pea Salsa
Bananas Foster Style over Rice Dream
Dinner: Jicama and Orange Salad
After Dinner Juice: Celery Apple Carrot Juice

Day Three

Breakfast Juice: Honeydew Melon Shake
1 scoop protein powder (optional)
Breakfast: Barley Cereal with Apples
Lunch: Wild Salmon with Snow Peas and Ginger
Braised Celery
Soy Yogurt and Butternut Parfait
Dinner: Celery Root and Lentil Soup
After Dinner Juice: Grandma's Mixed Vegetable Juice
1 scoop of protein powder (optional)

Day Four

Breakfast Juice: Date and Almond Smoothie
1 scoop of protein powder (optional)
Lunch: Hummus on Endive
Tilapia with Seaweed Vinaigrette
Vanilla Soy Pudding
Dinner: Roasted Tomato Soup
After Dinner Juice: Cauliflower, Celery, Carrot, Beet Juice

Day Five

Breakfast Juice: Chocolate Walnut Shake
1 scoop protein powder (optional)
Lunch: Mushrooms with Turmeric and Brown Basmati Rice
Pineapple Aloe Vera Jello
Dinner: Butternut Squash and Coconut Soup
After Dinner Juice: Iced Cinnamon and Spice Tea

Day Six

Breakfast Juice: Apple Strawberry Shake
1 scoop protein powder (optional)

Lunch: Pickled Asparagus with Jalapenos
Yukon Potato and Tempeh Stew
Dinner: Beet and Romaine Lettuce Salad
After Dinner Juice: 1 green mixed vegetable juice

Day Seven

Breakfast Juice: Very Nutty Shake
1 scoop of protein powder (optional)
Lunch: Cream of Salmon and Corn Soup
Dinner: Pear and Pine Nut Salad
Wakame and Soba Noodles
Roasted Onions with Aloe Vera and Rosemary
After Dinner Juice: Lemon Apple Juice

RECIPES FOR POWER AGING

Beverages/Juices

Pecan Shake
Peanut Butter Banana Shake
Very Nutty Shake
Iced Cinnamon and Spice Tea
Date and Almond Smoothie
Apple Strawberry Shake
Cauliflower Celery Carrot Beet Juice
Honeydew Melon Shake
Apple Grape Sprout Juice
Celery Apple Carrot Juice
Lemon Apple Juice
Lemon Apple Cucumber Juice
Grandma's Mixed Vegetable Juice
Chocolate Walnut Shake

Breakfasts

Sprout Toast with Spirulina and Sunflower Honey
Soy and Sunflower Pancakes
Barley Cereal with Apples

Appetizers/Snacks/Miscellaneous

Hummus on Endive
Roasted Portobello Mushrooms
Pickled Asparagus with Jalapenos
Brown Rice and Broccoli with Apricot Curry Sauce
Wakame and Soba Noodles

Salads

Sprouted Quinoa, Celery Root, and Carrot Salad
Beet and Romaine Lettuce Salad
Pear and Pine Nut Salad
Yucca Salad
Jicama and Orange Salad
Carrot and Currant Salad
Potato and Pea Salad
Sprout Bread and Tomato Salad
Sprouted Wheat Berries with Honey Mustard

Soups

Celery Root and Lentil Soup
Roasted Tomato Soup
Cream of Salmon and Corn Soup
Tropical Fruit Gazpacho
Butternut Squash and Coconut Soup
Apple and Curry Soup

Vegetables and Main Dishes

Braised Red Cabbage with Tofu and Dried Bing Cherries
Zucchini with Mint and Cumin
Mushrooms with Turmeric and Brown Basmati Rice
Spaghetti Squash with Tarragon
Fennel with Mustard
Roasted Onions with Aloe Vera and Rosemary
Braised Celery
Yukon Potato and Tempeh Stew

Fish

Tilapia with Seaweed Vinaigrette
Trout with Almonds and Parsley
Alaskan Halibut with Black-Eyed-Pea Salsa
Wild Salmon with Snow Peas and Ginger

Desserts

Bananas Foster Style over Rice Dream
Soy Yogurt and Butternut Parfait
Mango Jello
Pineapple Aloe Vera Jello
Vanilla Soy Pudding

Condiments

Honey Mustard Mayonnaise and Dressing
Curry Apricot Sauce
Wakame Vinaigrette
Turmeric Vinaigrette
Mint-Cumin Vinaigrette
Aloe Vera Vinaigrette
Simple Vinaigrette #7
Roasted Tomato Salsa

Many recipes can be made in advance, up to a day ahead of time. When cooking grains always cook extra; you can use the leftovers for salad, hot cereal, or other applications. Always take care in cooking your food and never forget the role of good nutrition.

BEVERAGES

PECAN SHAKE

¼ cup raw pecans, soaked overnight in water
1 each banana
1 ½ cups soy or rice milk
⅛ tsp ground cinnamon
2 T nondairy acidophilus
1 T flax oil
1 tsp green chlorophyll powder
1 serving vegetarian protein powder

Blend pecans, banana, soy/rice milk, cinnamon, acidophilus, and flax oil until smooth. While blender is on low, add green chlorophyll powder and protein powder.

PEANUT BUTTER BANANA SHAKE

1 ½ cups soy or rice milk
1 each banana (works well frozen)
2 T natural peanut butter
⅛ tsp ground cinnamon
1 T flax oil
2 T nondairy acidophilus
1 serving vegetarian protein powder

Blend soy/rice milk, banana, peanut butter, cinnamon, flax oil and acidophilus. While blender is on low add protein powder.

VERY NUTTY SHAKE

3 apples (¾ cup juice)
½ banana, mashed
2 T ground or whole—unsalted peanuts or peanut butter
¼ cup plus 2 T plain soy yogurt
1 T light colored honey
1 T pure unsweetened cocoa powder
½ tsp pure vanilla extract

Juice the apples. Set aside ¾ cup of the juice. In a blender or food processor, combine the juice with remaining ingredients until smooth.

ICED CINNAMON AND SPICE TEA

2 apples (½ cup juice)
1 orange (3 T juice)
1 Bengal Spice Tea Bag
1 cup boiling water
¼ tsp ground cinnamon
1 cup ice

Separately juice the apples and the orange. Steep the tea bag in boiling water for 4–6 minutes. Discard tea bag and set aside tea. In a blender or food processor, combine the juices with the cinnamon, tea and ice, and blend until smooth.

DATE AND ALMOND SMOOTHIE

¼ cup raw almonds, soaked overnight in water
2 large Medjol Dates, pitted and soaked overnight in water
1 each banana
1 ½ cups soy or rice milk
⅛ tsp ground cinnamon
2 T nondairy acidophilus
1 T flax oil
1 serving vegetarian protein powder

Blend almonds, dates, banana, soy/rice milk, cinnamon, acidophilus, and flax oil until smooth. While blender is on low add protein powder.

APPLE STRAWBERRY SHAKE

2 apples (½ cup juice)
1 banana (mashed)
3 T ground or whole—unsalted pecans or pecan butter
¼ cup fresh or frozen strawberries
½ cup unsweetened soy milk
¼ tsp pure lemon extract
½ cup ice

Juice the apples. In a blender or food processor, combine the juice with the remaining ingredients and blend until smooth.

CAULIFLOWER CELERY BEET CARROT JUICE

3 stalks celery (1 ¾ cup juice)
2 carrots (½ cup juice)
¼ head cauliflower, steamed and chilled
1 beet (¼ cup beet juice)
1 small ginger root (1 tsp juice)

Separately juice the celery, carrots, cauliflower, beet, and ginger. Combine the juices and blend immediately.

HONEYDEW MELON SHAKE

2 cups peeled honeydew melon chunks (⅔ cup juice)
1 banana, mashed
1 T unsweetened flaked coconut
2 T ground or whole—unsalted almonds or almond butter
1 T chopped dates
½ cup unsweetened soy milk
½ tsp pure almond extract
¾ cup ice

Juice the melon to create ⅔ cup juice. In a blender or food processor combine the juice with the remaining ingredients and blend until smooth.

APPLE GRAPE SPROUT JUICE

1 cup seedless red grapes
6 apples
4 carrots
1/2 cup sunflower or alfalfa sprouts

Separately juice the grapes, apples, carrots, and sprouts. Combine the juices and serve immediately.

CELERY APPLE CARROT JUICE

4 stalks celery
4 apples
4 carrots

Separately juice the celery, apples, and carrots. Combine the juices and serve immediately.

LEMON APPLE CUCUMBER JUICE

2 cucumbers
2 apples
1 yellow squash
1/2 zucchini
1 1/2 green bell peppers
1 tsp pure lemon extract
1 cup ice

Separately juice the cucumbers, apples, yellow squash, zucchini, and green peppers. In a blender or food processor, combine the juices with the lemon extract and ice. Blend until smooth.

GRANDMA'S MIXED VEGETABLE JUICE

2 apples
2 pears
2 carrots
1 cucumber
1 beet
1 small bunch Swiss chard
1 red bell pepper
1 small piece ginger root

Separately juice the apples, pears, carrots, cucumber, beet, Swiss chard, red pepper, and ginger. Combine the juices and serve immediately.

CHOCOLATE WALNUT SHAKE

4 apples
2 bananas, mashed
4 T whole or ground unsalted walnuts or walnut butter
1 cup unsweetened soy milk
1 ½ T pure unsweetened cocoa (or carob) powder
1 tsp pure almond extract
1 cup ice

Juice the apples. In a blender or food processor, combine the juice with the remaining ingredients, and blend until smooth.

BREAKFASTS

SPROUT TOAST WITH SPIRULINA AND
SUNFLOWER HONEY
(Serves 2)

This makes a great spread for a quick snack. Just toast some
sprout bread and use this as a spread. It is a good replacement for
the traditional toast and jelly for breakfast.

2 tsp tahini
2 T sunflower seeds
1 tsp powered spirulina
½ cup raw honey
2 pieces toasted sprout bread or bagel

Mix tahini, sunflower seeds, powered spirulina, and raw honey in
a bowl. Spread on toast and enjoy.

Chef's notes: This will hold for a month or more in the
refrigerator. Peanut butter can replace the tahini if you prefer.

SOY AND SUNFLOWER PANCAKES
(Serves 2)

½ cup soy flour
½ cup whole meal spelt flour
1 tsp baking powder
1 tsp baking soda
½ cup oats, pulsed in food processor to form a coarse meal
¼ cup sunflower seeds
2 T maple syrup
1 ¼ cup soy milk
2 T canola oil
1 Energy Egg Replacer

Mix flours, baking powder, and baking soda, and then sift. Add oats, sunflower seeds, maple syrup, soy milk, canola oil, and one powdered egg. Cook over medium heat in a nonstick pan.

APPETIZERS/SNACKS/MISCELLANEOUS

HUMMUS ON ENDIVE
(Serves 4)

2 cups garbanzo beans, cooked
4 lemons, juiced
1 T tahini
2 cloves garlic
½ cup olive oil
2 T cilantro, lightly chopped
1 tsp ground cumin
2 heads Belgium endive

In a food processor puree beans, lemon juice, tahini, garlic and olive oil. When the mixture is smooth add cilantro and cumin. Puree one last time to incorporate the ingredients. Cut one inch from the core of the endive and peel away the leaves. Spoon hummus onto the end of the endive. Serve as a snack or lunch with a salad.

ROASTED PORTOBELLO MUSHROOMS
(Serves 2)

2 Portobello mushrooms, stems and gills removed and
*   washed*
½ cup Simple Vinaigrette #7 (see page 279)
1 T fresh basil, chopped
1 T fresh rosemary, chopped
black pepper to taste

Steam mushrooms lightly for 3–5 minutes, then marinate them in vinaigrette, basil, rosemary and black pepper for two hours. Roast mushrooms in vinaigrette at 350° until they begin to brown, about 20 minutes. Serve alone or on sprout bread, with hummus or a salad.

PICKLED ASPARAGUS WITH JALAPENOS
(Serves 2)

2 cups water
1 cup raw unfiltered apple cider vinegar
½ cup succanat (whole, raw brown sugar)
1 sprig thyme
2 bay leaves
12 black peppercorns
2 jalapenos, split (optional)
1 lb asparagus

Bring water, vinegar, succanat, thyme, bay leaves, peppercorns, and jalapenos to a boil. Add asparagus and simmer for 30 seconds. Let asparagus cool in marinade. Serve cold.

BROWN RICE AND BROCCOLI WITH APRICOT CURRY SAUCE
(Serves 4)

3 cups vegetable stock
1 cup brown rice
½ head broccoli, washed, lightly steamed and chilled
½ cup Curry Apricot Sauce (see page 277)

In a small saucepot with lid bring stock to simmer. Stir in rice and reduce to a simmer. Place lid on pot and cook for one hour or according to package directions. When rice is cooked, let cool. Combine broccoli, rice and curry sauce.

Chef's notes: This is good served hot or cold. This salad will hold for at least three days in the refrigerator.

WAKAME AND SOBA NOODLES
(Serves 2)

$\frac{1}{2}$ *cup Wakame Vinaigrette* (*see page 277*)
$\frac{1}{2}$ *lb buckwheat noodles, cooked according to package directions and chilled*
3 green onions, thinly sliced
1 small cucumber, $\frac{1}{2}$ inch diced
1 medium carrot, shredded

Toss all ingredients and serve together.

SALADS

SPROUTED QUINOA, CELERY ROOT, AND CARROT SALAD
(Serves 2)

¼ cup organic quinoa, sprouted (takes one full day to pre-
  pare; see note below)
¼ cup celery root, shredded
¼ cup carrots, shredded
1 T pine nuts
1 T pumpkin seeds, raw
2 T apple cider vinegar
4 T canola oil
2 T pumpkin oil

Toss all ingredients and serve, or let marinate for up to 8 hours.

To make quinoa sprouts: Wash and rinse quinoa and soak in
purified water for two hours. Drain very well and let sit out on plate
for 8 to 16 hours. The quinoa will get little tails, which means they
have sprouted. You can place in the refrigerator for up to three days.
Wash and rinse every day with purified water to keep them fresh.

BEET AND ROMAINE LETTUCE SALAD
(Serves 2)

½ medium beet, grated
2 T raw sunflower seeds
1 small red onion, sliced thinly
½ head romaine lettuce, chopped
¼ cup Honey Mustard Mayonnaise and Dressing (see page
  277)

Toss all ingredients and serve.

PEAR AND PINE NUT SALAD
(Serves 2)

2 medium ripe pears, ½ inch diced
½ cup raw pine nuts
¼ cup onions, ¼ inch diced
½ head romaine lettuce, washed and 1-inch chopped
½ cup Simple Vinaigrette #7 (see page 279)

Toss all ingredients and serve.

YUCCA SALAD
(Serves 4)

2 lbs yucca, cut into 3 to 4 inch pieces, peeled and quar-
    tered
⅔ cup Mint-Cumin Vinaigrette (see page 278)
1 T fresh cilantro, chopped lightly

Place yucca in a pot of cool water. Bring to a boil and lower to a simmer. Cook until tender, about 20 minutes. Drain and cool. Pull the hard stringlike core from the yucca. Slice into ½-inch slices. Toss with Mint-Cumin Vinaigrette and cilantro.

JICAMA AND ORANGE SALAD
(Serves 2)

1 cup jicama, ½ inch diced
2 oranges, peeled and sliced
1 T apple cider vinegar
1 T fresh basil, lightly chopped
1 T fresh cilantro, lightly chopped
2 T raw sunflower seeds
1 T sunflower oil
¼ tsp ground cumin

Mix all ingredients and let marinate at least one hour before eating.

CARROT AND CURRANT SALAD
(Serves 2)

3 cups carrots, shredded
⅓ cup dried currants
⅓ cup Simple Vinaigrette #7 (see page 279)
⅓ cup Nayonaise (vegan mayonnaise substitute)
2 T raw pumpkin seeds

Mix all ingredients together and refrigerate for four hours.

POTATO AND PEA SALAD
(Serves 2)

½ lb Yukon potatoes, boiled, cooled and halved
½ cup fresh or frozen peas, boiled quickly and cooled
1 T fresh Italian parsley, lightly chopped
1 tsp fresh thyme, chopped
1 tsp fresh chives, chopped
¼ cup Turmeric Vinaigrette (see page 278)

Mix all ingredients and serve.

SPROUT BREAD AND TOMATO SALAD
(Serves 2)

4 slices sprout sandwich bread, 1 inch diced
2 large tomatoes, 1 inch diced with juices saved
2 tsp balsamic vinegar
2 T fresh basil, chopped lightly
1 tsp fresh thyme, chopped
2 T extra virgin olive oil

Toast bread in the oven at 400° for 5 minutes. Mix all ingredients in a bowl and serve.

SPROUTED WHEAT BERRIES WITH HONEY MUSTARD
(Serves 2)

1 cup wheat berry sprouts or organic wheat berries
¼ cup onion, ¼ inch diced
1 small cucumber, ½ inch diced
1 medium tomato, ½ inch diced
⅓ cup Honey Mustard Mayonnaise (see page 277)

To make wheat berry sprouts: Wash wheat berries with purified water. Soak them in two cups of purified water for three hours. Drain them very well. Let them sit twenty-four hours and rinse them with purified water again. Repeat this step as many times as necessary. You want them to sprout little tails the size of the berry itself. At this point they are done. They will keep in the refrigerator up to one week, as long as they are rinsed every day and have air.

To make the salad: Toss all ingredients and serve.

SOUPS

CELERY ROOT AND LENTIL SOUP
(Serves 4)

½ cup lentils, washed and drained
1 cup celery root, ½ inch diced
6 cups vegetable stock
¼ cup onions, ¼ inch diced
¼ cup celery, ¼ inch diced
¼ cup carrots, ¼ inch diced
1 tsp fresh thyme,chopped
1 tsp fresh rosemary, chopped

Place all ingredients in a soup pot with a lid. Simmer until lentils are tender. Puree in a blender or leave chunky. Or you may blend half and leave half whole and mix them.

ROASTED TOMATO SOUP
(Serves 4)

2 lbs tomatoes, washed and stemmed
½ cup vegetable stock
¼ cup fresh basil leaves
2 T extra virgin olive oil
Celtic sea salt to taste

Roast tomatoes in oven for ½ hour at 400°. Let tomatoes cool for 15 minutes. Add them and vegetable stock to a blender and puree until smooth. Add basil, olive oil, and a pinch of Celtic sea salt and serve.

Chef's notes: Make this soup when you have good-quality tomatoes. Add ½ cup cooked and chilled brown rice for tomato rice soup. You could serve this as a sauce for fish or rice as well. The addition of chopped onions and cilantro would turn this into salsa.

CREAM OF SALMON AND CORN SOUP
(Serves 4)

½ cup onion, ¼ inch diced
1 tsp garlic, chopped
1 tsp safflower or canola oil
2 cups vegetable stock
6 oz wild salmon filets, poached and crumbled
2 ears fresh corn, cut kernels off ears
2 T arrowroot, dissolved in 2 T of water
1 cup soy milk
½ tsp fresh thyme, chopped
½ tsp fresh tarragon, chopped

In a soup pot heat oil on medium and cook onions and garlic until tender. Add vegetable stock, salmon, and corn. Simmer for 10 minutes. Stir in arrowroot while simmering and add soy milk, thyme, and tarragon.

Chef's notes: The addition of diced potatoes would go well with this soup. The potatoes would actually help thicken the soup; rice would work the same way.

TROPICAL FRUIT GAZPACHO
(Serves 2)

1 mango, peeled, 1/2 inch diced
1 star fruit, 1/2 inch diced
1 prickly pear cactus, peeled, 1/2 inch diced
1/2 cup pineapple, 1/2 inch diced
1/4 cup onion, 1/2 inch diced
1 T fresh cilantro, lightly chopped
1 T fresh basil, lightly chopped
2 T apple cider vinegar
apricot nectar as needed

Mix all ingredients and refrigerate for four hours. The apricot nectar is used to adjust the consistency of the gazpacho; add as much nectar to make the soup as you like.

BUTTERNUT SQUASH AND COCONUT SOUP
(Serves 4)

2 lbs butternut squash, peeled and diced
5 cups vegetable stock
1 can (14 oz) coconut milk

Place all ingredients in a soup pot and cook until squash is tender. In a blender, puree soup until smooth.

APPLE AND CURRY SOUP
(Serves 4)

3 medium apples, cored and diced
1 medium onion, ½ inch diced
1 T curry powder
2 cups vegetable stock
2 cups coconut milk

Mix apples, onions, and curry powder and bake in a 300° oven for 20 minutes. Bring stock and coconut milk to a simmer, add apple mixture, and cook for 5 minutes. Puree in a blender and serve.

VEGETABLES AND MAIN DISHES

BRAISED RED CABBAGE WITH TOFU AND
DRIED BING CHERRIES
(Serves 4)

This recipe makes a lot, but this dish makes a great leftover.
Actually, it is at its peak after a couple of days.

8 oz firm tofu, 1-inch cubes
1 medium onion, ½ inch diced
2 cloves garlic
1 small head red cabbage, ½ inch slices
2 apples, cored and 1 inch diced
2 cups vegetable stock
2 T apple cider vinegar
1 tsp caraway seeds
3 T fresh horseradish, shredded
1 sprig thyme
1 cinnamon stick
½ cup dried Bing cherries

Combine all ingredients in a casserole dish with lid. Bake at 350°
for one hour or until cabbage is tender.

ZUCCHINI WITH MINT AND CUMIN
(Serves 2)

2 medium zucchini, split and ½ inch sliced
½ medium onion, split and ¼ inch sliced
⅓ cup Mint-Cumin Vinaigrette (see page 278)

Cook zucchini and onions in a 325° oven for 15 minutes. While
the zucchini and onions are hot, toss them with the vinaigrette.
Serve hot or enjoy chilled later.

MUSHROOMS WITH TURMERIC AND BROWN BASMATI RICE
(Serves 2)

3 cups vegetable stock
1 cup basmati brown rice
8 oz mushrooms, washed and stems removed, ¼ inch sliced
½ cup Turmeric Vinaigrette (see page 278)
1 T fresh mint, lightly chopped

In a small saucepot with lid bring stock to a simmer. Stir in rice and reduce to a simmer. Place lid on pot and cook for one hour or according to package directions. When rice is cooked, stir in mushrooms and cover for 20 minutes. The heat from the rice will cook the mushrooms and add some of the natural mushroom juices to the rice. Toss the rice with the vinaigrette and mint and serve warm or chilled.

SPAGHETTI SQUASH WITH TARRAGON
(Serves 2)

1 spaghetti squash, split lengthwise
1 T raw honey
1 T fresh tarragon, lightly chopped
½ tsp black pepper, cracked coarsely

Steam squash with skin on. If you do not have a steamer you can bake it cut side down on a baking sheet with a layer of water. Cook squash until meat is tender. Scoop out meat with a fork—this will cause the meat to come out in strings. Put squash in a bowl and mix with honey, tarragon and black pepper and serve. This can be served hot or cold.

FENNEL WITH MUSTARD
(Serves 2)

2 heads fennel, quartered and cores removed
1 onion, ½ inch sliced
2 cups vegetable stock
1 bay leaf
2 T grained Dijon mustard
1 T fresh basil, chopped

Mix all ingredients and place in a casserole dish with lid and bake at 375° for 45 minutes. Add basil and serve.

ROASTED ONIONS WITH ALOE VERA AND ROSEMARY
(Serves 2)

1 large onion, peeled and sliced ½ inch thick
1 T safflower oil
2 tsp fresh rosemary, chopped
⅓ cup Aloe Vera Vinaigrette (see page 278)

Toss onion with safflower oil and bake at 375° for 30 minutes. Remove onions and toss them with rosemary and Aloe Vera Vinaigrette; serve.

BRAISED CELERY
(Serves 2)

½ *head celery, cut into 4-inch-long pieces*
2 *cups vegetable stock*
1 *T curry powder*
1 *tsp cumin seeds*
½ *tsp celery seeds*
1 *sprig thyme*
1 *bay leaf*
4 *peeled garlic cloves cut in half*

Toss all ingredients and place in a casserole dish with lid. Bake at 350° for 45 minutes. Serve immediately. This makes a great leftover.

YUKON POTATO AND TEMPEH STEW
(Serves 2)

1 *package (8 oz) tempeh*
1 *lb Yukon potatoes, ¼ inch slices*
3 *cups vegetable stock*
½ *medium onion, sliced ¼ inch*
½ *tsp fresh thyme, chopped*
½ *tsp fresh rosemary, chopped*
2 *T grained Dijon mustard*
1 *T arrowroot, dissolved in 2 T water*

Steam potatoes and onions until tender. Simmer vegetable stock with tempeh, thyme, rosemary and mustard. Stir in arrowroot and return to a simmer. Add potatoes and onions to stock and place all into a casserole dish. Bake at 375° for 30 minutes.

FISH

TILAPIA WITH SEAWEED VINAIGRETTE
(Serves 2)

2 each 6-oz tilapia fillets
1 cup shiitake mushrooms, sliced
½ cup Wakame Vinaigrette (see page 277)

In a nonstick sauté pan lightly sear tilapia fillets and shiitakes.
You may need to rub a light layer of safflower oil on the pan. Flip
the filets and top with vinaigrette. Turn heat on low and cover for
5 minutes. This fish cooks quickly.

TROUT WITH ALMONDS AND PARSLEY
(Serves 2)

1 T Dijon mustard
2 T fresh lemon juice
2 6-oz trout fillets
¼ cup sliced raw almonds
1 T fresh parsley, chopped lightly

Mix the mustard with 2 tsp of the lemon juice. Coat the trout
fillets with the mustard and coat with the almonds. Bake trout at
350° for 10 minutes. Remove trout and top with parsley and
remaining lemon juice.

ALASKAN HALIBUT WITH
BLACK-EYED-PEA SALSA
(Serves 2)

2 6-oz halibut fillets
2 T organic white wine
2 T fresh lemon juice
1 cup cooked black-eyed peas
1 tsp garlic, chopped
¼ cup onion, ¼ inch diced
¼ cup red bell pepper, ¼ inch diced
½ tsp fresh thyme, chopped
¼ tsp fresh rosemary, chopped
pinch ground cumin
1 tsp fresh cilantro, lightly chopped
⅓ cup Simple Vinaigrette #7 (see page 279)

Bake halibut in casserole dish with lid at 350° with wine and lemon juice for about 20 minutes or until cooked through. Mix the remaining ingredients. This can be served warm or chilled. Top halibut with salsa and serve.

WILD SALMON WITH SNOW PEAS
AND GINGER
(Serves 2)

2 6-oz wild salmon fillets
2 cups vegetable stock
1 T Bragg Liquid Aminos
1 T ginger, chopped
2 tsp garlic, chopped
1 T fresh basil, lightly chopped
1 T fresh cilantro, lightly chopped
1 tsp toasted sesame oil
snow pea shoots, for garnish

Place salmon in a casserole dish with vegetable stock, Bragg, ginger, and garlic, and cover. Bake at 400° for 20–25 minutes, until salmon is cooked through. Garnish with basil, cilantro, sesame oil, and pea shoots.

Chef's note: This dish works well with buckwheat soba noodles.

DESSERTS

BANANAS FOSTER STYLE OVER
RICE DREAM
(Serves 2)

2 bananas, peeled and sliced 1/2 inch thick
1/4 cup maple syrup
1/4 cup fresh orange juice
1/4 tsp cinnamon
Vanilla Rice Dream

In a small sauté pan combine bananas, maple syrup, orange juice, and cinnamon. Cook for 2 minutes. Pour bananas over a scoop of Rice Dream.

SOY YOGURT AND BUTTERNUT PARFAIT
(Serves 2)

1/2 cup butternut squash or pumpkin puree
1 cup soy yogurt
1 T maple syrup
1/8 tsp cinnamon
1 tsp vanilla extract

First peel, seed, and dice squash or pumpkin, then steam until soft. Puree in a food processor until smooth. Chill puree. Whisk all ingredients in a bowl until smooth, and serve.

MANGO JELLO
(Serves 2)

2 cups mango juice
2 vanilla beans, split and scraped
1 tsp agar flakes
⅓ cup maple syrup
2 T arrowroot, dissolved in 2 T of water

Blend mango juice with vanilla beans, agar, and maple syrup for 10 seconds. Simmer mixture for 5 to 10 minutes on very low heat. Then drizzle arrowroot in while stirring and return to simmer. Pour into small cups or molds. Refrigerate for four hours and serve.

PINEAPPLE ALOE VERA JELLO
(Serves 2)

1 ½ cups pineapple juice
½ cup whole leaf aloe vera juice
2 vanilla beans, split and scraped
1 tsp agar flakes
⅓ cup maple syrup
2 T arrowroot, dissolved in 2 T of water

Blend pineapple and aloe vera juices with vanilla beans, agar, and maple syrup for 10 seconds. Simmer mixture for 5 to 10 minutes on very low heat. Then drizzle arrowroot in while stirring and return to simmer. Pour into small cups or molds. Refrigerate for four hours and serve.

VANILLA SOY PUDDING
(Serves 2)

2 cups soy milk
1 tsp agar flakes
2 vanilla beans, split and scraped
⅓ cup maple syrup
2 T arrowroot, dissolved in 2 T water

Blend soy milk and agar. Add vanilla beans and maple syrup, and simmer for 5 minutes over low flame. Drizzle in arrowroot while simmering for one more minute. Pour into a bowl and refrigerate for six hours. Remove from refrigerator and puree.

CONDIMENTS

HONEY MUSTARD MAYONNAISE AND DRESSING

⅓ cup raw honey
⅓ cup Dijon mustard
⅓ cup unfiltered raw apple cider vinegar
1 ½ cups canola oil

Blend honey, mustard, and vinegar for 10 seconds. Slowly add oil to blender while on low. For vinaigrette add ⅓ cup water to thin consistency.

CURRY APRICOT SAUCE

2 cups apricot nectar
½ cup raw honey
2 T curry powder
½ cup unsulfured apricot, soaked in water overnight

Blend all ingredients well.

WAKAME VINAIGRETTE

¼ cup wakame, prepared, drained and chopped
½ cup brown rice vinegar
2 T toasted sesame oil
1 cup canola oil
2 T Bragg Liquid Aminos
3 scallions, sliced
1 T fresh mint, chopped

Blend wakame, vinegar, oils, and Bragg. Add scallions and mint to mixture; store in refrigerator for up to three days.

TURMERIC VINAIGRETTE

1 T tahini
1 T Dijon mustard
¼ cup raw unfiltered apple cider vinegar
2 tsp turmeric
¾ cup canola oil

Blend tahini, mustard, vinegar, and turmeric in a blender. Slowly drizzle in oil while blender is on low. Store in airtight container for up to one month. Shake before serving.

MINT-CUMIN VINAIGRETTE

½ tsp ground cumin
2 T tahini
⅓ cup raw unfiltered apple cider vinegar
⅛ tsp Celtic sea salt
⅔ cup canola oil
3 T fresh mint, chopped

Blend cumin, tahini, vinegar, and sea salt. Drizzle in oil while blender is on low and add mint.

ALOE VERA VINAIGRETTE

½ cup whole leaf aloe vera juice
3 T Dijon mustard
1 T fresh rosemary, chopped
1 ½ cups canola oil

Blend aloe vera juice, mustard, and rosemary in blender. While blender is on low, slowly drizzle in oil. Store in refrigerator for up to one week; shake before serving.

SIMPLE VINAIGRETTE #7

1 T tahini
1 T Dijon mustard
¼ cup raw unfiltered apple cider vinegar
1 T raw honey
¾ cup canola oil

Blend tahini, mustard, vinegar, and honey in an upright blender.
Slowly drizzle oil while blender is on.

ROASTED TOMATO SALSA

2 lbs tomatoes, washed and stemmed
¼ medium onion, peeled and ¼ inch sliced
¼ cup fresh basil leaves

Roast tomatoes and onions in oven for ½ hour at 400°. Let
tomatoes and onions cool for 15 minutes. Add them to a blender
and puree, leaving some whole pieces in. Add basil and use hot
or cold.

CHAPTER 11

COUNTERING COMMON CONDITIONS

Specific Supplementation Plans

America's baby boomers and senior citizens, who number over 150 million, are spending over a trillion dollars a year to diagnose and treat their diseases. This situation will only accelerate. Annual expenses to take care of this group's ailments will increase to around three trillion dollars in the coming decade. The sad—but also promising—thing is, the diseases are basically preventable and frequently reversible. We're going to look at some ways to do that in this chapter. But first, let's step back and gain a little perspective.

THE WELLNESS MODEL

Let's review some general health goals, i.e., things we can do that will help all of our systems across the board as we continue our journey to optimal health and longevity. We can:

- Relieve stress
- Help nourish the cells
- Help get the by-products of that nourishment out of the cells
- Use antioxidants to guard the cells against free radicals

- Keep our intestines clean
- Keep our blood clean
- Keep our liver functioning properly

If we do all that, and we certainly can, then a lot of conditions usually treated separately will be alleviated. In addition, a lot of conditions usually considered hopeless will not be. In other words, by being proactively oriented toward health, we're actually attacking a whole slew of conditions at once. I call this the Wellness Model of health maintenance.

Let me elaborate. Recently, I conducted a year-long health support group for people with a variety of conditions, ranging from the merely irritating to the very serious. But I never once mentioned a single illness. I never gave a single individual a protocol for a single condition. There were people in the group with eye problems, bowel problems, cancers, and Parkinson's disease, but I did not allow questions about their particular illnesses. Instead, the focus was entirely on wellness. At the end of the year, people had remarkable positive changes, as proven by their blood chemistries and medical evaluations, taken before and after the study. Across the board, people from every walk of life, with every stage of illness, showed improvements or the total elimination of their particular illness.

How is it possible to eliminate or ameliorate an illness when it is never specifically treated? I was, it turned out, promoting a new concept: In the absence of anything that will feed a disease, wellness is promoted. This is not a common idea for the average American, who thinks he or she is "well" as long as he or she has not been diagnosed with an illness. I disagree. The average person, by means of the unhealthy life he leads, is in the process of creating disease, for which a specific illness is just one of the end stages in the process. By the time a cancer manifests in that individual's body, he could have been hurting himself for twenty or thirty years. By the time he has a heart attack or stroke, he might have been doing the wrong things for twenty, thirty, or forty years. If you see the logic behind this concept, I have a question for you: Why wait to end up with the unwelcome symptoms of a disease process that develops because you have been making incorrect choices, when you can make the right choices and prevent or reverse that process in the first place?

When we eat and drink the nutrients that will rejuvenate, cleanse, and detoxify, we are helping the body's natural immune system to fight on our behalf. In that way, when the body comes in contact with a cold or flu virus, for example, it is able to destroy it. When we are in a polluted environment our body is able to recover from it. We can keep on going, despite an assault on our system. In effect, we are rejuvenating our cells.

A WELLNESS PROTOCOL

Before we begin exploring specialized treatments for individual ailments, I want to offer a baseline wellness protocol. This one-size-fits-all program of supplementation is based on the work I did in the health support groups and represents one of the pillars of my Wellness Model. Note: Although the following guidelines are appropriate for most Power Agers, you should work with your doctor to make sure that the supplements listed below are right for you. This is particularly important if you are taking any medications. Moreover, you should not be taking all these supplements at once.

Baseline Wellness Program

Vitamin A	15,000 IU
Vitamin C	10,000 mg
Magnesium	400 mg
Vitamin D	300 IU
Vitamin E	500 IU
Vitamin B_1	75 mg
Vitamin B_2	50 mg
Vitamin B_3	150 mg
Vitamin B_6	102 mg
Folic Acid	800 mcg

Vitamin B_{12}	250 mcg
Biotin	400 mcg
Pantothenic Acid	500 mg
Calcium	282 mg
Iodine	10 mcg
Magnesium	800 mg
Zinc	20 mg
Manganese	25 mg
Chromium	200 mcg
Selenium	100 mcg
Molybdenum	125 mcg
Potassium	50 mg
Copper	2 mg
Astaxanthin	25 mg
L-Carnosine	100 mg
Rosemary Leaf Powder	25 mg
Tocotrienols	25 mg
Raspberry Leaf Powder	5 mg
Citrus Bioflavonoid	300 mg
Rutin	25 mg
Red Wine Concentrate	25 mg
Grape Skin Extract	150 mg
China Green Tea Leaf Powder	200 mg
Licorice Root	25 mg
Cabbage Leaf	25 mg
Carrot Root	25 mg
Para Amino Benzoic Acid	200 mcg
Mushroom Complex	50 mg
Milk Thistle Leaf Extract	25 mg
Bilberry Fruit Powder	25 mg
Lycopene	20 mg
Grape Seed Extract	50 mg
Coenzyme Q10	50 mg
Quercetin	50 mg
Ginkgo Biloba Leaf Powder	60 mg

Broccoli	75 mg
Acerola	100 mg
Hesperedin	100 mg
Glutathione	100 mg
Linolenic Acid	100 mg
Ginger Rhizome Extract	100 mg
Superoxide Dismutase	25 mg
Alpha-Lipoic Acid	150 mg
Trimethylglycine	200 mg
Phosphatidylserine	200 mg
Isoflavone Genistein	200 mg
Inositol	250 mg
Lutein	25 mg
Citrus Bioflavonoids	300 mg
Methylsulfenyl Methane	400 mg
L-Taurine	500 mg
N-Acetyl Cysteine	500 mg
L-Lysine HCI	500 mg
Orthinine Alpha Ketoglutarate	500 mg
Choline Bitartrate	500 mg
Phosphatidyl Choline	500 mg
Acetyl-L-Carnitine	500 mg
Bromelain	15 mg

THE IMPORTANCE OF EXERCISE

When we talk about wellness, I have to say that many baby boomers and senior citizens have a distorted notion of what it means to live a healthy lifestyle. In part because they have become, to put it bluntly, physically lazy. This was apparent when I recently visited West Palm Beach, Ft. Lauderdale, and Boca Raton, Florida, where there is a culturally mixed group of senior citizens and boomers. They are somewhat physically active, eat a standard diet, take their medications, and think they are fine. However, they are doing almost nothing that really contributes to their health.

Yes, they are active, in that they play golf and tennis and bicycle, but these activities aren't doing them much good because when engaged in casually, the activities do not constitute resistance training. These are perfectly enjoyable games, but people should not delude themselves into thinking that casual exercise will get them into shape. Truly effective programs include aerobic, nonstop resistance exercise, such as power walking or swimming for at least forty-five minutes to an hour a day, plus lifting weights. Of course, you want to get the go-ahead from your physician before you embark on this program.

It is regrettable that senior citizens, especially women, are reluctant to weight train. Heading to the gym to lift weights seems antithetical to their culturally conditioned idea of what is appropriate for older ladies. However, that is precisely what they need to do. Any muscle that is not used is abused, and it becomes a repository for toxins and fat.

Furthermore, older Americans' standard diets result in weight gain. We've said this earlier in the book, but it bears repeating: We generally have to eat less as we get older because we have slower metabolisms. If we eat the same amount of food at age sixty as we did at forty, we will gain twelve pounds. So begin by reducing your caloric intake, but do not stop there. Switch to eating more living and raw foods, which supply healthy energy, because as we get older, mitochondrial activity—that is, the activity of the cells' "energy factories"—slows down. Thus, you really want to maximize your nutrition. Some of the ways you can do that are by eating two to three servings of sea vegetables every week, eating proteins that are easy to digest, keeping your blood sugar down, and drinking up to thirteen glasses of organic vegetable and fruit juices daily. And don't forget the daily nutritional supplements we talked about in Chapter 9.

Also, the following procedures are recommended: Have your thyroid gland checked to make sure it is not underactive. An underactive thyroid causes weight gain, depression, and fatigue. Get a good cardiovascular checkup to make sure you are capable of doing vigorous exercise. Get an SMAT-24, which is a basic blood chemistry test, a lipid profile, and an inflammatory profile to check if you have any inflammation or cytokine activity, which contributes to degenerative diseases. And you might consider having the mercury fillings removed from your teeth, because this metal is a dangerous toxin that can undermine your health.

There is no reason for us to be overweight in America. We just have to exercise, eat healthfully by eliminating refined carbohydrates and excessive protein, eat sparingly with a reduced caloric input, and cleanse our systems.

THE CONDITIONS

Read This First: In the discussions of specific conditions that follow, I sometimes provide a very long list of recommended supplements. But it is important to stress that if you have more than one condition, you should not be taking every single supplement and treatment that I suggest. That would simply overwhelm your system. The idea is to use my listings as a taking-off point when you work with a holistic health practitioner to determine a regimen that's right for you. Start with just a few nutrients, and then, after several weeks, evaluate the impact they have. You can then reconfigure your protocol.

And if you have a diagnosed illness, always make sure you are in the hands of a competent holistic, board-certified clinician. Let him or her guide you, and, if you desire, show him some of the relevant sections in this book or another, or say, for instance, "I heard Gary Null suggest that we use vitamin C in a dosage of . . ." This way you can work constructively with your clinician to tailor an individualized program.

Also, remember that protocols are designed to be followed in an incremental fashion—that is, dosages should be gradually worked up to over time; they should be taken under medical supervision; and they should be followed only one at a time. By this I mean that if you're taking a certain amount of a nutrient for one condition, but you have another illness as well, don't add on the recommended dosage for the second condition! This warning may seem like common sense, but I want to make it crystal-clear that you should not be adding together dosages. The body does not work like that.

Finally, these suggestions for specific diseases are given with the understanding that you are already juicing, eating, cleansing, and detoxifying according to the general plan discussed in Chapter 9. This combination approach is the best way to get positive results.

Allergies. Allergies are some of the most common conditions experienced by people both young and old. An allergy is more often than not due to an immune system that is in a hypervigilant response mode. Your body is responding to something you have eaten, imbibed, inhaled, or made skin contact with. The more challenge there is to your immune system, the greater the response will be, although each individual's body responds differently. One person can walk into a dusty, moldy room and sneeze, cough, and get red eyes and a runny nose. Another person can walk into that same room, and nothing happens. If you have a really strong immune system, your lymphocytes and phagocytes are able to engulf and digest antigens such as dust. But many today do not have this advantage. Therefore, to eliminate allergic responses we must strengthen our immune systems.

Probably 40 million Americans suffer from hay fever. During the hay fever season, ragweed germination fills the air with billions of microscopic particles. They enter your body and immediately combine with the immune system cells known as immunoglobulins, specifically the type called IgE. A series of chemical transformations occur that release the substance called histamine. That is the immediate cause of the annoying allergic responses. If they continue for too long, they can actually develop into asthmatic conditions.

Allergies to food are probably the most common type, since we tend to overindulge in the foods that we really like, but which we are allergic to—foods such as wheat bread, dairy products, orange juice from nonorganic oranges, meat, sugar, and corn. If you are allergic to a food it does not matter what form of it you eat—you will get the same reaction. For example, if you are allergic to corn, you will get a reaction from cornbread, cornflakes, or corn on the cob. The solution is to go on an allergen-free program; simply eliminate all the causes of the reactions.

Chemical sensitivities are allergic reactions to substances in the environment, such as fumes from a photocopy machine at work, molds in your home, or pesticide residues on lawns and flowerbeds. IgE-mediated allergy tests are used to detect what the offending substance or condition is. (IgE, as we've mentioned, is an antibody, or immune cell, that binds to an allergy-causing substance in your system.) Once a test helps you determine what you're allergic to, you can eliminate it whenever possible. Sometimes, of course, it's not possible, such as when your neighbors spray a noxious chemical right outside your window. At such times, we must turn to other things that can help.

Adding bentonite clay to your cleansing drink at night can help because it has a negative charge, and therefore attracts positively charged particles. Toxins are drawn to the clay and then eliminated through the body. The generally used amount is one teaspoon in about 10 to 12 oz of water. Another thing you can do is spray the room with extracts of orange and lemon, which has an air-purifying effect.

We also know that lemon juice and watermelon juice are great drinks for helping people eliminate allergies. Plus the more "live," completely unprocessed food you have in the diet, the better it is for you if you are allergic. You should make sure that your soaps are without artificial scents, and your shampoos are made with natural oils and without contaminants. Do not use artificial deodorants or talcum powder. Use natural moisturizers that contain aloe, vitamin E, and sesame oil. When using exfoliating cleansers for the skin, make sure that you use a soft loofah to remove the dead epithelial cells. Don't use artificial room deodorizers, because they are frequently toxic. Instead, try the ones made from the natural skins of fruit—they are terrific for killing viruses and bacteria without harmful side effects.

Supplements to Combat Allergies. Concerning nutrients to counteract allergies, it's always best, as we've mentioned several times elsewhere in this book, to consult your own holistic health care practitioner before embarking on any regimen. This is important because each person has his or her own individual needs, and some things may be contraindicated for people with certain conditions. That said, you should know that the chief nutrient for fighting allergies is vitamin C, and that using divided doses throughout the day is the most effective way of benefiting from this nutrient. Vitamin C reduces histamine levels in the blood and helps strengthen the immune system, both of which are important benefits. Grape seed extract is another recommended antiallergy supplement. You generally have to use at least 200 mg of both vitamin C and grape seed extract two to three times a day. With allergies, however, I usually suggest that people start at 1,000 mg (1 gram) and go up to 5,000 mg (5 grams).

Mast cells, which are part of your connective tissue, contain histamine, the trigger of allergic reaction. If you take the bioflavonoid quercetin you will be strengthening the membranes of these cells, thus preventing their bursting and hence avoiding the release of histamine.

Eating the wrong way can help set the stage for food allergies. People generally eat until they are full. This is wrong. In addition, as we discussed in Chapter 9, they drink too many beverages while they eat. This is another bad habit. Plus they drink carbonated beverages, a really bad mistake. And, finally, from a health standpoint, caffeinated beverages are terrible accompaniments to a meal. I think of the typical American meal of a hamburger, fries, and a cola, followed by a cup of coffee. This is not—to understate the facts—doing you any good.

To somewhat counteract such bad habits and thus lessen your susceptibility to allergies, the following may be helpful to know: GLA, a fatty acid (generally at 1,000 mg), borage seed oil, black currant oil, or oil of primrose are important aids in digesting food. This is especially so if you've been eating the wrong way for a long time: too fast, or the wrong combinations of foods, or highly processed foods, or simply too much food.

If you absolutely have to have liquids with your meal, try to have just herbal teas or fresh juices. Also, when we suspect there is impaired digestion, we recommend digestive enzymes. While ideally you want to flood the body with the natural enzymes found in fresh food and juices, for extra help the enzymes you get at the health food store can be valuable. Take the amount directed with each meal to facilitate better digestion.

A variety of herbs can help with allergies. In my opinion, garlic is the number-one herb for building immunity and acting as a natural antiseptic agent. It is fine to take an odorless garlic pill, obtainable at health food stores, if you need to remain socially active. Astragalus is a crucial herb for allergies. It is one of the very best immune builders because it increases the number and activity of immune cells. It can be taken on a daily basis, generally at 100 mg. Echinacea, taken only for two to three weeks at a time, boosts the immune system as well. It's known mostly as an aid to quicker recovery from the flu and colds, but it also helps ameliorate allergic responses. Ginseng—a builder of endurance and stamina, and a traditional stabilizer of the chi, or life energy—also helps build the immune system. Wild cherry bark helps with hay fever and common allergies. If you have allergies that manifest in the lungs, mullein leaf and horehound can help.

I would also suggest stinging nettle, capsicum, ginger root, peppermint leaf, burdock root, dandelion root, grapefruit seed extract, and at least 6 oz of aloe vera consumed throughout the day. Make sure that you are getting 1 tsp of miso in soup daily.

One more strategy to knock out allergies: Look for a combination capsule with the following broad-spectrum nutrients: glucosamine sulfate, pantothenic acid, B complex, vitamin C, vitamin E, coenzyme Q10, glutathione, bromelain, quercetin, and garlic.

Arthritis. Very many people suffer from arthritis, a local inflammatory process. Chronic infections lead to inflammation, and there are a whole variety of things in our environment that lead to both. If you have Epstein-Barr virus, herpes, or cytomegalovirus, you have infection and inflammation. If you have chronic infections from yeasts and fungi, you have inflammatory process. If you have been exposed to pesticides, food colorings, preservatives, chlorine, fluoride, noxious fumes, excessive electromagnetic radiation, or allergens specific to you, you may get an inflammatory result. In short, poisons, allergens, viruses, and bacteria all produce infections leading to inflammation. Put these together with a low-functioning immune system and you have the basis for arthritis. Our world can really be a negative influence on our bodies!

First, we should focus on juicing. The phytochemicals in the organic juices help heal because they rejuvenate the cell and repair the damage done to the DNA. Some beneficial juices include: pineapple (especially good with juiced alfalfa sprouts); a combination of aloe vera, star fruit, and cabbage juices; cucumber juice; fresh apricot juice; and cantaloupe juice. Ginger has been known for a very long time for its anti-inflammatory nature and should be added to many juices.

An important goal with arthritis is to eliminate anything that is creating uric acid. Meat is a primary suspect here, and arthritis sufferers are urged to become vegetarians, if they have not done so already. Dandelion greens, parsley, and alfalfa are particularly good for fighting uric acid, as is the herb devil's claw. Tofu, tempeh, and miso, which are high in methionine, also help. Cold-water fish is good, as are folic acid and folic acid–rich foods such as oats and lentils. Recommended also are avocados and the use of olive oil.

Some recommended herbs are boneset; boswellia (one of the best natural remedies for arthritis); burdock root, a great blood cleanser; cayenne pepper, long known for its antiarthritis power; devil's claw, which we've already mentioned as a uric-acid fighter and thus one of the best herbs to help our joints; stinging nettle; prickly ash bark; white willow bark; yucca; garlic; sea cucumber; ginger, as we've mentioned; buchu leaf; and turmeric. Use these all as directed.

The following nutritional supplements are recommended for arthritis: chondroitin sulfate (generally at 500 to 1,000 mg), glucosamine sulfate (1,000 mg), silica (50 mg), manganese (25 mg), L-cysteine (500 mg), boron (5 mg), B complex (100 mg), vitamin E (400 units), calcium and magnesium citrate (1,200 mg), coenzyme Q10 (400 mg), DMG (150 mg), TMG (150 mg), folic acid (1,000 mcg), zinc (25 mg), MGM3 (1,500 mg), and a tablespoon of emulsified cod liver oil on an empty stomach when you wake up in the morning. In addition, take oil of primrose (2,000 mg), vitamin C (between 5 and 15 grams divided throughout the day), and MSM (1,000 mg).

Candida. An overgrowth of yeast in the body is known as candidiasis, or candida. Candidiasis in the intestines or vagina is quite common. Many of the causes are conditions we have become familiar with: our diet, our overconsumption of sugar and acid foods, and the great stress in our lives; all lead to a lowered immune system, and all of these things can cause candida.

A protocol similar to the one given for cancer (see Chapter 6) is good for candida as well. A list of actions that will help combat candida includes things in both the emotional and physical realms: We have to concentrate on getting rid of bad feelings such as frustration and anger. We want to avoid untrusting relationships, and to stop draining our energy. We have to stop using cortisone and antibiotic hormone imbalancers. We have to really conquer the depression caused by a low immune state, because when we are depressed, candida manifests. Go on a diet without alcohol, cheese, mushrooms, refined carbohydrates, and baked goods. Many of these foods contain some form of yeast, which fuels this condition. In addition to the usual healthful nutrients, we should add extra acidophilus and extra fish oils, as well as evening primrose oil, vitamin C, echinacea, vitamin A, and zinc (great for building immunity and helping increase mucous membrane integrity). Also, those fighting candidiasis should consider selenium, molybdenum, magnesium (a great detoxifier), folic acid, citrus seed extract from grapefruit, berberine, tea tree oil, bromelain, aloe vera, pau d'arco, black walnut extract, astragalus, and hawthorn extract.

Chronic Fatigue. How many Americans would feel better if they just weren't so tired? So many factors can contribute to this problem. Any time you have a weakened immune system, there is fatigue. Any time your body has been attacked by free radicals, heavy metals, viruses, or bacteria, you are going to sustain damage to the cells' energy factories, the mitochondria. Hence, you are going to be fatigued.

There is a lot that can be done with natural substances to restore vim and vigor to every moment of your waking life. For one thing, add more fresh juices to your day: Green juices are, as usual, very beneficial, but also include lemon, lime, watermelon, and grape juice—not white grape juice but the juice from grapes of darker hues. Include soy (for the isoflavones) and aloe vera in your food selections. Helpful herbs include garlic, St. John's wort, turmeric, echinacea, bee propolis, astragalus, skullcap, burdock, red clover, milk thistle, and kombucha. As we've mentioned before, you do not have to take all of these, and you most likely should not. They are listed here to show all that benefit the body, but your healthcare practitioner will work with you to determine your personal regimen.

For chronic fatigue, the following supplements have been found to help people: MGM3, quercetin, coenzyme Q10, L-carnitine, lecithin, digestive enzymes, vitamin E, DMG, the B complex, B_6, B_{12}, GABA, sea vegetable capsules, anti-parasitic formulas, and medically given intravenous bio-oxidative therapies, including vitamin C.

Chronic Pain. Unfortunately, chronic pain, like chronic fatigue, is an especially common condition. Just imagine how much better many Americans would feel if they weren't in pain and fatigued. Overcoming pain and fatigue really is possible, and it gives people their quality of life back!

Caveat. First, keep in mind that pain is a signal that something is wrong in your body. So you should seek medical help with pain problems.

Once you have sought medical help, you should know that the following will work against pain: the same elimination and detoxification regimens we used for many other conditions (see Chapter 9), bio-oxidative methylating agents such as vitamin C and juices, and living (raw) foods. I find that juicing is the single most important measure you can take, but you must also remember to choose foods that do not make your blood sugar fluctuate too greatly—i.e., avoid simple sugars.

Once you get rid of the source of the pain, here are the things that can really make a difference: Dl-phenylalanine or DLPA, the B complex, and vitamin C.

Proteolytic enzymes cause inflammation after an injury, and thus, pain. By halting the production of protease, the effects of inflammatory processes can be reduced. The essential fatty acids help with this task. They can turn off or minimize prostaglandin E2, the "bad" prostaglandin. Prostaglandin E1 helps to do this, as do the omega fatty acids DHA, generally recommended at 500 mg; and EPA at 1,000 to 1,500 mg.

Flaxseed oil, borage oil, salmon oil, and cod liver oil can help in turning off pain, as can wild ginger, as well as cinnamon. To help with what the Chinese call the "energy flow," there is bupleurum. For headache pains we can use the herbs feverfew, cayenne, valerian, and skullcap, and theanine, an amino acid found in the leaves of green tea. Again, you are not expected to use all of these. For example, just take theanine, at 100 mg, two or three times a day. That can frequently turn off a headache and give a calming feeling. Calcium-magnesium at 1,500 mg can also do that. Feverfew is very good for stopping migraine headaches because it affects blood vessel dilation. Magnesium is one of the single most important things to take for any kind of local pain, muscle pain, or headache pain. Dong quai, together with ginger and mint, is often effective. You can make a tincture with all of these combined. You can even juice some ginger and drink it straight, or diluted by celery juice. White willow bark is useful in alleviating headache pain. In fact, that is what aspirin was originally made from, but with white willow bark the negative side effects are minimized.

If you have stomach pain, use mints: peppermint, spearmint, and winter mint, with some cinnamon, anise, and fennel. Make a tea out of these. This tastes great with some raw honey, and it is very good for you. For pain from urinary tract infections, the alkaloid berberine is extremely good. Oregon grape root is used to help this condition as well, together with the Chinese herb coptis and marshmallow. Rosemary is recommended for general pain all over the body, including fibromyalgia, arthritis, lupus, and some of the diabetic neuropathies.

Sometimes we can apply rosemary oil. Alternatively, try almond oil, which may be applied by diluting it: Take one drop of almond oil and ten drops of canola oil, mix them and massage into the painful areas. The herb blue vervain contains anti-inflammatory and analgesic properties, as does curcumin, a bright yellow compound derived from turmeric. Curry has turmeric in it. It is used all over India to help with generalized pain.

More Pain-Busters. Increasing circulation always helps alleviate pain, because you are increasing the nutrients getting into the area, and the debris getting out. Circulation help is provided by vitamin E, vitamin C, glutathione, N-acetyl-cysteine, and alpha-lipoic acid. Exercise is important because it releases endorphins, and promotes release of natural cortisone. Since pain and discomfort are frequently accompanied by excessive anxiety and stress, it is important to find ways to relax. Here are some suggestions: deep breathing; exercise of all types, including walking, biking, and swimming; reading; entertainments such as plays, movies, and concerts; watching television (selectively!); playing a musical instrument; and doing any sort of hobby. Magnets can be very effective at alleviating pain; for example, magnetic leg wraps help with leg pain. I have seen biofeedback be of great benefit to people with pain. Therapeutic touch is also important, as is the increasingly mainstream practice of chiropractic adjustments.

When you have pain you want to make sure that you are balancing your pH, because the pH of the body can directly impact pain. Therefore, stay away from salted foods, vinegar, and mayonnaise. Cut down on salt and, of course, have no sugar, alcohol, coffee, or other beverages containing caffeine. All of these can worsen pain. The B complex vitamins have a natural analgesic effect. Vitamin C alleviates gum sensitivity. And, above all, our basic program, set forth on these pages, is going to make a difference.

Colds and Flu. Colds and flu have reached near-epidemic proportions among senior citizens and baby boomers. Here are some suggestions for both aggressively preventing the illnesses and shortening their duration.

Take more green tea, possibly three times a day. Use MGM3 and IP6, the mushroom complexes that increase killer cell activity, three times a day. Eat sea vegetables twice daily. Have a protein shake two to three times a day. Remove mercury fillings with a holistic dentist. Take grape seed extract (from 200 to 2,000 mg), germanium (150 mg), and reduced L-glutathione (300 mg). Do aromatherapy with lavender and rosemary. Take DMG, L-arginine with MSM, and lots of vitamin C, quercetin, and herbal teas. Juice throughout the day, concentrating particularly on garlic, onion, ginger, and aloe vera juices—the juices that are most helpful with colds and flu. Cleanse the colon and stimulate the liver to flush and release its toxins so it can properly metabolize and detoxify the body. Practice stress management.

And remember to keep hydrated at all times, drinking plenty of pure water and juice!

Digestive Disorders. Acid disorders of the stomach, such as burping, flatulence, distension, diarrhea, and constipation, stem from eating the wrong foods in the wrong combinations, eating too much, eating at the wrong times, or eating under stress. Foods we eat begin to putrefy and cause acid indigestion and, therefore, bad digestion. Constantly eating highly processed foods, together with other factors, can lead to Crohn's disease, constipation, bad breath, diarrhea, diverticulitis, flatulence, food allergies, gastric reflux, irritable bowel syndrome, malabsorption syndrome, peptic ulcers, and ulcerative colitis.

However, you can improve these conditions or make sure they do not develop in the first place, if you eat healthy clean foods and drink plenty of fresh juices, especially the green juices containing chlorophyll. Other measures include taking lots of aloe vera, lots of enzymes, chamomile tea, fennel (which helps stop the cramping and indigestion), ginger, nettles, and oats. Eating smaller portions of food also helps. For cleaning out parasites and fungi, there are natural antibiotics such as grape seed extract, pau d'arco tea, garlic, and artemisia. Your doctor may give you some Nystatin or Diflucan, anti-fungal medications.

If you are following this book's advice in general, you are already doing good things for your digestive system, such as keeping to a yeast-free, non-mucus-generating, properly alkaline diet with plenty of fiber, to help move things along, so to speak! Here are two important nutrients that should be taken in high doses: vitamin C, generally at 5 to 20 grams; and glutamine, generally at 1 to 5 grams. Glutamine nourishes and heals the entire lining of the upper and lower intestines. As always in these cases, the high doses should be arrived at in gradual steps. Other nutrients needed include: glutathione, coenzyme Q10, digestive enzymes with each meal, magnesium, especially for people who are constipated (magnesium is a natural laxative), the omega-3 fatty acids, and peppermint oil (good at killing harmful bacteria and parasites and reducing colonic spasms). Stress reduction will, of course, help your digestion.

Colon therapy and hydrotherapy use water to flush out the intestines, to eliminate stored waste and restore proper tissue and organ function, and are extremely important. These treatments, in essence, are detoxifying the bowels. Intestinal massage is another treatment available.

When we get rid of harmful bacteria in the intestines, we should always replace them with beneficial organisms. These are called probiotics.

Emphysema. Another major problem for senior citizens and some baby boomers is emphysema. This is a kind of chronic obstructive pulmonary disease that results from long-standing insults to the lung tissue such as cigarette smoking and environmental irritants, coupled with a toxic lifestyle: poor nutrition, sedentary habits, alcohol consumption, and high stress.

Our usual healthy protocol applies to this condition, with a few specific recommendations: Increase your intake of green juices, going up to thirteen glasses of vegetable juice a day, and include garlic/onion juice. Dilute the garlic and onion with aloe vera, cabbage, celery, or apple juice. Remember—work your way up to the thirteen glasses gradually and in small amounts. For example, start with one juice every day for the first month, proceed to two glasses daily during the second month, and so on up to thirteen juices a day at the end of thirteen months.

Start the day with a 12 oz protein shake of quality predigested vegetable protein. Use fenugreek tea and comfrey tea throughout the day. You may benefit from the medically supervised treatments of chelation therapy, intravenous vitamin therapy, and hyperbaric oxygen therapy. Take vitamin C at 5,000 to 15,000 mg; DMG at 300 mg, three times a day; TMG (use as directed); and MSM (as directed). The sulfur in MSM binds to allergens, thus preventing allergic reactions. It also coats the intestinal lining to prevent dust mites from causing asthmatic reactions. Take 300 mg of coenzyme Q10 (100 mg three times a day); cayenne (10 to 30 mg); NADH (5 mg twice a day); L-taurine (1,000 mg twice a day); L-cysteine and L-methionine; amino acids, in divided doses; and vitamin A (25,000 units, as an emulsion).

Additional suggestions: Take N-acetyl-cysteine at 1,000 mg; acetyl-L-carnitine at 1,000 mg; vitamin K at 10 mg; magnesium at 1,500 mg; IP6, to increase natural killer cells; and MGM3, as directed. Take pantothenic acid and zinc for adrenal support, and eat sea vegetables twice a day. Use breathing exercises, colon cleansing, Amma therapy, air purifiers, water purifiers, and castor oil packs applied to the back and chest areas to enhance breathing. The best results come when the full elimination program is followed, together with the foregoing protocol.

Eye Disorders. Eye disorders, such as macular degeneration, glaucoma, and cataracts, are common ailments in the senior population. These conditions have the same underlying causes as many other diseases, and hence, the same remedies, which is the main idea in these pages. There are some nutrients, however, that work especially well for the eyes. At the top of the list are two superstar nutrients that are known to help the lens of the eye, namely, reduced glutathione and vitamin C. By using these we can do more good for our eyes than by using anything else. It is most important to get intravenous vitamin C. This can only be given by a physician. An intravenous drip of vitamin C and glutathione together will do the maximum amount of good. Orally, we can take vitamin C throughout the day, if it is buffered. Always build up the amount of C gradually to just about bowel tolerance and then take it back down to where your bowels have no trouble with it.

The regular healthy diet we have been promoting, plus the essential fatty acids, will be fine for your eyes. We should emphasize the juices of broccoli, spinach, and beet greens, and eat yellow, orange, and green fruits (using only organic produce, of course!). Sulfur-rich foods, such as garlic, onion, and asparagus, are particularly helpful for our vision.

Chelation therapy is appropriate because toxic metals in the body, including cadmium, mercury, and aluminum, cause oxidative stress in the eyes.

In Chapter 3 we mentioned circulatory deficit as a facet of aging that is, unfortunately, not kind to our eyes. The fact is that decreased circulation is, in effect, starvation of your body's tissues. Your body needs blood supplying oxygen and nutrients to the cells all day long. When this doesn't happen efficiently, either due to sedentary habits and lack of aerobic exercise, or due to our not taking methylating agents, we end up experiencing oxidative stress and nutrient deficiencies. The combination also produces free radicals and inflammatory agents such as cytokines. This in turn is a major detriment to the eyes.

The circulation to the eyes (and to the whole body, of course) must be kept in tip-top shape! For circulatory system help, the following apply: Ginkgo biloba, gotu kola, hawthorn berry, vitamin E, cayenne pepper, ginger, marjoram, and garlic. Bilberry is an extremely important nutrient, a superstar for the eyes. Pine bark extract and grape seed extract (generally between 100 to 500 mg a day) are also good because they fortify the capillaries that furnish the eyes with fluid, and aid in the prevention of lens impairment. Two Chinese herbs useful for healing dry and inflamed eyes are daigaku eyedrops and shehu. If you have cataracts, the following are important: acetyl-L-carnitine at

1,000 mg, alpha-lipoic acid at 500 mg, vitamin E at 800 units, N-acetyl-cysteine at 1,000 mg, the bioflavonoids at 2,000 mg, and reduced glutathione at 500 mg.

Various vision therapies are available. Dr. Robert Michael Kaplan, author of *The Power Behind Your Eyes*, shows how proper visual hygiene can help to enhance vision. There are books on eye exercises. Acupuncture and acupressure are frequently used to lessen tension and improve vision. Pressure point therapy and reflexology are also used for eye problems. Practitioners of this technique explain that there are reflex points in the foot, generally between the second and third toe, that, when touched, will help the eyes. Massage can clear nerve blockages in the eyes. Biofeedback can help in re-regulating eye focus, muscle movement, and control.

Research has found that artificial sweeteners are terrible for the eyes, as are caffeine, sugar, and alcohol. Steroids and mercury from dental fillings are capable of causing oxidative stress to the eyes. In short, staying away from any kind of environmental toxin is good "sight insurance."

Foot and Leg Problems. Foot and leg problems are often dismissed as trivial nuisances. They are minimized and misunderstood, and therefore inadequately treated or ignored. There seems to be an assumption in our culture that these conditions are inevitable. It is only when our ability to walk is impaired that we pay attention to them. We rarely think about what we can do to prevent the problems, but this is a shame because our feet are literally the way we get anywhere in the world! So we should maintain foot and leg health diligently.

To this day I remember an experience from a college class. The teacher asked, "If you were to take off your shoes and socks, would your feet look normal?" Almost everyone said they had normal feet. The teacher proceeded to describe the appearance as well as the mechanics of a normal foot. He showed the metatarsals, which are bones that allow the toes to wiggle, and the normal span of the toes. He demonstrated that with each step the toes spread apart and the balance shifts from the heel to the ball when pushing off. Finally, he had us look at our feet, and he repeated his question. What a surprise! Now, almost no one said they had normal feet.

This experience came to mind years later during conversations with a friend who is a podiatrist. He had wondered why so many women in their thirties and forties all exhibited the same phenomenon—very ugly and deformed feet. In each case, he discovered that the cause was the same: They wore high-heeled shoes with pointed toes, and stuffed wide feet into narrow shoes.

Physics provides a simple explanation for the problems that result. Wherever the greatest amount of pressure is applied, something gives. In the foot, it is the big toe that gives and moves, pointing inward. Some people have their big toes not only pointing inward, but actually overlapping their second toes. This distortion affects the entire walking mechanism and fosters the development of corns, calluses, bunions, and fungus under the nails.

Women are not the only ones prone to this problem. When men wore pointed shoes and cowboy boots, which were considered hip in the seventies, they were prime targets for toe problems. I myself almost fell into this fashion trap. I wanted a pair of cowboy boots, so I went to a store, tried on a pair, and walked around. They looked great, but they were uncomfortable. The college class image of a normal foot burst into my mind. I chose the health of my feet over the look of the boots.

Just recently I had occasion to see deformed feet in an unexpected situation when I was in Florida participating in a national championship race. While we were getting ready, I watched the other athletes put on their shoes and socks. Every single one of them had foot deformities. Can you imagine the discomfort they experience during training and racing? It has to be particularly painful for athletes to have feet with deformities. And what was the probable cause? Incorrectly designed shoes.

Shoe styles are often the initial cause of distortions of the normal anatomy of the foot. Then, once our feet are distorted in this way, other problems can ensue. In addition, problems in different parts of the body can create foot problems. For example, if we have poor circulation, which is likely if we are very sedentary or overweight, any problem occurring in our feet will be exacerbated. Most people neglect exercising and caring for their feet, even though these activities can improve circulation. When was the last time you exercised or massaged your feet?

Peripheral Neuropathy. Peripheral neuropathy is a condition that can affect the feet; some symptoms are sensations of burning, pins and needles, tingling, and itching. These unpleasant sensations may have significant causes and severe consequences. The problem stems from either sensory dysfunction or malfunction in the motor nerves, which can be induced by metabolic disorders such as diabetes. Patients with diabetes tend to suffer from extreme cases of neuropathy, which can be characterized by complete numbness. A snowball effect of damage can be set into motion by this condition. Due to the numbness in their feet, patients have stepped on sharp objects and gotten cuts that became infected and even gangrenous before they were given attention. Furthermore, healing is more difficult because of the lack of adequate circulation. Not only can a variety of abrasions, wounds, and sores result, but amputations are also common. In fact, amputations are more common in diabetics with neuropathy than in people with any other condition.

Peripheral neuropathy may also be caused by thyroid hyperactivity and hypoactivity, kidney disease, and liver disease.

It is vital to realize that to overcome these painful nerve conditions we need to cleanse and detoxify our bodies. Drinking lots of clean liquids is extremely helpful for neuropathy. Removing metals from the body is another important step. The body accumulates metals and the nerves in the lower extremities begin to degenerate as the levels of metals in the body rise. For example, the longer one is exposed to lead, the more it accumulates in the body, and the more the nerves in the lower body respond by degenerating. Even mercury fillings in our teeth are problematic. The good news is that metals can be removed from the body by the removal of mercury fillings and by undergoing chelation therapy. Large numbers of people report that after these two processes, not only do the pins and needles sensations disappear, but also circulation improves throughout the body.

Vitamin C, especially as an intravenous drip, is another important measure. Go to a knowledgeable holistic doctor for this treatment. It will generally start with 35,000 mg of vitamin C and will gradually increase. The doctor will probably include, as part of your protocol, calcium, magnesium, glutathione, and other nutrients known to go into cells to feed, nourish, and enhance methylation and proper oxygen utilization.

Juices are also useful. One or two glasses daily of red fruit juices such as cherry, cranberry, raspberry, and blueberry, spiked with vitamin C and aloe vera, are extremely beneficial. Lycopene, the bioflavonoids, and lutein taken at least three times a day are also extremely important.

Blisters, Wounds, Warts, and Dry Skin. Blisters, wounds, warts, or dry skin on feet and legs are often due to imbalances in our biochemistry. The more toxic we are, the more bacteria and viruses we have. The more stress on the metabolic mechanisms inside our bodies, the more likely it is to manifest as some kind of problem on the feet or legs. If wounds do not heal, it is usually an indication that the immune system is depressed; therefore, building up your immunity is necessary to relieve the problem.

To boost your immunity, do a complete cleansing and detoxification. Eat lots of fruits, vegetables, and grains. Eat very pure and clean food. Also, use ozone therapy, which can be given only by a doctor and is currently only available in certain states. Ozone therapy is extremely beneficial in killing bacteria and viruses. High levels of a water-soluble form of vitamin A, administered intravenously with glutathione, can also build the immune system and help heal the body.

Alpha-lipoic acid is a superstar nutrient for building the immune system. Other nutrients that help fight viruses and bacteria are St. John's wort, bitter melon, astragalus, pau d'arco, echinacea, red clover, Chinese green tea, and vitamin C. It is extremely important to take them on a regular basis in a disciplined fashion.

Bedsores (and ulcers) develop on bedridden people because there is no circulation in their bodies. To stimulate circulation, magnetic leg wraps can be applied, or magnetic mattress pads, placed on top of one's regular mattress, can help. Another useful technique is the leg massage—especially with aloe vera and an essential oil—administered at least once a day. With massage you stimulate lymph glands and help bring energy and nerve sensation to the tissue, which, in turn, allows muscles to contract and relax.

Calluses and Corns. Calluses, another omnipresent foot problem, are caused by thick accumulations of dead skin over a period of time. Neglect is partly responsible for their formation. When most people take a shower or bath, they do not wash the bottoms of their feet. Whether you know it or not, you have dead skin accumulating there. Corns, on the other hand, originate from calcified protrusions on the bone that either press against the skin from inside the foot or receive extreme pressure from shoes, the ground, or another toe. Fortunately, since calluses and corns consist primarily of dead skin, they are not terribly dangerous. To remove them, you can gently use a pumice stone or other grating apparatus. If you cannot do it yourself, go to a salon that specializes in foot care. But make sure proper hygienic conditions are met. The salon should sterilize the pumice stone to kill viruses and bacteria, by cleaning it with hydrogen peroxide before using it on you. If the client before you had any kind of infection, it can be directly transmitted to you. Since metal can cut through the skin, resulting in infection, no metal tool should be used in a salon. By gently removing calluses and corns, you will improve the balance, hygiene, and, of course, aesthetics of your feet.

To reiterate, do not wear shoes that squeeze your feet. Why wear shoes that are supposed to make your feet look sexy only to take the sexy shoe off to reveal a horror-film foot? In fact, always go barefoot when you are at home. Going barefoot is healthier, more hygienic, and better balanced, and it feels better. Have you ever walked in the sand barefoot? Then, you know it feels good, and it massages the whole foot. It is easy to see that wearing shoes that keep feet constricted and sweaty inside makes no sense.

Rashes. Rashes, including blistering types, are frequently due to what we put on our skin. One cause is soap because it may contain an artificial chemical that produces an adverse reaction. If you have a rash problem, it is advisable to use the type of soap that is 100 percent natural, or at least one that is unscented. A rash can be cleaned with a mixture composed primarily of aloe vera, along with colloidal silver, bee propolis, pau d'arco, and purified water. Then, wrap the area with gauze that is kept somewhat moist, so the mixture remains on the rash. After four or five hours, the rash should begin to heal.

You should know that besides being externally induced, rashes can be the body's response to an internal condition. Therefore, you need to clean up the body and stimulate the immune system. With vitamin C therapy, rashes will often clear up.

Athlete's Foot. Athlete's foot is a fungal skin infection that is almost always due to a highly acidic diet and a warm, moist environment, such as that created by shoes, and sneakers in particular. Sneakers do not breathe the way regular shoes breathe, because of their rubber content. Therefore, sneakers are a perfect environment for the growth of skin fungus, especially if you have a weakened immune system. Lower levels of T-cells are associated with athlete's foot. Ozone therapy and immune stimulation can reverse the problem. Also, it is essential to keep feet cool and dry. The bottoms of the feet and the areas between toes should be dried after getting out of the shower or bath. Most people dry only the upper parts of their feet. Your feet must certainly be dry before putting them into socks, and it is wise to avoid socks made of synthetic fibers, because they do not breathe. Avoid acid-producing foods such as meats, foods high in phosphates such as sodas, sugary foods, and fried foods, since athlete's foot is an acidic condition. Instead, eat the alkaline foods that are components of a healthy vegetarian diet. Watermelon juice with lemon and lime is wonderful for rebalancing an overly acidic system.

Hemorrhoids. A lot of Americans have hemorrhoids and do not give them much thought other than, "What's the big deal? We've got them." And they start taking medications and creams. Hemorrhoids, also known as piles, are swollen blood vessels that cause the mucous membranes of the lower rectum or anus to protrude. When they are on the outside of the anus they are referred to as external hemorrhoids. They can be on the inside, or internal, as well. Generally, people with sedentary lifestyles are more prone to this affliction, and those who exercise, less prone. A dairy-free diet makes one less prone. People with a sedentary lifestyle who eat dairy and other high-protein foods are much more likely candidates for hemorrhoids because high-protein diets have little fiber in them. Without fiber, it is hard to move wastes through the lower rectum and anus. This leads to constipation and straining to defecate, a direct cause of hemorrhoids.

A living-foods, high-fiber diet will help. Eat plenty of sprouts. Have sea vegetables such as chlorella or spirulina twice a day, and about five ounces total of aloe vera. Drink ten glasses of vegetable juice a day (working up to this total gradually). Magnesium, vitamin C, and bioflavonoids are important, as are the essential fatty acids, olive oil, and flaxseed oil. Drink green tea two to three times a day. Topical application of papaya skin is important in the inflamed areas, and raw potato slices can also be used.

Aloe vera is the superstar of hemorrhoid protocol because this substance, with its mucopolysaccharides, will increase the circulation. It has a natural laxative effect and soothes the alimentary canal. Start with one teaspoon of the gel and work up to two or three teaspoons a day. This should be quite helpful. Also, use some Cyprus oil, a so-called venous tonic, applied externally or in bathwater, with chamomile and nettle. You can bathe in Epsom salts to reduce swelling effectively.

Other useful hemorrhoid fighters are: topically applied calendula ointment, and, taken internally, vitamin E, butcher's broom tea, vitamin C, quercetin, bromelain, and grape seed extract. Vitamin B_6 is a very important, generally underutilized nutrient; take about 25 to 50 mg a day. Use vitamin K at 5 mg, and cat's claw. Also useful are warm sitz baths, homeopathy, and acupuncture. Exercise, especially good resistance workouts about four days a week, can help. There is also a psychological component to this that we should pay attention to: Try not to be "anal" (in the colloquial sense of "retentive"). Let yourself flow.

Hypoglycemia. Hypoglycemia, unrecognized and undiagnosed in most people with the condition, can lead to diabetes and obesity. It is a malfunction of carbohydrate metabolism whereby blood glucose (blood sugar) reaches lower than normal levels. Glucose is the number-one nutrient needed by the brain. Therefore, when your blood sugar is too low, you can end up with brain fog or nervous system disorders. The main cause of low blood sugar is a diet high in refined carbohydrates. Unfortunately, when people get tired, they reach for sugary foods. That is the worst thing they can do, because all they will get will be a momentarily high blood sugar rush. After that, the blood sugar level becomes unstable, resulting in a roller-coaster ride of up and down levels. The end results will be fatigue, weakness, headaches, visual disturbances, allergy susceptibility, anxiety and mood swings, depression, yeast infections, and even asthma.

The protocol for hypoglycemia consists of cleansing the system and doing the other healthful things generally recommended on these pages. But you really have to be very careful: Any carbohydrate that goes into the body must be a quality complex carbohydrate. There can be no exceptions! Eat high-fiber foods. Vegetables and whole grains are good. Beans and nuts are extremely good. Sea vegetables, eaten several times a day, are recommended. And fish is valuable for its contributions in terms of protein, oils, and minerals. Also, with hypoglycemia it is very important to eat many small meals, rather than three large ones.

In addition, the healthy support of the liver is crucial. The liver stores glucose as glycogen and breaks it down in a process called glucogenesis. Certain botanicals, such as dandelion root, Siberian ginseng, and beet leaf, aid in the process. Celandine, methionine, and choline are other substances that help ensure the efficacy of the liver. Lipotropic factors help control blood sugar, as does chromium picolinate.

Adrenal support is also very important. The adrenal glands secrete stressor hormones. Vitamin C (in a large dosage) and pantothenic acid are important adrenal supporters; they also support the pancreas, which, involved as it is in insulin creation, plays a central role in sugar-level balancing.

A hypoglycemic individual definitely needs emotional support. If you have this condition, try different methods of calming yourself, from meditation to exercise to talking with supportive friends. Do not consume caffeine, which exacerbates low blood sugar, and may tend to make you nervous. Take B complex vitamins at 100 mg; this is needed and beneficial at this unusually high dosage, but after one month, bring the dosage down to 50 mg. Niacin, vitamin E, and the essential fatty acids are all important.

But above all, you must stay away from anything that will create a quick fix! Do not ever eat the simple carbohydrate foods that are absorbed too rapidly into the bloodstream.

Impotence. Impotence is a big problem for men. While cleaning up the body, rejuvenating the cells, and re-creating a vital life force will help, also try something perhaps a little esoteric: Get your chi rebalanced. Focus on what you want to do from this day forward in your life that honors your real self. Men in particular seem to suffer in silence. They hold in their emotions. They are not honoring their life. If asked, "Would you do everything over again, just the way you did it, if you had to start from scratch?" most people say "No. I'd do some things differently, but I made the choice. I made my bed; I've got to lie in it." This need not be true.

Today is a new day. So let us get our chi honored. Open up your chi, or life energy, to the reality that you can do what you want to do. You should be thinking in terms of future potential. Most baby boomers and senior citizens have had families and careers. This doesn't mean that one's career is now over. It doesn't mean the family is all gone. It means that now one can focus a primary amount of one's time on honoring oneself in a healthy way.

Start to include these nutrients: L-arginine at 10,000 mg a day, phosphatidyl choline at 1,000 mg a day, mura puama, oat ashwagandha, saw palmetto, ginkgo biloba, cinnamon, cardomom, anise, and yohimbe bark. Also, sunflower and other seeds, soaked in water for several hours, and lots of green juices, will help. All of these foods and nutrients can enhance circulation and libido. I have seen some major improvements in that area when people have used this protocol properly. Men with prostate conditions should follow this program, and, in addition, consider taking stinging nettle, pygeum africanum, cat's claw, marshmallow, hydergine, garlic, cayenne, and lemon juice.

Menopausal Problems. I would direct women going through menopause to the book *For Women Only*, by Barbara Seaman and me. It has probably got the most definitive information on menopause imaginable. Another helpful book by Barbara Seaman is *Women's Health Solutions*. It is in your local library or available at bookstores, and has an enormous amount of information on natural hormone balancing. But let's summarize. Herbs that can help rebalance hormones, thereby reducing hot flashes, include dong quai, angelica, licorice root, chaste berry (Vitex), black cohosh, skullcap, wild yam, motherwort, valerian, burdock root, damiana, gotu kola, Siberian ginseng, hops, ginger, shizandra, and muira puama.

Other aids when you have menopausal problems are vitamin C—from 5 to 10 grams a day, and flax and borage seed oil. Also, you want to drink lots of berry juices, because all the berries—raspberries, cherries, blueberries, cranberries, and blackberries—taken in a 16 oz juice every morning, are very rich in phytochemicals and low in calories. In addition, watermelon juice is wonderfully healthy!

Other supplements to discuss with your health care practitioner include vitamin E (400 to 800 units); primrose oil (500 mg); pantothenic acid (500 mg); and boron (3 mg). In addition, consider SAMe, calcium magnesium from citrate, L-arginine, L-lysine, selenium, DHEA at 25 mg, aloe vera, and alpha-lipoic acid at 500 mg.

Make sure your supplementation is added onto the good foundation of a vegetarian diet that includes some soy products. That way, you'll be maximizing the condition of your skin and hair, your muscle strength, your libido, and your energy level, as well as minimizing hot flashes.

Finally, exercise makes all the difference in the world.

Muscle and Nerve Problems. People with muscle and nerve health problems should eat potassium-rich foods, such as broccoli, beans, whole grains, and bananas. Sea vegetables are very important, as are the herbs horsetail, oat straw, valerian, and passionflower. Also helpful are: quercetin (2,000 mg); vitamin C (5 to 10 grams); arnica mantana (a homeopathic supplement); B complex vitamins (50 mg); pantothenic acid; grape seed extract; N-acetyl-cysteine; phosphatidyl choline (1,000 mg); phosphatidyl serine (1,000 mg); acetyl-L-carnitine (1,000 mg); and L-carnosine (1,000 to 2,000 mg). I find that magnet therapy, yoga, meditation, biofeedback, and chiropractic adjustment also help with this.

Muscle fatigue can be lessened with red clover, squaw vine (200 mg), magnesium (1,500 mg), vitamin K (generally at 10 mg), potassium (500 mg), and cayenne (10 to 15 mg). The Epsom salt bath is an old standby technique that can help, and deep tissue massage is beneficial as well.

Osteoporosis. We often hear about older people who fall down and break their hips. For people with osteoporosis, it is more of a compound snapping of the hips, which are already disintegrating before the fall. With osteoporosis, bones are porous, the skeletal system is very weakened, and so fractures are particularly serious. This situation is common in postmenopausal women, but it is totally unnecessary.

To deal with osteoporosis a balanced form of calcium must be put into our bodies, our hormones must be rebalanced, and our musculoskeletal systems strengthened. We have to have an alkaline pH level in the blood because acidic blood—induced by eating excess sugar, refined carbohydrates, animal protein, and caffeine, as well as by stress and hazardous waste products in our environment—fosters osteoporosis. This occurs because if the pH level of the blood is too acidic, the parathyroid glands are forced to balance this level by releasing calcium from the bones.

A family history of osteoporosis predisposes people to this condition, but there is a preventive program you can undertake that entails changes in diet, the addition of nutrients, and exercise.

The Anti-Osteoporosis Diet. In order to preserve your bones, meat, caffeine, sugar, and refined carbohydrates should be eliminated from your diet, because these substances chelate calcium out. On the other hand, green vegetables, sea vegetables, root vegetables, sunflower and sesame seeds, and nuts need to be included, to add calcium. At least five servings of green vegetables, such as broccoli, kale, brussels sprouts, collard greens, and arugula, should be eaten daily. It is interesting to note that women in Asia rarely have osteoporosis, because their calcium and magnesium come from sea vegetables. Contrary to popular belief, dairy products, which are hardly ever consumed by these women, are not the best sources of calcium. Large quantities of green juices are an important component of the preventive diet.

The significance of water is not to be underestimated. Ideally, water should constitute 70 to 74 percent of our body weight. Taking an impedance test will enable you to determine what percentage of your body is water. Many people with osteoporosis have a very low moisture content, resulting in a loss of strength and energy, a weakening of the immune system, and an increase in inflammation, as well as an increase in the osteoporotic condition.

Bone-Saving Nutrients. The following nutrients are great for assimilating calcium into our bones: vitamin D_3 at 300 units, vitamin B_6 at 20 mg, folic acid at 200 micrograms, calcium and magnesium from citrate at 500 mg, oat straw at 15 mg, and trimethylglycine (TMG) at 100 mg. Also, make sure you have 10 mg of vitamin K and 50 mg of fiber in your diet daily. With a good vegetarian diet, you will.

Vitamin C is crucial to the health of the bones. Herbs that are valuable sources of calcium and vitamin C are nettle, dandelion, and horsetail. Also, alpha-lipoic acid at 300 to 400 mg and N-acetyl-cysteine are valuable because they contribute greatly to building a strong immune system.

To balance our hormones, DHEA, at about 25 mg, is crucial because this master hormone diminishes in the later years of life. For women, synthetic hormones have been widely prescribed; however, natural progesterone, often obtained from wild yams, is preferable. It can be rubbed on the soft tissue of the spinal region for a period of approximately two weeks each month. Also, eating a lot of vegetables and red fruits, and drinking a lot of vegetable and fruit juice, will provide you with the phytonutrients that feed the phytoestrogens that in turn help produce the hormones needed to achieve hormonal balance as we age.

Homeopathy can also help osteoporosis. Calcarea phosphorica can be relied upon for extended periods of time for the treatment of soft, weak, and brittle bones. This homeopathic remedy should be administered at a potency of 200 C for acute pain; people with chronic symptoms should begin treatment with about 12 to 30 C. The recommended potencies should be administered in groups of three to four pellets placed under the tongue and consumed on an empty stomach. I am opposed to all types of steroids that are given because they are traumatic to the body and depress the immune system.

Exercise for Skeletal Health. Weight-bearing exercises are very important to help avoid osteoporosis. Weight lifting, including curls and bench presses, is a beneficial activity. Women should not resist going to gyms as they age. But even if you don't go to a gym, you can still profit from taking a little one-pound weight and curling it throughout the day. In fact, you can take a five-minute break every hour to do exercises. Dancing, stair-climbing, and brisk walking are all weight-bearing exercises, which promote mechanical stress in the skeletal system, contributing to the placement of calcium in the bones. Aerobic exercises such as biking, rowing, and swimming do not strengthen the bones, although they do promote cardiovascular fitness and enhance flexibility and range of motion, which are important too. Warming up, cooling down, and taking your time while stretching should be integral parts of a workout.

If you're concerned about preventing falls, remember that yoga is effective at extending range of motion, stretching muscles, and promoting relaxation, all of which are going to help keep you balanced and on your feet.

Urinary Tract Infections. Urinary tract infection (UTI), also known as bladder infection, is another condition that does not get the attention it deserves. It is a large problem for people in the baby boomer to senior citizen age range, for young sexually active women, and for people with multiple sclerosis and other neurological disorders. Studies show that 8 to 10 percent of women over sixty contract bladder infection at some time in their later years. Although many sexually active women contract bladder infections at some point in their lives, there are large numbers of females who seem to magically escape this irritating problem.

A cause for UTI is trapped bacteria that develop in the large intestines and contaminate the nearby urethra and vagina. An explanation for this condition is hormonal imbalance. Estrogen and progesterone, which reinforce the urethral cells, attract and entrap bacteria that are propelled into the region. Under normal circumstances the invasive bacteria are expelled during urination, but in women with hormonal imbalances the bacteria are not discharged effectively, thus setting the stage for bladder infections. Therefore, women who have experienced menopause are often susceptible to this condition. Their reduced levels of estrogen tend to enhance the adhesive qualities of the urethral lining, which prevents proper bacterial emissions.

A weakened immune system is another factor in the development of UTI. In this scenario widespread reproduction of bacteria is encouraged because the immune system cannot effectively combat the growth. Faulty nutritional habits, prolonged exposure to stress, or the occurrence of a traumatic situation can debilitate the immune system, increasing the chances of illness.

Another prominent cause of UTI is weakened pelvic muscles, which often result after childbirth. The bladder, as a consequence, protrudes closer to the vagina and the rear position of the bladder sags below its neck. The bladder cannot drain properly, so stagnant urine accumulates and bacterial communities grow.

Persistent bowel problems have been correlated with recurrent UTIs. Our bodies eliminate wastes in several ways, including the excretion of feces by the bowels, the expulsion of carbon dioxide by the lungs, perspiration by the skin, and the discharge of urine by the kidneys and bladder. If any of these processes is malfunctioning, an excessive burden is placed upon the other systems. I do not believe that antibiotics are the proper treatment for UTIs because they do not get to the underlying cause. The proper approach is to rebalance the system by switching from an acidic diet to an alkaline one. Unsweetened cranberry juice with cherries and raspberries, four to five times a day, can ameliorate the severe pain. Pomegranate juice, two times a day, and grapefruit juice with the seeds and the skins are valuable too. Lemon, lime, and bee propolis with 10 drops of colloidal silver are also helpful. Because of the vitamin C content, these juices will create acidic urine (but not acid in the body), which creates an unfavorable environment for bacteria in the urine and bladder. Chlorophyll from spirulina is exceptionally good for the body as well.

Recommended vitamins and minerals are vitamin C, vitamin A, and zinc. Actually, the best treatment is intravenous vitamin C, for which you have to go to a doctor. An extremely high dose of up to 50,000 or 75,000 mg streaming through the body will eliminate a lot of negative bacteria. Buffered vitamin C, taken daily in doses as high as 20,000 mg, will also create the necessary acidity in the urine. But if you're going to do this, start with 1,000 mg, increase the dosage gradually, and be sure to use a buffered vitamin to avoid the diarrhea or upset stomach that sometimes accompanies large doses of vitamin C. Vitamin A fortifies the mucous membranes lining the bladder, and zinc, at a dose of 25 to 50 mg, stimulates the proper amount of white blood cell production and eliminates bacteria.

Other nutrients that are crucial to this process are alpha-lipoic

acid, N-acetyl-cysteine, cysteine, and glutathione. Garlic and onion in massive quantities cannot be underestimated. Antiseptic herbs such as buchu, uva ursi, and juniper help stop the onset of cystitis. Marshmallow root, which is actually corn syrup, is also good because it is a demulcent, which soothes the mucous membranes of the urethra. Natural diuretics such as parsley, cabbage and celery juices, burdock, fennel, and slippery elm taken two to three times a day are also helpful. Teas—and green teas in particular—taken two or three times a day, are especially good.

Participating in an aerobic activity such as jogging, race walking, swimming, or bicycling will enhance circulation, which aids in eliminating blood congestion in the pelvic area. Inverted-position exercises such as yoga headstands and shoulder stands, and rotating the legs in a bicycle-like motion while lying on the back also provide improved circulation in that region. If performing these exercises causes back or neck pain, support the body with an old door or a couple of wooden boards that are braced with one end on your couch and the other end on the floor. Lying on the board with your legs and feet at the higher end will transport the blood from the pelvic region to the head. Additional treatments that both enhance blood flow and allow for the removal of toxins from the pelvic region are sitz baths, hot compresses, and therapeutic massage.

Varicose Veins. Varicose veins are almost always due to circulatory problems. And these circulatory problems are, in turn, connected to liver problems, in the following way: Blood circulates through the liver, and so if the liver is congested, the entire venous system can back up, which, in turn, adds pressure on the veins, damages heart valves, and results in varicose veins.

Milk thistle is an extremely beneficial herb for the liver. Other herbs helpful for this organ are dandelion root, bilberry extract, red clover, and gotu kola. Foods that support the liver are burdock root, artichoke, and dark-skinned fruits and berries. So eating dark-skinned fruits such as blueberries, cherries, and grapes, and drinking cherry juice, are ways to tackle circulatory problems. Horse chestnut, butcher's

broom, vitamin E with tocotrienols, and vitamin C with quercetin are beneficial for veins and feet.

Alternative therapies such as chelation therapy, massage of the legs, and magnetic wraps are helpful for varicose veins. Since so many people suffer from varicose veins, it is unfortunate that they remain unaware of the varied alternative treatments available. Even Epsom salts can make a difference.

Deep varicose veins are characterized by red and brownish markings, white dots, and especially dark concentrated areas above the ankle and on the lower leg. Skin discolorations are warning signs of serious circulatory problems or heart valves that are not functioning properly. Varicose veins can be both a result of other problems, and accompanied by them.

As the veins swell, the legs and feet can become plagued by itching, and sores can develop that become open or ulcerated wounds, a serious problem. Another common outcome of varicose veins is phlebitis, characterized by inflammation within veins and clotting of blood. If a blood clot breaks away from a vein, a sudden stroke or heart attack can ensue. Vitamin E, vitamin C, and chelation therapy can all alleviate the suffering associated with varicose veins.

A NOTE ON FINDING THE RIGHT ALTERNATIVE HEALTH PRACTITIONER

Throughout the book, I've constantly advised people to work in concert with their doctors. Thus, finding the right holistic practitioner is absolutely key to wellness. Deciding on a practitioner could be one of the most important decisions that you make, one that could affect—and enrich—the rest of your life. A good alternative practitioner is invaluable in determining where the weaknesses are in your body, and essential in creating your optimal personalized program of care.

There are approximately 88,000 holistic practitioners in the United States. These include chiropractors, herbalists, naturopaths, medical doctors, homeopaths, and nutritionists. They should be certified, and insured as well, and must understand how to work with you. Do not

be afraid to ask all the questions you have to to get the information you want. This is your right, and your responsibility to yourself.

You may consider the following issues when you are shopping for an alternative practitioner:

- Are you seeking a practitioner who believes in noninvasive diagnostic treatments, i.e., administered intravenously or orally?
- Does the practitioner offer alternative treatments with recommendations and insights?
- Does this practitioner recognize the importance of even the smallest symptoms regardless of whether they seem directly/ indirectly related to the condition at hand?
- Does the practitioner strive to rebalance and to build up the immune system in his/her program to strengthen the overall bodily systems?
- Does this practitioner take a thorough family history?
- Does the practitioner demonstrate a sensitivity and awareness as to the role of an individual's attitude toward health and wellness?

PART IV

MORE HELP

CHAPTER 12

TECHNIQUES TOWARD TRANSFORMATION

Affirmations for Bringing the Magic and Passion Back to Life

U p until this point I have covered mostly physical approaches toward optimal health and wellness. Now let us look at an equally important aspect of well-being: psychological conditioning through affirmations and goal-setting. If you are suffering from stress, anxiety, or depression, or are just a constant worrier, please pay extra attention to this section. Reread it on a monthly basis to help refocus.

Each day, we are bombarded with commercial advertisements that tell us what to wear, what to eat, and worst of all, how we should feel about ourselves depending on whether or not we are using the product that is being promoted. For example, how are senior citizens being portrayed in television advertisements? From what I've seen, if the ads aren't trying to sell them a drug, medical insurance, or legal services in case they fall, they're portraying seniors as people on the last leg of their journey through life who are now in need of diapers (for themselves) as they experience their single joy in life—their grandchildren. And these images surround us wherever we look. I'm a grandfather and I love my grandchildren, but my life remains ever-expanding with purpose because I know in my heart, as well as intellectually, that if I'm not growing, I'm dying.

So this multibillion-dollar industry of advertising has been built on the precept that clever repetition of thoughts can manipulate human behavior for profit. And to put it simply: It works like a charm! In addition to this power of words and images, we have a store of impressions from throughout our lives that impact every move and breath we take. Even our physical postures are often imitations of examples that surround us. You might think: What's wrong with the way I breathe or the way I stand? Well, you might be emulating someone else's slouch, which would then be negatively affecting your spine. Are you aware of why you breathe or stand the way you do? What if you were born and raised on the other side of the globe, let's say—if you are in the United States—in China? Do you think that your walking, breathing, and eating habits would be the same as they are now? Or do you think that you would have grown up subconsciously trying to emulate one or both of your parents, your friends, or leading authorities and idols of your native land? And if these icons were Chinese, would your ingrained physical patterns then not be more Chinese than American in form? I believe they would be, regardless of your genetic makeup.

In other words, we are the way we are largely due to a lifelong battery of subconscious conditioning from our surroundings and impressions. This is actually a powerful testament to the strength of the human survival instinct. The brain has an ability to seek out whatever it concentrates its focus on, subconsciously, especially if one's survival is connected to it. Why do you think sex in advertisements sells products so well? It's because the reptilian core of the brain controls our sex drive. And it is at that core level of reaction that people are being influenced by advertisements, which commonly connect sex with survival. The idea in those ads is that if we don't use the product advertised, then our attraction to the opposite sex, which we need in order to procreate, will be diminished. On the other hand, if we use the product suggested, we will be fulfilling our aim of survival through procreation. It's a clever trick!

IT'S TIME FOR "INNER ADVERTISING"!

So how do we overcome unwanted commercial influences? We simply have to create our own "inner advertising." By doing so, we override the nonstop external bombardment that keeps trying to manipulate our lives. And by doing so, we can direct our lives in the way that we want instead of just accepting assumptions and circumstances that are dictated to us. But in order to create this personal, inner advertising, daily work is required. First of all, we must get clear on what our aims are in life on all levels—personal, business, emotional, and spiritual. And the best way to do this is to *begin writing*! Here's what I recommend:

Outlining Goals

1. On three separate pages (ideally three sections in a notebook), outline what your goals are personally, professionally, and financially. Try to dedicate ten minutes to each category. Do it now!
2. Don't continue beyond this point if you haven't done step one.
3. Put deadlines next to each aim. Categorize your aims into one-year or shorter goals, two-year goals, five-year goals, ten-year goals, and twenty-year goals. Take about three minutes to complete each category.
4. Finally—and this is probably the most important step—state a reason in writing why you *must* attain the aims that you've set forth. Try to look deep inside yourself and ask yourself: What might my life be like if I don't attain my goals? Create *on paper* a "have to" situation. It's only when you really have to do something that you can put all of yourself into its attainment. Now, if you're thinking, I'm too old to set goals, well, then remember—if you're not growing, you're dying! And one way to ensure growth is to plan on it.

So let's review the steps to take in more detail, from a slightly different viewpoint.

Getting started:

- Prepare an outline of what you want to change or achieve, whether in your health, finances, relationships, etc.
- Do due diligence—research—do homework. Know exactly what you want to achieve and the magnitude of the achievement in relation to where you are right now. Devise a "procedure list" of steps that you *must* take in order to attain your aim. Review these steps on a daily basis and take individual steps from your procedure list as part of your daily tasks. Do not tackle more than three tasks per day. And if you find that you slip one day and don't even remember to look at your list, that's OK. Just hop back on track the next day. Don't shoot for perfection—perfection does not exist in our world. Just look around in nature. Nature isn't perfect. This can be observed by the fact that there are no straight lines in nature. Look at the leaf of a tree or the ridge of a mountain. These objects are as unique as you or I. And while their physical forms seem almost abstractly beautiful, perfection would indicate a consistency in form, so they are most certainly not perfect—just like you or me. Try to look at life in a similar light; perhaps it can't be perfect in its results, although you may get close to your aim (if you have one), but each step through life can be as objectively beautiful as a mountain view or a virgin river if we see it for what it is.
- Prepare yourself for the challenges by committing to your goal on a daily basis. Keep your outline in front of you daily and review it, knowing full well that distractions may come your way in that day.
- Create a process of confidence by using positive affirmations.
- Begin with small changes. Remember to always "group" your

steps—meaning, do not overwhelm yourself with too many things. Try to keep your steps to no more than the three most important goals for the day. Consider three steps as one group of achievements.

• Accept that you cannot control all results and that, possibly, you will make mistakes most of the time. Realize that that's OK, mistakes are a way that we can learn what not to do in the future. It's been said that success is a result of good judgment. Good judgment is the result of experience. And experience is the result of bad judgment! So don't be afraid to mess up because it can ultimately lead to success.

• Look at the gains, even when the results are *not* what you expected or wanted.

• Be flexible—refocus, reformulate. If something isn't working, notice what is not working. Refocus on your goal and find another path with the realization that it's not the path that you must focus on but the achievement of your goal that you *must* attain.

• Remember that when you commit to something positive in life, there will always be equal and opposite energy coming your way. The more you try to achieve a result the more obstacles will appear. This is a law of nature! These obstacles are life's tests, which are not the same as "life's failures"—unless you decide to just not take the tests of life. Remember: If you don't take the test, you instantly fail. In a sense, these obstacles are saying: Let's see if you can keep with your goal! Let's see if you're awake to the *real* forces in life. If you can see obstacles as gifts that help you push to a higher level, then life can be a miraculous and deeply fulfilling experience in the hardest of times.

• Change the way you see yourself to a more "can-do, will-do, will-learn, can-grow" self. Ask yourself, What can I do next? What can I do today? These can be aims in and of themselves.

Resolving Pain and Resentment

In order to be in the moment, you must let go and resolve past pain. The following exercises are helpful in resolving pain and resentment.

- Don't make excuses for the person who hurt you.
- Don't use shame, guilt, or revenge. Just forgive them.
- Forgive—and gain. Once again, when you for-*give*, an equal and opposite energy will come your way. This is just a rule in life that must be accepted and observed. So when you give, you will receive. You have no control over when and what you will receive but rest assured that there is no wasted energy in this universe. The universe is very ecological. This is the ecology of Karma.

Following are affirmation and meditation suggestions. Of course the best affirmations come from you. And remember to write down your affirmations in a specially devoted notebook. Or if you don't have a notebook, write on a piece of paper that your first affirmation is: "I have a dedicated notebook where I write my aims and desires. I review this book, daily." Get the picture? Then go out and buy the notebook! There should be no excuses to not move forward in attempts at growth. You just need to reach down inside and begin with the emotions of *must change*! Review your aims, desires and affirmations, daily, for at least fifteen minutes. Then, during your daily workout (power walking, weight lifting or your choice of fitness), you can focus on your affirmations while gaining energy through the exercise. This may result in the ability to emote your desire(s) for your aim as you push through your physical activity. Don't just repeat your thoughts, put emotions behind them. If you can't find the emotions to put behind them, then either your aim is not important enough to you, in which case you need a new aim, or you need to really search for other reasons why you "have to" attain your aim.

Please begin your journal now! Don't put it off. Think about what you want in your life.

Do you want:

- Joy every day?
- Loving relationships?
- More money—how much more?
- To help feed the hungry?
- Powerful friendships?
- Passion in your work?
- To write music?
- To write a novel?

Make your list today! Please believe in the powerfully transformative process of "getting clear" with yourself in all areas of your life and organizing your thoughts on paper. I wish you much success on your journey. . . .

AFFIRMATIONS AND THOUGHTS

I am powerfully silent.

I easily release negativity from my life.

Each morning I repeat—ten times, out loud, with passion—
   my goals and dreams as if they have already happened.

I expect the best from life.

I see and feel myself as financially prosperous.

I am full of life.

I live with integrity.

My honesty brings me great fortune, peace of mind, and
   rewards.

I am a person who always chooses to see the good in others, as
   I know we are all individuals on our own spiritual journey.

I approach every action I take as responsibly as if I were being
   paid money to do it!

I am only in competition with myself.

Every day in every way I'm getting better and better.

Investing love and caring in what I do adds to the quality of my work.

The real measure of my wealth is how much I would be worth if I lost all my money.

Every night I give thanks for everything I now have and for all the blessings I am receiving.

I take care of my physical well-being and strive toward balance and serenity.

I visualize success! If I can see it, I can achieve it.

Now more than ever before, I add positive energy into the world consciousness.

My thoughts are powerful!

I use my power for myself, my loved ones, and our world!

When I look in the mirror I see beauty, grace, and strength.

I am willing to do whatever it takes to transform my life.

I am willing to release all my resistance to change.

I vow to eliminate all toxic circumstances from my life.

I value my body and commit to only nourishing it with healthy living foods.

I wake up each day with optimism and joy.

I look at each crisis in my life as an opportunity for growth and learning.

CHAPTER 13

VOICES OF EXPERIENCE

Testimonials of Life Change

Over the past ten years I've conducted numerous health studies with more than ten thousand participants throughout the country. The programs that led to the following testimonials are simple, systematic approaches to living life more naturally. And although we had great successes even in the first few years of our groups, new techniques and information have become available during the past decade, making the programs progressively more effective. For example, potent antiaging nutrients have emerged during this span of time. I am glad to have been able to present that information in this material. This book is the culmination of new technologies and approaches toward life extension and overall wellness. I hope you are inspired by the sincere words offered in this chapter.

Job/ / / / 71 years old

My mother introduced me to good diet and healthy living. Although I listened to Gary Null for twenty-three years I did not actualize. I weighed 210 pounds, smoked three packs of cigarettes a day, drank alcohol, felt de-

pressed, and had knee pains and upper respiratory infections. One day I looked at the very aged man in the mirror and was shocked.

Today I follow the protocol and use green chlorophyll powder and red fruit powder. The shakes keep me feeling full and satisfied all day. I drink "clean" water, use supplements, and feel terrific. I did not get a cold in five years—no more upper respiratory infections. I am organic-vegan. I do not take vaccines. My neighbors tell me I look forty-five years old. They admire my changes. I appreciate my healthy lifestyle. It makes me quite aware of the tremendous amount of obesity today. I am confident and pleased with my life.

Jessie////86 years old

I am an eighty-six-year-old woman. My blood pressure was high. My energy was very low. I felt old. My hands were full of age spots. I felt quite discouraged. I joined a Gary Null support group. Once I felt the impact of group interaction I began to feel optimistic about my future.

I keep to Gary's protocol. My emotional and physical changes are wonderful. I feel younger and free. I eat organically; I juice and exercise multiple times a week. My blood pressure has lowered and energy has increased. The age spots are lighter. My physical improvements created emotional improvements.

I am grateful for this second chance.

Charles////69 years old

My journey toward improving my health began when I attended a Gary Null seminar. I worked in construction as an ironworker and had several accidents. During my younger years I held several jobs at a time and developed hypertension. It was time to rebuild my physical system. I considered my energy to be adequate for an aging man.

I gradually investigated organic foods and vegetarian replacements for flesh foods. My health is maintained with supplements, lifting weights, gar-

dening, and drinking power shakes with red and green powders. I still work in building and construction and just built a playhouse for my grandchildren.

Listening to health programs on the radio gave me some information; however, following today's healthier lifestyle and taking proper products supplies me with more energy than I have ever had. I bounce back easily from exhaustion. Except for a constant knee condition, I do not feel the consequences of falling off buildings. I do not have hypertension anymore.

My family does not follow or cooperate with my food preparation. I prepare my meals separately and enjoy them. Hopefully, one day my grandchildren will open to this healthy concept. I feel younger than my sixty-nine years and look forward to a happy future.

Alice////73 years old

When I came into a Gary Null health support group, I had an acute allergy from cortisone injections into my scalp for alopecia. I had many upper respiratory infections during the year. I needed to sleep long hours to feel rested. My eyes were dry, a condition which was annoying and uncomfortable.

It took a while to adjust to my new eating plan. I never realized true taste before. My body felt cleaner after a month. Best of all, I no longer have alopecia. Symptoms of the cortisone allergy are subsiding. My eyes are healthier. I wake up refreshed, full of energy, with less sleep.

I am uncluttering my home environment, drinking green drinks, and rereading the group class assignments. When I think of where I was before, I am ecstatic about where I am now.

Alston////90 years old

I retired from the merchant marine at age sixty-five. I have always been very active and healthy but considered my future health. I heard Gary Null on the radio and began to read books on health and nutrition.

I follow a vegetarian diet and juicing. I use a rebounder every morning.

I get on the train and travel to Manhattan to buy supplements. Most people my age cannot do this. As a matter of fact, I do not see many people my age these days. Most of them have caretakers and are dependent. I am totally self-sufficient. I care for my home, shop, wash my clothes, even remove my curtains to wash, and stand on a ladder to replace them. I do not need anyone to take care of me. I can accomplish my tasks alone.

I believe my diet and nutritional supplements are responsible for maintaining my health.

Warnetta////78 years old

I listened to Gary's show many years before I actualized the information.

My cholesterol and blood pressure were elevated but my primary concern was obesity—my weight was 209. I wore a size 22 and was diagnosed with an underactive thyroid, low energy, osteoporosis, osteoarthritis, cataracts, and carpal tunnel syndrome. Gary explained that detoxification must precede dieting to be effective. That made a lot of sense to me so I went with the protocol.

Today I weigh 150 pounds and maintain it. Recent physical examinations ruled out an abnormal thyroid, carpal tunnel syndrome, and cataracts. I take lutein and blueberry capsules and threaded a fine needle today without difficulty. My cholesterol and blood pressure are slightly elevated but not abnormal. I have no symptoms of osteoarthritis or osteoporosis. I exercise three times a week with a senior class in a Buddhist temple. I buy organic food, and stopped eating meat and eat fish. Ingredient labels shocked me. I am more aware of the unnecessary amount of salt in products. I explain these concepts to people interested in regaining their health.

I am determined to enjoy life in good health and with positive energy.

Athena////60 years old

I had premenstrual syndrome, which caused fatigue, pain, and depression. I also had cystic breasts and eye floaters. My hair was getting gray. I chose bad relationships and had an unpleasant job. I decided to join a health support group. [Previously] nothing seemed to improve my life and current group members spoke of improvements and regaining health.

Today I have no signs of premenstrual syndrome. I do not feel cysts in my breasts. Although I do get tired, the fatigue has lessened, and feelings of depression were gone within six weeks on the protocol. My eye floaters seem to be diminishing and I notice fewer new gray hairs.

I uncluttered all bad relationships, and I allow myself to be close to people and found a new job at a higher wage that I enjoy.

Joanne////64 years old

I was diagnosed with chronic fatigue syndrome. I was always exhausted and had many allergies. I did not follow any food plan and was a coffee drinker. I listened to Gary Null on the radio and read Who Are You Really? *When an allergy support group opened up, I joined. At that time I took time away from work to recover.*

I have had excellent results following Gary's protocol. I need less sleep, and am alert and aware of nutrition. I no longer drink coffee. My allergies are practically neither nonexistent nor are signs of chronic fatigue present.

Writing forgiveness letters relieved the weight of anger I held and I detached from a painful past. I live in the present. Uncluttering was unpleasant but helped me think clearly. I am actualizing my sense of community responsibility. I now give "professionalism and quality of life" seminars. My husband is supportive of my new lifestyle.

Dolly////61 years old

Although we considered ourselves nutritionally aware and healthy for seniors, my husband and I felt "something" was missing. I had Bell's palsy and low energy. We knew our lives and health could improve but found no satisfaction in traditional guidelines. We did not want our vitality to diminish as we aged. After hearing Gary Null on the radio we decided to join one of the first Reversing the Aging support groups.

We easily followed the protocol cold turkey. We also had vitamin drips. We eliminated all meat, dairy, and chicken in our diet. We are now organic and vegetarian, using air, water, and shower filters. We have magnetic appliances. Our amalgam fillings were removed and our home is healthier by removing our shoes at the door. When a neurologist confirmed I had Bell's palsy I had a consult with Gary.

We meditate, practice yoga, and run. Our physician daughter now runs. I am a nurse teacher and busier than ever. We feel great by juicing, using green, red, and protein powders. Bell's palsy symptoms subsided within ten days of the protocol. Our energy is strong and our bodies feel vital and healthy. We use alternative physicians.

The program was very successful for us.

Fran////67 years old

I joined a health support group and followed Gary Null's protocol when obvious and unpleasant signs of aging became too uncomfortable. My skin was sagging and moles grew on it. There were dark age spots on my body. Energy decreased. My LDL and HSL elevated. My hair changed color and I felt my mental function was slowing. The group was a total lifestyle enhancement. The people were optimistic. I influenced them. They influenced me.

Today my skin is tight and great; I am more youthful in looks and attitude. The moles fell off. Age spots are gone. My new hair growth is dark brown. LDL and HDL went to zero risk. I have energy galore and my mental function improved from the protocol.

I feel absolutely wonderful.

Gloria////73 years old

I was hypoglycemic. I used dairy and wheat, and ate flesh foods. My concentration and mental clarity were poor. My energy was low and I suf-

fered from many upper respiratory infections. I joined the year and a half support group because I was a college senior and required extra energy to complete my degree.

Today things are quite different. I lost eight pounds and am now size 4 or 6. I feel energetic and do not experience frequent upper respiratory infections. My physician confirmed I do not need stronger glasses. My skin has fewer wrinkles and appears to be brighter. My hair is thicker. I use juices throughout the day without a desire for meals. I learned to honor myself and develop solutions for daily problems by keeping a positive outlook. I am an active walker. I convinced my daughter to use an alternative physician for my granddaughter who was diagnosed psychotic. The child returned to school within two weeks.

Jean////64 years old

I was diagnosed with lung cancer. I was anemic and had arthritis, almost no energy, and elevated blood pressure. Pain went through me when I walked. I underwent radiation, chemotherapy, and body scans. I was ready for a life change but was not certain where to go or whom to see. After hearing Gary Null on television and radio I was curious and joined a health support group.

I ate flesh foods and used dairy. Today I am vegan. I drink green juices and follow the protocol. I am cancer free without medication. My arthritis has diminished and I can use and enjoy my body by walking, doing yoga, and working in the wardrobe department of a theatrical company. I look forward to a good season with the crew. I am delighted with the results of each new blood test.

The class homework motivated me to go forward, made me understand my former pitfalls and myself. I have personal insight. Sounds good to me!

John////71 years old

I developed psoriatic arthritis thirty years ago and had surgery to fuse my right wrist. My knees and neck were deteriorating. I used heavy medications and over the counter analgesics. The physician advised me to change careers. My daughter motivated me to join a health support group.

I am vegan (no sugar or wheat). I make and drink green vegetable and fruit juices. I was pain free within four weeks. I do not need medication. The swelling subsided. My doctor commented that my knee joints are the best he has observed. My blood pressure is normal and at last I can take long walks. I have reclaimed life.

My neighbors now follow the protocol. One couple, a diabetic and his wife with multiple sclerosis, report physical improvements. My cousin lost ten pounds in two weeks and no longer has heartburn.

Lillian////76 years old

I was a sculptor and inhaled chemicals and clay dust. I also smoked and was exposed to asbestos. I was adjusting to a new life after my husband's death but I had many physical disabilities. I needed a leg brace for torn ligaments in my knee. My energy was slowly declining, my hair thinning, I was obese and ate flesh foods, dairy, and sugar. I was diagnosed with emphysema, Epstein-Barr, and bronchiocytosis. Life was getting very difficult.

I listened to Gary's radio show for ten years. The world of alternative health and healing opened to me. I began to take supplements and change my diet, and I underwent chelation therapy. I joined a support group and listened to the wonderful speakers at each meeting. My response to the food on the protocol was immediate and positive.

Today I am organic and vegan. Everything tastes so good; I create wonderful desserts with fresh fruit, honey and nuts. I no longer need a leg brace. My hair is thicker, my skin is lovely, and my pulmonary problems have lessened. I lost eight pounds and will continue the loss. I work several days a week and exercise by swimming and walking. I huff and puff during the walks but continue and congratulate myself when it is over. Without this protocol I would have been taking an antibiotic one week per month for the rest of my life.

Marcia////77 years old

I was overweight. My thinning hair turned white. I lost pubic and under-arm hair after menopause. My energy was low and I felt unhappy about entering "old age." I thought: "Is this me? Is this my body?"

I heard members of Gary's support groups speak of their experiences on his radio show and immediately made plans to join a group. I followed the protocol and did my journals and homework. Group members and I created an atmosphere for success.

Today the hair on my head is thick and my original color returned. Hair on my body parts is returning. My libido is as strong as it was in my early forties. I experience phenomenal energy and require only four to five hours of sleep a night. I teach love and sex workshops in two local colleges and lecture to singles groups. The health support group and protocol cer-tainly gave me an optimistic, healthy future.

Michael////62 years old

In 1989 I attended a Gary Null retreat. I learned the benefits of vegetar-ianism, juicing, taking supplements, and meditation.

In 1994 I became disabled because of carbon monoxide poisoning. I am still in the process of recovery. I no longer work. I cannot see computer screens. Surgery for two detached retinas affected my eyesight. My blood pressure was extremely high. My heartbeat accelerated to a dangerous level. I took several pharmaceutical drugs to control these conditions. A few years later seizures began with Alzheimer's-like symptoms. Abnormally severe edema in my legs incapacitated me. I was in a coma for sixty days. Nursing home care was considered. However, I rationally reconsidered and joined Gary's health support group.

My health soon improved as I followed the protocol. Juicing, stress management, and homework revealed my potentials and purpose in life. I discovered the best of what works and realized I was not doing anything worthwhile.

Today I no longer need a compressor for leg edema. My leg size decreased

30 percent. I sleep less, lost 23 pounds, and exercise with hand weights. I recently received a Bowflex to build my upper body. My blood pressure is lower. My brain speed seems to be faster. I feel like a teenager, just blossoming. Parts of my future plans include researching natural life energies.

Pat////72 years old

"I am a walking miracle."

I weighed 225 pounds. I was hospitalized three times for congestive heart disease. I also suffered from arthritis, diabetes, sciatica, and glaucoma. I lived in a wheelchair twenty-four hours a day on oxygen using steroids for emphysema. It was in this condition that I was wheeled into the Los Angeles Gary Null health support group to turn this unhappy life around.

Today I am not in pain from arthritis or discomfort with emphysema. I take long walks daily. I am an organic vegan carefully keeping to the protocol that revitalized my life. I lost weight and most of all I lost contact with the toxic situations and people that formerly kept me in the sick mode.

Rick////77 years old

I am following Gary Null's protocol for the past ten years now. My health has been severely challenged during that time and I have survived each assault. I had surgery many years ago for a hiatic hernia. My diet of vegetables and juices controls this condition.

My father and two sisters died from aortal abdominal aneurisms. My brother had one repaired successfully. I was diagnosed with this condition. Surgery was indicated. I prepared myself for six months with a specific protocol. This included a good vitamin regimen, mental and attitudinal insights, and healthy food.

During that time I obtained a copy of the surgical procedure from a medical library and realized it was an extensive operation. My internal *organs would be removed from my ribs to my pubic bone. My aorta had a balloon type defect, which would be opened and patched. My organs would then be replaced.*

I meditated on every organ in my body several times before surgery. I was relaxed before and after the procedure. I demanded my body to heal itself. My immune system was at its peak. I survived the surgery well, in excellent condition. I left intensive care in two days and took a bus home a few days later. My physicians were amazed. I explained how I obtained my strong immune system with diet, supplements, and respect for my body.

I am now in the process of creating the biggest project of my life: building the world's largest wind farm. Following the Gary Null protocol gave me the strength and energy I must call upon to complete this mission.

I encourage seniors to build your energies, both mental and physical, and create new goals, exercise, build your immune system, study, and be a part of your environment.

Ruth////75 years old

I have always been a busy person with an active career but I was plagued with frequent illnesses, especially upper respiratory infections.

I participated in a health support group two years ago. Before that my diet was quite unhealthy. I ate flesh foods, dairy, sugar, desserts, confections, and breads without regard for health or weight gain. I did not exercise. It was time to correct this imbalance of career and family vs. frequent illnesses. I wanted my energy back and decided to improve my life.

The initial phase of the detox was interesting. Eliminating "comfort" foods was difficult but so were my options. I stayed with the program. It was uncomfortable at times in restaurants. My friends devoured their toxic food while commenting on my fish and vegetable plate.

My hair and skin greatly improved. I have no more upper respiratory infections.

Today I am a person holding the tools for healthy aging. My eating companions are rapidly getting old. I work several days a week. I use a stationary bike and lift weights. It's wonderful to hear this positive feed-back. My grandson is proud of his attractive, vital grandmother. I am proud of myself.

Irene////66 years old

I lived in a very large home surrounded by years and years of lovely but nonessential objects. It was difficult keeping up with chores. My husband and I lived alone because our children are adults. I was overweight. I had high blood pressure, cardiac arrhythmia, high cholesterol, weak nails, and low energy. I felt this huge, cluttered space around me. I thought that it would be difficult changing my life. I grew accustomed to the way things were but I wanted to be free of physical disabilities and I wanted to feel healthy.

I joined a support group and lost thirty pounds. Changes came week by week. My blood pressure normalized. My cholesterol lowered. Energy began to move me mentally and physically. Eventually my arrhythmia ceased.

We sold our large home and gave our family the unessential, nostalgic items. We now live in a four-room home. We are much happier and I feel wonderful.

I let go of objects and let our future in.

Lino////78 years old

My life was going nowhere. I held myself back with bad habits and attitudes. I overused alcohol. I was overweight. Eating fatty flesh foods gave me an almost constant heartburn and fatigue. I felt anxious and angry and not at all content with myself. Gary's protocol was really a radical change. I never drank green juices. In fact, I never ate healthy food. I was not aware of nutrition or meditation. I did not care to look inward or deal with past angers and pain.

My life is very different today. I am vegan and organic. I gave alcohol up quickly. The green juices filled an empty space with vitality instead of dulling emotions. I lost thirty pounds. For some reason I feel less or no anger and am relaxed, even content. My eating plan is satisfying and there is no after heartburn.

I feel and act younger. I look back into my past and wonder why. It was not a lack of self-esteem; it was a lack of body cleansing, natural foods. I found myself.

Lou/ / / /76 years old

I had an unsuccessful quadruple bypass and five years later I was told that I had one month to live without another operation. Now, without the bypass, I underwent chelation therapy, vitamin C drips, and lifestyle changes that have all made a drastic improvement in my quality of life. I am very active now, walking five miles a day. I also dance two to three hours a day. And best of all I have no chest pains.

Alice/ / / /61 years old

I had my ovaries removed when I was in my forties. That caused extremely severe menopausal symptoms. I was told it would continue for the rest of my life. I felt extreme abdominal pain, which put me in a depression. Wrinkles and bags developed under my eyes. My energy was low and I had brain fog.

The support group and protocol changed all of the above. Because I followed the protocol, used juices, became vegan and organic and looked within, this woman is brand-new. My depression lifted. No more abdominal pain. My skin is less wrinkled and the under-eye bags are gone. I have an enormous amount of energy; the brain fog and cloudy thinking are gone. I realize I am more intelligent than I thought I was. It's as if vitamins and juices washed my brain. I can recommend the protocol with much love and enthusiasm.

Bob////80 years old

I seem to be one of those people who had to get sick before seeking a healthier lifestyle.

Before I heard of Gary Null's support groups I suffered headaches, allergies, and several colds and flus a year. Cholesterol and blood pressure were elevated. I ate junk food, pretending everything would work out. Personalitywise I was tense and often irritable.

Something had to change; I wanted that thing to be me.

I followed the protocol carefully. After a week my energy returned, I slept less, my headaches were gone, and blood pressure and cholesterol levels dropped.

I am calmer and more patient, far less irritable. My wife of forty years was a great support. We both benefited with my new health and are thankful we participated in this life-changing process.

Brian////60 years old

I was not certain vegetarianism and nutrients could help me. I was one of those tense corporate people having unpleasant personal relationships. There were pockmarks and eczema on my face. My hair was graying. My eye color changed to a darker shade. I was diagnosed with hypertension. My nails grew slowly. I also had a scar from an old wound that did not lighten.

My wife and I joined a support group with amazing results. Hypertension is a thing of the past. My skin had amazing results; no more eczema or facial pockmarks. My gray hair is growing new hair the color of my childhood blond and the receding hairline is reversing. My eyes returned to their blue color. Nails grew in quickly and the scar disappeared. I left the corporate world for a happier life and improved relationships.

Charles////64 years old

I ate the typical American diet: meat, dairy, sugars. I thought my primary health concern was not being able to gain weight.

One day I heard Gary Null on the radio and continued to listen to Gary's radio show. Gary presented valid research. Guests explained scientific evidence on issues I never before thought about. Support group members explained their experiences and life changes. They seemed energetic and happy. Many of these people were my age or older. Their testimonials influenced me to change my life.

I follow the protocol on my own from a book. I use green, red, and protein powders. I no longer put poison in my system by eating meat. Mine is a natural way of eating. I walk six to eight miles a day and use supplements.

The radio program "Natural Living with Gary Null" is my classroom on the air. I gather information daily and put it to use. My health is better today than it was during my younger years.

Doug////69 years old

I was overweight but considered myself healthy until an abnormal pre-op EKG for gall bladder surgery indicated cardiac problems. I had a quadruple bypass March 2000.

I saw Gary on television and purchased one of his videos and a book. After reading and watching the tape I joined a health support group. I investigated alternative methods to reclaim my health. I had twenty EDTA chelation treatments, became vegan, eliminated sugar, wheat, sodas, and gluten. I shop in a health food store to eliminate sprayed vegetables. I enjoy new information regarding healthier lifestyles.

Today I need only six hours of sleep per night, wake up to exercise each morning, and have my large meal midday. I enjoy sharing new insights with others. I am healthy without symptoms of cardiac disease or sinus problems. I am in a new business. I use green and red powders, supplements, protein powders, and magnets. I eliminated carpeting from my home.

I plan to study vegeterian cooking and create new recipes.

Thomas////70 years old

I was very interested in Gary Null's radio guests. Some of the people began their juicing and organic protocol because they had illnesses. They spoke about belonging to a group that gave them the strength to change. I needed that.

I am a Parkinson's patient. I had hypertension, B-simplex outbreaks, arthritis, and skin problems. I became aware of the importance of nutrition and studied various theories but my physical problems continued. Parkinson's symptoms caused shame in public. I could not write and I typed with two fingers. My hands trembled when I put food in my mouth. I was prescribed medications but past experiences were unpleasant so I refused them.

I began Gary's detoxification protocol and learned the specifics of diet and organics, the biochemical necessity of green juices and grasses, the importance of attitude and beliefs.

Things began to look up. I uncluttered my life of people and objects and I now honor myself and share my knowledge with others. I am alert without past negative influences. Green and red drinks keep me going.

These are my happiest and proudest times. I intend to live another seventy years.

References and Selected Bibliography

CHAPTER 1
1. Univ of CA—San Diego. Preliminary study shows high-dose of CoQ10 slows functional decline in Parkinson's patients. 2002 Oct 15.

CHAPTER 2
1. "The Holy Grail of Scientific Certainty." Rachel's Environment & Health Weekly #440. 1995 May 4.
2. Lancet. 1995 Jan 21;345.
3. Ramey, Paul F. Univ of FL. Medical experts war against carbon monoxide poisoning. 1998 Feb 11.
4. Pimentel, D, et al. Environmental & economic costs of pesticide use. Bioscience 42(10).

CHAPTER 3
1. Can the Human Lifespan Be Extended? LE Mag. www.lef.org/research.lifespan.html
2. DHEA and Aging, Aging. 1995 Dec 29;774:1-350.
3. Proc Natl Acad Sci USA. 2000 Feb 1;97(3):1202-5.
4. Zheng, W, et al. Well done meat intake and the risk of breast cancer. J Nat Cancer Inst. 1998 Nov 18 90:1724.

5. Ader, Robert, Felton, David L., Cohen, Nicholas, eds. *Psychoneuro-immunology*, 2nd ed. Academic Press, 1991.

6. Vaillant, GE, MD. The Study of Adult Development. Brigham & Women's Hospital. Boston, MA.

CHAPTER 4

Replenish Testosterone Naturally. LE Mag. Jan 2000.

BPH: The Other Side of the Coin. LE Mag. Feb 1999.

Male Hormone Modulation Therapy, www.lef.protocols/prtcls-txt/t-ptrcl-130.html

Journal of Steroid Biochemical Molecular Biology 46(3).

The Life Extension Foundation has designed a scientific program to counteract all the known biochemical processes proposed (by gerontologists) as primary causes of aging. To access this information free of charge, log on to www.lef.org. You may also call 1-800-544-4440 to request a copy of The Directory of Life Extension Technologies.

Further Reading

Araghi-Niknam, M; Ardestani, SK; Molitor, M; Inserra, P; Eskelson, CD; Watson, RR. Dehydroepiandrosterone (DHEA) sulfate prevents reduction in tissue vitamin E and increased lipid peroxidation due to murine retrovirus infection of aged mice. Proc Soc Exp Biol Med. 1998 Jul;218(3):210-7.

Araneo, BA; Ryu, SY; Barton, S; Daynes, RA. Dehydroepiandrosterone reduces progressive dermal ischemia caused by thermal injury. J Surg Res. 1995;59:250-62.

Arlt, W; Callies, F; van Vlijmen, JC et al. Dehydroepiandrosterone replacement in women with adrenal insufficiency. N Engl J Med. 1999 Sep 30;341(14):1013-20.

Barrett-Connor, E; von Muhlen, D; Laughlin, GA; Kripke, A. Endogenous levels of dehydroepiandrosterone sulfate, but not other sex hormones, are associated with depressed mood in older women: the Rancho Bernardo Study. J Am Geriatr Soc. 1999 Jun;47(6):685-91.

Bellino, FL; Daynes, RA; Hornsby, PJ et al. DHEA and aging. Aging 1995 Dec 29;774:1-350.

Bloch, M, et al. Dehydroepiandrosterone treatment of midlife dysthymia. Biol Psychiatry 1999 Jun 15;45(12):1533-41.

Brincat, M, et al. Sex hormones and skin collagen content in post-menopausal women. Br Med J. 1983;287(6402):1337-8.

Christeff, N, et al. Changes in cortisol/DHEA ratio in HIV-infected men are related to immunological and metabolic perturbations leading to malnutrition and lipodystrophy. Ann NY Acad Sci. 2000;917:962-70.

Cutolo, M. Sex hormone adjuvant therapy in rheumatoid arthritis. Rheum Dis Clin North Am. 2000;26:881-95.

Danenberg, HD; Ben-Yehuda, A; Zakay-Rones, Z; Friedman, G. Dehydroepiandrosterone (DHEA) treatment reverses the impaired immune response of old mice to influenza vaccination and protects from influenza infection. Vaccine 1995;13(15):1445-8.

Danenboerg, HD, et al. Dehydroepiandrosterone (DHEA) increases production and release of Alzheimer's amyloid precursor protein. Life Sci. 1996;59(19):1651 7.

Diallo, K et al. Inhibition of HIV-1 replication by immunor (IM28), a new analog of DHEA. Nucleosides Nucleotides Nucleic Acids 2000;19:2019-24.

Du, C; Khalil, MW; Sriram, S. Administration of dehydroepiandrosterone suppresses experimental allergic encephalomyelitis in SJL/J mice. J Immunol. 2001 Dec 15;167(12):7094-7101.

Ferraccioli, G; Casatta, L; Bartoli, E. Increase of bone mineral density and anabolic variables in patients with rheumatoid arthritis resistant to methotrexate after cyclosporin A therapy J Rheumatol. 1996 Sep;23(9):153-42.

Ferrucci, L, et al. Serum IL-6 level and the development of disability in older persons. J Am Geriatr Soc. 1999 Jun;47(6):639-46.

Folsom, AR; Aleksic, N; Catellier, D; Juneja, HS; Wu, KK. C-reactive protein and incident coronary heart disease in the Atherosclerosis Risk in Communities (ARIC) study. Am Heart J. 2002 Aug;144(2):233-8.

Friess, E, et al. DHEA administration increases rapid eye movement sleep and EEG power in the sigma frequency range. Am J Physiol. 1995 Jan;268 (1, Pt.1):E107-13.

Futterman, LG; Lemberg, L. High-sensitivity C-reactive protein is the most effective prognostic measurement of acute coronary events. Am J Crit Care. 2002 Sep;11(5):482-6.

Genazzani, AD et al. Oral dehydroepiandrosterone supplementation modulates spontaneous and growth hormone-releasing hormone-induced growth hormone and insulin-like growth factor-1 secretion in early and late post-menopausal women. Fertil Steril. 2001 Aug;76(2):241-8.

Glaser, JL, et al. Elevated serum dehydroepiandrosterone sulfate levels in practitioners of the (TM) and TM-Sidhi programs. J Behav Med. 1992 Aug;15(4):327-41.

Goodyer, IM, et al. Adrenal secretion during major depression in 8- to 16-year-olds. I. Altered diurnal rhythms in salivary cortisol and dehydro-epiandrosterone (DHEA) at presentation. Psychol Med. 1996 Mar;26(2): 245-56.

Haden, ST; Glowacki, J; Hurwitz, S, et al. Effects of age on serum dehy-droepiandrosterone sulfate, IGF-I, and IL-6 levels in women. Calcif Tissue Int. 2000 Jun;66(6):414-8.

Hastings, LA; Pashko, LL; Lewbart, M.L; Schwartz, AG. Dehydroepian-drosterone and two structural analogs inhibit 12-O-tetradecanoylphorbol-13-acetate stimulation of prostaglandin E2 content in mouse skin. Carcinogenesis 1988 Jun;9(6):1099-1102.

Heinz, A, et al. Severity of depression in abstinent alcoholics is associated with monoamine metabolites and dehydroepiandrosterone-sulfate concen-trations. Psychiatry Res. 1999 Dec 20;89(2):97-106.

Herrington, DM, et al. Dehydroepiandrosterone and coronary atherosclerosis. Ann. NY Acad Sci. 1995 Dec 29;774:271-80.

Inagaki, M, et al. Effect of acute and chronic administration of dehydro-epiandrosterone on (+/-)-1-(2,5-dimethoxy-4-iodophenyl)-2-aminopropane-induced wet dog shaking behavior in rats. J Neural Transm. 1999; 106(1):23-33.

Inserra, P, et al. Modulation of cytokine production by dehydroepiandros-terone (DHEA) plus melatonin (MLT) supplementation of old mice. Proc Soc Exp Biol Med. 1998 May;218(1):76-82.

James, K, et al. IL-6, DHEA and the ageing process. Mech Ageing Dev. 1997 Feb;93(1-3):15-24.

Jesse, RL, et al. Dehydroepiandrosterone inhibits human platelet aggrega-tion in vitro and in vivo. Ann NY Acad Sci. 1995 Dec 29;774:281-90.

Khorram, O, et al. Activation of immune function by dehydroepiandros-terone (DHEA) in age-advanced men. J Gerontol A Biol Sci Med Sci. 1997 Jan;52(1):M1-M7.

Kim, SH; Han, HM; Kang, SY, et al. Modulation of chemical carcinogen-induced unscheduled DNA synthesis by dehydroepiandrosterone (DHEA) in the primary rat hepatocytes. Arch Pharm Res. 1999 Oct;22(5):474-8.

Kipper-Galperin, M; Galilly, R; Danenberg, HD, et al. Dehydroepiandrosterone selectively inhibits production of tumor necrosis factor alpha and interleukin-6 in astrocytes. Int J Dev Neurosci. 1999 Dec;17(8):765-75.

Labrie, C; Flamand, M; Belanger, A; Labrie, F. High bioavailability of dehydroepiandrosterone administered percutaneously in the rat. J Endocrinol. 1996;150:S107-118.

Lavie, CJ, et al. Effects of cardiac rehabilitation and exercise training programs in women with depression. Am J Cardiol. 1999 May 15;83(10):1480-3,A7.

Maurice, T, et al. Dehydroepiandrosterone sulfate attenuates dizocilpine-induced learning impairment in mice via sigma 1-receptors. Behav Brain Res. 1997 Feb;83(1-2):159-64.

Metzger, C; Mayer, D; Hoffmann, H; Bocker, T; Hobe, G; Benner, A; Bannasch, P. Sequential appearance and ultrastructure of amphophilic cell foci, adenomas, and carcinomas in the liver of male and female rats treated with dehydroepiandrosterone. Toxicol Pathol. 1995 Sep-Oct;23(5):591-605.

McCraty, R, et al. The impact of a new emotional self-management program on stress, emotions, heart rate variability, DHEA and cortisol. Integr Physiol Behav Sci. 1998 Apr-Jun;33(2):151-70.

Morales, AJ, et al. Effects of replacement dose of dehydroepiandrosterone in men and women of advancing age. J Clin Endocrinol Metab. 1994 Jun; 78(6):1360-7.

Morales, AJ, et al. The effect of six months treatment with a 100 mg daily dose of dehydroepiandrosterone (DHEA) on circulating sex steroids, body composition and muscle strength in age-advanced men and women. Clin Endocrinol. 1998 Oct;49(4):421 32.

Murialdo, G, et al. Hippocampal perfusion and pituitary-adrenal axis in Alzheimer's disease. Neuropsychobiology 2000;42:51-7.

Oberbeck, R; Dahlweid, M; Koch, R; van Griensven, M; Emmendorfer, A; Tscherne, H; Pape, HC. Dehydroepiandrosterone decreases mortality rate and improves cellular immune function during polymicrobial sepsis. Crit Care Med. 2001 Feb;29(2):380-4.

Pashko, LL, et al. Inhibition of 7,12-dimethylbenz(a)anthracene-induced skin papillomas and carcinomas by dehydroepiandrosterone and 3-beta-methylandrost-5-en-17-one in mice. Cancer Res. 1985 Jan;45(1):164-6.

Rhodes, ME, et al. Enhancement of hippocampal acetylcholine release by the neurosteroid dehydroepiandrosterone sulfate: an in vivo microdialysis study. Brain Res. 1996 Sep 16;733(2):284-6.

Schwartz, AG; Pashko, LL. Food restriction inhibits [3H] 7,12 dimethyl-benz(a)anthracene binding to mouse skin DNA and tetradecanoylphorbol-13-acetate stimulation of epidermal [3H] thymidine incorporation. Anticancer Res. 1986 Nov-Dec;6(6):1279-82.

Schwartz, AG; Pashko, LL. Cancer prevention with dehydroepiandrosterone and non-androgenic structural analogs. J Cell Biochem Suppl. 1995;22:210-7.

Simile, M, et al. Inhibition by dehydroepiandrosterone of growth and progression of persistent liver nodules in experimental rat liver carcinogenesis. Int J Cancer 1995 Jul 17;62(2):210-5.

Straub, RH; Konecna, L; Hrach, S, et al. Serum dehydroepiandrosterone (DHEA) and DHEA sulfate are negatively correlated with serum interleukin-6 (IL-6), and DHEA inhibits IL-6 secretion from mononuclear cells in man in vitro: possible link between endocrinosenescence and immunosenescence. Clin Endocrinol Metab. 1998 Jun;83(6):2012-7.

Straub, RH; Scholmerich, J; Zietz, B. Replacement therapy with DHEA plus corticosteroids in patients with chronic inflammatory diseases-substitutes of adrenal and sex hormones. Z Rheumatol. 2000;59(Suppl. 2):II/108-18 (in German).

Swierczynski, J; Kochan, Z; Mayer, D. Dietary alpha-tocopherol prevents dehydroepiandrosterone-induced lipid peroxidation in rat liver microsomes and mitochondria. Toxicol Lett. 1997 Apr 28;91(2):129-36.

Uozumi, K, et al. Serum dehydroepiandrosterone and DHEA-sulfate in patients with adult T-cell leukemia and human T-lymphotropic virus type I carriers. Am J Hematol. 1996 Nov;53(3):165-8.

Van Vollenhoven, RF, et al. Treatment of systemic lupus erythematosus with dehydroepiandrosterone: 50 patients treated up to 12 months. J Rheumatol. 1998 Feb;25(2):285-9.

Watson, RR, et al. Dehydroepiandrosterone and diseases of aging. Drugs Aging 1996 Oct;9(4):274-91.

Wellby, ML; Kennedy, JA; Pile, K; True, BS; Barreau, P. Serum interleukin-6 and thyroid hormones in rheumatoid arthritis. Metabolism 2001 Apr;50(4):463-7.

Wolkowitz, OM, et al. Dehydroepiandrosterone (DHEA) treatment of depression. Biol Psychiatry 1997 Feb 1;41(3):311-8.

CHAPTER 5

The Silent Stroke Epidemic. LE Mag. May 2001.

Inflammation and Heart Disease. LE Mag. Jan 2001.

"Homocysteine protocol" http://www.lef.org/protocols/prtcl-122.shtml

Nature. 1996;381:6584.

Petrie, K; Dawson, A; Thompson, L; Brook, R. A double-blind trial of melatonin as a treatment for jet lag in internation cabin crew. Biological Psychiatry 1993 33(7):526-530.

Hyperhomocysteinemia and low pyridoxal phosphate: common and independent reversible risk factors for coronary artery disease. Circulation. 1995 Nov 15:2825-2830.

The American Journal of Epidemiology. 1996 143(9);845-859.

Further Reading

Packard, CJ, et al. Lipoprotein-associated phospholipase A2 as an independent predictor of coronary heart disease. West of Scotland Coronary Prevention Study Group. N Engl J Med. 2000 Oct 19;343(16):1148-55.

Lindahl, B, et al. Markers of myocardial damage and inflammation in relation to long-term mortality in unstable coronary artery disease. FRISC Study Group. Fragmin during Instability in Coronary Artery Disease. N Engl J Med. 2000 Oct 19;343(16):1139-47.

Rader, DJ. Inflammatory markers of coronary risk. N Engl J Med. 2000 Oct 19;343(16):1179-82.

Ridker, PM, et al. Plasma concentration of interleukin-6 and the risk of future myocardial infarction among apparently healthy men. Circulation. 2000 Apr 18;101(15):1767-72.

Bordia, AK. The effect of vitamin C on blood lipids, fibrinolytic activity and platelet adhesiveness in patients with coronary artery disease. Atherosclerosis. 1980 Feb;35(2):181-7.

Kipper-Galperin, M, et al. Dehydroepiandrosterone selectively inhibits production of tumor necrosis factor alpha and interleukin-6 [correction of interlukin-6] in astrocytes. Int J Dev Neurosci. 1999 Dec;17(8):765-75.

Haden, ST, et al. Effects of age on serum dehydroepiandrosterone sulfate, IGF-I, and IL-6 levels in women. Calcif Tissue Int. 2000 Jun;66(6):414-8.

Reddi, K, et al. Interleukin 6 production by lipopolysaccharide-stimulated human fibroblasts is potently inhibited by naphthoquinone (vitamin K) compounds. Cytokine. 1995 Apr;7(3):287-90.

Teucher, T, et al. [Cytokine secretion in whole blood of healthy subjects following oral administration of Urtica dioica L. plant extract]. Arzneimittelforschung. 1996 Sep;46(9):906-10.

Obertreis, B, et al. Ex-vivo in-vitro inhibition of lipopolysaccharide stimulated tumor necrosis factor-alpha and interleukin-1 beta secretion in human whole blood by extractum urticae dioicae foliorum. Arzneimittelforschung. 1996 Apr;46(4):389-94. Published erratum appears in Arzneimittelforschung 1996 Sep;46(9):936.

Bossavy, JP, et al. A double-blind randomized comparison of combined aspirin and ticlopidine therapy versus aspirin or ticlopidine alone on experimental arterial thrombogenesis in humans. Blood (U.S.). 1998 Sep 1; 92(5):1518-25.

Willoughby, S, et al. The use of aspirin in polycythaemia vera and primary thrombocythaemia. Blood Rev (Scotland). 1998 Mar;12(1):12-22.

Lopez-Farre, A, et al. Thrombosis and coronary disease: neutrophils, nitric oxide and aspirin. Rev Esp Cardiol (Spain). 1998 Mar;51(3):171-7.

Kim, YH, et al. Prophylaxis for deep vein thrombosis with aspirin or low molecular weight dextran in Korean patients undergoing total hip replacement. A randomized controlled trial. Int Orthop (Germany). 1998;22(1):6–10.

Shiflett, SC. Overview of complementary therapies in physical medicine and rehabilitation. Physical Medicine and Rehabilitation Clinics of North America. 1999;10(3):521-529.

Stocker, A, et al. Specific cellular responses to alpha-tocopherol. J Nutr. 2000 Jul;130(7):1649-52.

Rahman, K, et al. Dietary Supplementation with Aged Garlic Extract Inhibits ADP-Induced Platelet Aggregation in Humans. J Nutr. 2000 Nov; 130(11):2662-2665.

Kang, WS, et al. Antithrombotic activities of green tea catechins and (-)-epigallocatechin gallate. Thromb Res. 1999 Nov 1;96(3):229-37.

Logani, S, et al. Actions of Ginkgo Biloba related to potential utility for the treatment of conditions involving cerebral hypoxia. Life Sci. 2000 Aug 11;67(12):1389-96.

Clostre, F. [Ginkgo biloba extract (EGb 761). State of knowledge in the dawn of the year 2000]. Ann Pharm Fr. 1999 Jul;57 Suppl 1:1S8-88.

Akisu, M, et al. Platelet-activating factor is an important mediator in hypoxic ischemic brain injury in the newborn rat. Flunarizine and Ginkgo biloba extract reduce PAF concentration in the brain. Biol Neonate. 1998 Dec;74(6):439–44.

Lagente, V, et al. Effects of the platelet activating factor antagonists BN 52021 and BN 50730 on antigen-induced bronchial hyperresponsiveness and eosinophil infiltration in lung from sensitized guinea-pigs. Clin Exp Allergy. 1993 Dec;23(12):1002–10.

Ceriello, A, et al. Total plasma antioxidant capacity predicts thrombosis-prone status in NIDDM patients. Diabetes Care (United States). 1997 Oct; 20(10):1589-93.

Vyshevskii, ASh, et al. [The role of platelets in the protective effect of a combination of vitamins A, E, C and P in thrombinemia]. Gematol Transfuziol. 1995 Sep-Oct;40(5):9-11.

Back, O, et al. Retinoids and fibrinolysis. Acta Derm Vencreol. 1995 Jul; 75(4):290-2.

Van Bennekum, AM, et al. Modulation of tissue-type plasminogen activator by retinoids in rat plasma and tissues. Am J Physiol. 1993 May;264 (5 Pt 2):R931-7.

Thompson, EA, et al. Effect of retinoic acid on the synthesis of tissue-type plasminogen activator and plasminogen activator inhibitor-1 in human endothelial cells. Eur J Biochem. 1991 Nov 1;201(3):627–32.

Kooistra, T, et al. Stimulation of tissue-type plasminogen activator synthesis by retinoids in cultured human endothelial cells and rat tissues in vivo. Thromb Haemost. 1991 May 6;65(5):565–72.

Oosthuizen, W, et al. Both fish oil and olive oil lowered plasma fibrinogen in women with high baseline fibrinogen levels. Thromb Haemost. 1994 Oct; 72(4):557–62.

Flaten, H, et al. Fish-oil concentrate: effects on variables related to cardiovascular disease. Am J Clin Nutr. 1990 Aug;52(2):300-6.

Midorikawa, S, et al. Enhancement by homocysteine of plasminogen activator inhibitor-1 gene expression and secretion from vascular endothelial and smooth muscle cells. Biochem Biophys Res Commun. 2000 May 27;272(1):182-5.

Sandrick, Karen. Teasing out the value of new C-reactive protein test. In CAP Today. 2000 Jan:43-47.

Kaneko, K, et al. C-Reactive protein in dilated cardiomyopathy. Cardiology. 1999;91(4):215-9.

Lindahl, B, et al. Markers of myocardial damage and inflammation in relation to long-term mortality in unstable coronary artery disease. FRISC Study Group. Fragmin during Instability in Coronary Artery Disease. N Engl J Med. 2000 Oct 19;343(16):1139-47.

CHAPTER 6

1. Everyday Carcinogens: Stopping Cancer Before it Starts. March 26 & 27, 1999. McMaster University, Hamilton, Ontario, Canada. (transcripts online: http://www.stopcancer.org)

2. The National Cancer Institute's Annual National Cancer Report, May 15, 2002. http://www.cancer.gov/newscenter/2002reportnation

3. Epstein, Samuel S. *The Politics of Cancer.* New York: Anchor Books, 1979.

4. Lichtenstein, P, et al. Environmental and heritable factors in the causation of cancer—analyses of cohorts of twins from Sweden, Denmark, and Finland. N Engl J Med. 2000;343:78-85,135-136.

5. Haber, D. Roads leading to breast cancer. N Engl J Med. 2000 Nov 23; 343(21).

6. Steinmetz, KA; Potter, JD; Folsom AR. Vegetables, fruit, and cancer in the Iowa Women's Health Study. Cancer Res. 1993 Feb 1;53(3):536-43.

7. Sellers, TA; Kushi, LH; Cerhan, JR; Vierkant, RA; Gapstur, SM; Vachon, CM; Olson, JE; Therneau, TM; Folsom AR. Dietary folate intake, alcohol, and risk of breast cancer in a prospective study of postmenopausal women. Epidemiology. 2001 Jul;12(4):420-8.

8. Smith, GD; Gunnell, D; and Holly, J. British Medical Journal. 2000 October 7;321:847-848.

9. Http://cat007.com/cansug.htm

10. Franceschi, S, et al. Dietary glycemic load and colorectal cancer risk. Ann Oncol. 2001 Feb;12:173-8.

"Sugar and Prostate Cancer." Health Express, October 1982, p. 41.

Bostick, RM; Potter, JD; Kushi, LH; et al. Sugar, meat, and fat intake, and non-dietary risk factors for colon cancer incidence in Iowa Women. Cancer Causes and Controls. 1994;5:38-52.

Moerman, C, et al. Dietary sugar intake in the etiology of biliary tract cancer. International Journal of Epidemiology. 1993;22(2):207-214.

Cornee, J, et al. A case-control study of gastric cancer and nutritional factors in Marseille, France. European Journal of Epidemiology. 1995; 11:55-65.

11. Cantor, KP; Lynch, CF; Hildesheim, ME; Dosemeci, M; Lubin, J; Alavanja, M; Craun, G. Drinking water source and chlorination byproducts. I. Risk of bladder cancer. Epidemiology. 1998 Jan;9(1):21-8.

   Hildesheim, ME; Cantor, KP; Lynch, CF; Dosemeci, M; Lubin, J; Alavanja, M; Craun, G. Drinking water source and chlorination byproducts. II. Risk of colon and rectal cancers. Epidemiology. 1998 Jan;9(1):29-35.

12. Woznicki, Katrina. The Washington Post. May 17, 2000.

13. Porta, M; Malats, N; Jariod, M; Grimalt, JO; Rifa, J; Carrato, A; Guarner, L; Salas, A; Santiago-Silva, M; Corominas, JM; Andreu, M; Real FX. Serum concentrations of organochlorine compounds and K-ras mutation in exocrine pancreatic cancer. PANKRAS II Study Group. Lancet. 1999 Dec 18-25;354(9196):2125-9.

   Hoyer, AP; Grandjean, P; Jorgensen, T; Brock, JW; Hartvig, HB. Organochlorine exposure and risk of breast cancer. Lancet. 1998 Dec 5;352(9143):1816-20.

14. "Exposure to Pesticides Linked to Pancreatic Cancer." Reuters Health Information, December 21, 1999.

15. "Do Pesticides Cause Lymphoma?" http://www.lymphoma.org

16. Sherman. JD. "Life's Delicate Balance: The Causes and Prevention of Breast Cancer." New York and London: Taylor and Francis, 2000.

17. Ferrie H. New Perspectives in the War on Cancer. Vitality Magazine, Fall 1999. Toronto, Canada.

18. Brandes, LJ; Warrington, RC; Arron, RJ; Bogdanovic, RP; Fang, W; Queen, GM; Stein, DA; Tong, J; Zaborniak, CL; LaBella, FS. Enhanced cancer growth in mice administered daily human-equivalent doses of some H1-antihistamines: predictive in vitro correlates. Natl Cancer Inst. 1994 May 18;86(10):770-5.

19. Cotterchio, M; Kreiger, N; Darlington, G; Steingart A. Antidepressant medication use and breast cancer risk. Am J Epidemiol. 2000 May 15; 151(10):951-7.

20. 35th Annual Meeting of the Society for Epidemiologic Research, Seattle, June 2000.

21. Fitzpatrick, AL; Daling, JR; Furberg, CD; Kronmal, RA;, Weissfeld, JL. Use of calcium channel blockers and breast carcinoma risk in post-menopausal women. Cancer. 1997 Oct 15;80(8):1438-47.

22. Newman, TB; Hulley, SB. Carcinogenicity of lipid-lowering drugs. JAMA. 1996 Jan 3;275(1):55-60.

23. Simons, M. Molecular multitasking: statins lead to more arteries, less plaque. Nat Med. 2000 Sep;6(9):965-6.

    Kureishi, Y; Luo, Z; Shiojima, I; Bialik, A; Fulton, D; Lefer, DJ; Sessa, WC; Walsh, K. The HMG-CoA reductase inhibitor simvastatin activates the protein kinase Akt and promotes angiogenesis in normocholesterolemic animals. Nat Med. 2000 Sep;6(9):1004-10.

24. Akagi, K; Ikeda, Y; Miyazaki, M; Abe, T; Kinoshita, J; Maehara, Y; Sugimachi, K. Vascular endothelial growth factor-C (VEGF-C) expression in human colorectal cancer tissues. Br J Cancer. 2000 Oct;83(7):887-91.

25. Chiarelli, F; Santilli, F; Mohn, A. Role of growth factors in the development of diabetic complications. Horm Res. 2000;53(2):53-67.

26. Brinton, LA; Lubin, JH; Burich, MC; Colton, T; Hoover, RN. Mortality among augmentation mammoplasty patients. Epidemiology. 2001 May;12(3):321-6.

    Brinton, LA; Lubin, JH; Burich, MC; Colton, T; Brown, SL; Hoover, RN. Cancer risk at sites other than the breast following augmentation mammoplasty. Ann Epidemiol. 2001 May;11(4):248-56.

27. Stolberg, Sheryl Gay. "Associated Press Study Links Breast Implants to Lung and Brain Cancers." Washington Post, April 25, 1998.

    Stolberg, Sheryl Gay. "'Silicone Survivors' Take Fight Over Implants to Capital." New York Times, July 26, 1998.

28 Everyday Carcinogens: Stopping Cancer Before it Starts. March 26 & 27, 1999. McMaster University, Hamilton, Ontario, Canada. (transcripts online: http://www.stopcancer.org)

29. "What Causes Breast Cancer?" Rachel's Environment and Health News #723, April 26, 2001.

30. Journal of the National Cancer Institute. 2000 Feb 16;92.

31. Nordenskjold, B; Hatschek, T; Kallstrom, A-C; et al. Results of prolonged adjuvant tamoxifen therapy of breast cancer correlated to steroid receptor, S-phase and ERBB2 levels. The South-East Sweden Breast Cancer Group. Proc Am Soc Clin Oncol. 1999;18:70a.

32. Http://www.NCI.org

33. Ferrie, H. New Perspectives in the War on Cancer. Vitality Magazine, Fall 1999, Toronto, Canada.

34. Preobrazhenskaya, MN; Bukhman, VM; Korolev, AM; Efimov, SA. Ascorbigen and other indole-derived compounds from Brassica vegetables and their analogs as anticarcinogenic and immunomodulating agents. Pharmacol Ther. 1993 Nov;60(2):301-13.

    Arnao, MB; Sanchez-Bravo, J; Acosta, M. Indole-3-carbinol as a scavenger of free radicals. Biochem Mol Biol Int. 1996 Aug;39(6):1125-34.

    Diaz, GD; Li, Q; Dashwood, RH. Caspase-8 and apoptosis-inducing factor mediate a cytochrome c-independent pathway of apoptosis in human colon cancer cells induced by the dietary phytochemical chlorophyllin. Cancer Res. 2003 Mar 15;63(6):1254-61.

    Egner, PA; Wang, JB; Zhu, YR; Zhang, BC; Wu, Y; Zhang, QN; Qian, GS; Kuang, SY; Gange, SJ; Jacobson, LP; Helzlsouer, KJ; Bailey, GS; Groopman, JD; Kensler, TW. Chlorophyllin intervention reduces aflatoxin-DNA adducts in individuals at high risk for liver cancer. Proc Natl Acad Sci USA. 2001 Dec 4;98(25):14601-6.

35. Kamat, JP; Boloor, KK; Devasagayam, TP. Chlorophyllin as an effective antioxidant against membrane damage in vitro and ex vivo. Biochim Biophys Acta. 2000 Sep 27;1487(2-3):113-27.

36. Kumar, SS; Devasagayam, TP; Bhushan, B; Verma, NC. Scavenging of reactive oxygen species by chlorophyllin: an ESR study. Free Radic Res. 2001 Nov;35(5):563-74.

37. Boloor, KK; Kamat, JP; Devasagayam, TP. Chlorophyllin as a protector of mitochondrial membranes against gamma-radiation and photosensitization. Toxicology. 2000 Nov 30;155(1-3):63-71.

38. Dennert, G, et al. Retinoic Acid Stimulation of the Induction of Mouse Killer T-cell in Allogeneic and Syngeneic Systems. Journal of the National Cancer Institute. 1979;62:89.

39. DiSorbo, DM; Litwack, G. Vitamin B_6 Kills Hepatoma Cells in Culture. Nutrition and Cancer. 1982;3(4):216-222.

40. Riordan, D. Nutrition therapy for Cancer Patients. Adjuvant Nutrition in Cancer Treatment Symposium. Tampa, Florida, Sept. 30, 1995.

41. Schauzer, GN. Selenium in Nutritional Cancer Prophylaxis: An Update. Vitamins, Nutrition and Cancer, edited by Prosad, KN. Basel, Switzerland: Karger, 1984.

42. Zinc, Boik J.: Dietary Micronutrients and Their Effects on Cancer. Cancer and Natural Medicine. Princeton, MN: Oregon Medical Press, 1995, 147.

43. Simopoulos, AP. The Mediterranean diets: What is so special about the diet of Greece? The scientific evidence. J Nutr. 2001 Nov;131(11 Suppl):3065S-73S.

44. Fortes, C; Forastiere, F; Farchi, S; Rapiti, E; Pastori, G; Perucci, CA. Diet and overall survival in a cohort of very elderly people. Epidemiology. 2000 Jul;11(4):440-5.

45. Meydani, M. The Boyd Orr lecture. Nutrition interventions in aging and age-associated disease. Proc Nutr Soc. 2002 May;61(2):165-71.

46. Bonnefoy, M; Drai. J; Kostka, T. Antioxidants to slow aging, facts and perspectives. Presse Med. 2002 Jul 27;31(25):1174-8.

47. Bouic, PJ. The role of phytosterols and phytosterolins in immune modulation: a review of the past 10 years. Curr Opin Clin Nutr Metab Care. 2001 Nov;4(6):471-5.

48. lminen, E; Heikkila, S; Poussa, T; Lagstrom, H; Saario, R; Salminen, S. Female patients tend to alter their diet following the diagnosis of rheumatoid arthritis and breast cancer. Prev Med. 2002 May;34(5):529-35.

49. Marchand, JL; Luce, D; Goldberg, P; Bugel, I; Salomon, C; Goldberg, M. Dietary factors and the risk of lung cancer in New Caledonia (South Pacific). Nutr Cancer. 2002;42(1):18-24.

50. Harnack, L; Nicodemus, K; Jacobs, DR Jr; Folsom AR. An evaluation of the Dietary Guidelines for Americans in relation to cancer occurrence. Am J Clin Nutr. 2002 Oct;76(4):889-96.

51. Lahmann, PH; Lissner, L; Gullberg, B; Olsson, H; Berglund, G. A prospective study of adiposity and postmenopausal breast cancer risk: The Malmo diet and cancer study. Int J Cancer. 2003 Jan 10;103(2):246–52.

52. Kasim-Karakas, SE; Almario, RU; Gregory, L; Todd, H; Wong, R; Lasley, BL. Effects of prune consumption on the ratio of 2-hydroxyestrone to 16alpha-hydroxyestrone. Am J Clin Nutr. 2002 Dec;76(6):1422–7.

53. Burdette, JE; Chen, SN; Lu, ZZ; Xu, H; White, BE; Fabricant, DS; Liu, J; Fong, HH; Farnsworth, NR; Constantinou, AI; Van Breemen, RB; Pezzuto, JM; Bolton, JL. Black cohosh (Cimicifuga racemosa L.) protects against menadione-induced DNA damage through scavenging of reactive oxygen species: bioassay-directed isolation and characterization of active principles. J Agric Food Chem. 2002 Nov 20;50(24):7022–8.

54. Parcell S. Sulfur in human nutrition and applications in medicine. Altern Med Rev. 2002 Feb;7(1):22-44.

55. Lengacher, CA; Bennett, MP; Kip, KE; Keller, R; LaVance, MS; Smith, LS; Cox, CE. Frequency of use of complementary and alternative medicine in women with breast cancer. Oncol Nurs Forum. 2002 Nov-Dec;29(10):1445-52.

56. Powell, CB; Dibble, SL; Dall'Era, JE; Cohen, I. Use of herbs in women diagnosed with ovarian cancer. Int J Gynecol Cancer. 2002 Mar-Apr; 12(2):214-7.

57. Tough, SC; Johnston, DW; Verhoef, MJ; Arthur, K; Bryant, H. Complementary and alternative medicine use among colorectal cancer patients in Alberta, Canada. Altern Ther Health Med. 2002 Mar-Apr; 8(2):54-6,58-60,62-4.

58. Zhao, AG; Zhao, HL; Jin, XJ; Yang, JK Tang, LD. Effects of Chinese Jianpi herbs on cell apoptosis and related gene expression in human gastric cancer grafted onto nude mice. World J Gastroenterol. 2002 Oct;8(5):792-6.

59. Hsieh, TC; Lu, X; Guo, J; Xiong, W; Kunicki, J; Darzynkiewicz, Z; Wu, JM. Effects of herbal preparation Equiguard on hormone-responsive and hormone-refractory prostate carcinoma cells: mechanistic studies. Int J Oncol. 2002 Apr;20(4):681-9.

60. Kapadia, GJ; Azuine, MA; Tokuda, H; Hang, E, Mukainaka, T; Nishino, H; Sridhar, R. Inhibitory effect of herbal remedies on 12-o-tetradecanoylphorbol-13-acetate-promoted Epstein-Barr virus early antigen activation. Pharmacol Res. 2002 Mar;45(3):213-220.

61. Abdullaev. FI. Cancer chemopreventive and tumoricidal properties of saffron (Crocus sativus L.). Exp Biol Med (Maywood). 2002 Jan;227(1):20-5.

62. Carnesecchi, S; Schneider, Y; Ceraline, J; Duranton, B; Gosse, F; Seiler, N; Raul, F. Geraniol, a component of plant essential oils, inhibits growth and polyamine biosynthesis in human colon cancer cells. J Pharmacol Exp Ther. 2001 Jul;298(1):197-200.

63. Surh, YJ; Han, SS; Keum, YS; Seo, HJ; Lee, SS. Inhibitory effects of curcumin and capsaicin on phorbol ester-induced activation of eukaryotic transcription factors, NF-kappaB and AP-1. Biofactors. 2000;12(1-4): 107-12.

64. Tatman, D; Mo, H. Volatile isoprenoid constituents of fruits, vegetables and herbs cumulatively suppress the proliferation of murine B_{16} melanoma and human HL-60 leukemia cells. Cancer Lett. 2002 Jan 25;175(2):129-39.

65. Wargovich, MJ; Woods, C; Hollis, DM; Zander, ME. Herbals, cancer prevention and health. J Nutr 2001 Nov;131(11 Suppl):3034S-6S.

66. Sadava, D; Ahn, J; Zhan, M; Pang, ML; Ding, J; Kane, SE. Effects of four Chinese herbal extracts on drug-sensitive and multidrug-resistant small-cell lung carcinoma cells. Cancer Chemother Pharmacol. 2002 Apr;49(4):261-6.

67. Pirani. JF. The effects of phytotherapeutic agents on prostate cancer: an overview of recent clinical trials of PC SPES. Urology. 2001 Aug; 58(2 Suppl 1):36-8.

68. Chenn. S. In vitro mechanism of PC SPES. Urology. 2001 Aug;58 (2 Suppl 1):28-35, discussion 38.

69. Huerta, S; Arteaga, JR; Irwin, RW; Ikezoe, T; Heber, D; Koeffler, HP. PC-SPES inhibits colon cancer growth in vitro and in vivo. Cancer Res. 2002 Sep 15;62(18):5204-9.

70. Schwarz, RE ; Donohue, CA; Sadava, D ; Kane, SE. Pancreatic cancer in vitro toxicity mediated by Chinese herbs SPES and PC-SPES: implications for monotherapy and combination treatment. Cancer Lett. 2003 Jan 10;189(1):59-68.

71. Thomson, JO; Dzubak, P; Hajduch, M. Prostate cancer and the food supplement, PC-SPES. Minireview. Neoplasma. 2002;49(2):69-74.

72. Hsieh, TC; Lu, X; Chea, J; Wu, JM. Prevention and management of prostate cancer using PC-SPES: a scientific perspective. J Nutr. 2002 Nov;132(11 Suppl):3513S-3517S.

73. Terry, P; Baron, JA; Bergkvist,L; Holmberg, L; Wolk, A. Dietary calcium and vitamin D intake and risk of colorectal cancer: a prospective cohort study in women. Nutr Cancer. 2002;43(1):39-46.

74. Wu, K; Willett, WC; Fuchs, CS; Colditz, GA; Giovannucci, EL. Calcium intake and risk of colon cancer in women and men. J Natl Cancer Inst. 2002 Mar 20;94(6):437-46.

75. Rahman, K. Garlic and aging: new insights into an old remedy. Ageing Res. Rev 2003 Jan;2(1):39-56.

CHAPTER 7

1. Martin, A; Cherubini, A; Andres-Lacueva, C; Paniagua, M; Joseph, J. Effects of fruits and vegetables on levels of vitamins E and C in the brain and their association with cognitive performance. J Nutr Health Aging. 2002;6(6):392-404.

2. Halliwell, B. Role of free radicals in the neurodegenerative diseases: therapeutic implications for antioxidant treatment. Drugs Aging. 2001; 18(9):685-716.

3. Drewnowski, A; Shultz, JM. Impact of aging on eating behaviors, food choices, nutrition, and health status. J Nutr Health Aging. 2001;5(2):75-9.

4. Cantuti-Castelvetri, I; Shukitt-Hale, B; Joseph, JA. Neurobehavioral aspects of antioxidants in aging. Int J Dev Neurosci. 2000 Jul-Aug;18(4-5):367-81.

5. Joseph, JA; Shukitt-Hale, B; Denisova, NA; Bielinski, D; Martin, A; McEwen, JJ; Bickford, PC. Reversals of age-related declines in neuronal signal transduction, cognitive, and motor behavioral deficits with blueberry, spinach, or strawberry dietary supplementation. J Neurosci. 1999 Sep 15;19(18):8114-21.

6. Galli, RL; Shukitt-Hale, B; Youdim, KA; Joseph, JA. Fruit polyphenolics and brain aging: nutritional interventions targeting age-related neuronal and behavioral deficits. Ann N Y Acad Sci. 2002 Apr;959:128-32.

7. Perrig, WJ; Perrig, P; Stahelin, HB. The relation between antioxidants and memory performance in the old and very old. J Am Geriatr Soc. 1997 Jun;45(6):718-24.

8. Casadesus, G; Shukitt-Hale; B; Joseph, JA. Qualitative versus quantitative caloric intake: are they equivalent paths to successful aging? Neurobiol Aging. 2002 Sep-Oct;23(5):747.

9. Fioravanti, M; Ferrario, E; Massaia, M; Cappa, G; Rivolta, G; Grossi, E; Buckley, AE. Low folate levels in the cognitive decline of elderly patients and the efficacy of folate as a treatment for improving memory deficits. Archives of Gerontology and Geriatrics. 1997;26(1):1-13.

10. La Rue, A; Koehler, KM; Wayne, SJ; Chiulli, SJ; Haaland, KY; Garry, PJ. Nutritional status and cognitive functioning in a normally aging sample: a 6-year reassessment. Am J Clin Nutr. 1997 Jan;65(1):20-9.

11. Abou-Saleh, MT; Coppen, A. The biology of folate in depression: implications for nutritional hypotheses of the psychoses. J Psychiatr Res. 1986;20(2):91-101.

12. Deijen, JB; van der Beek, EJ; Orlebeke, JF; van den Berg, H. Vitamin B-6 supplementation in elderly men: effects on mood, memory, performance and mental effort. Psychopharmacology. 1992;109(4):489-96.

13. Carmel, R. Prevalence of undiagnosed pernicious anemia in the elderly. Arch Intern Med. 1996 May 27;156(10):1097-100.

14. Lindenbaum, J; Healton, EB; Savage, DG; Brust, JC; Garrett, TJ; Podell, ER; Marcell, PD; Stabler, SP; Allen, RH. Neuropsychiatric disorders caused by cobalamin deficiency in the absence of anemia or macrocytosis. N Engl J Med. 1988 Jun 30;318(26):1720-8.

15. Villeponteau, B; Cockrell, R; Feng, J. Nutraceutical interventions may delay aging and the age-related diseases. Exp Gerontol. 2000 Dec;35(9-10):1405-17.

16. Villeponteau, B; Cockrell, R; Feng, J. Nutraceutical interventions may delay aging and the age-related diseases. Exp Gerontol. 2000 Dec;35(9-10):1405-17.

17. Vatassery, GT; Bauer, T; Dysken, M. High doses of vitamin E in the treatment of disorders of the central nervous system in the aged. Am J Clin Nutr. 1999 Nov;70(5):793-801.

18. Kontush, A; Mann, U; Arlt, S; Ujeyl, A; Luhrs, C; Muller-Thomsen, T; Beisiegel, U. Influence of vitamin E and C supplementation on lipoprotein oxidation in patients with Alzheimer's disease. Free Radic Biol Med. 2001 Aug 1;31(3):345-54.

19. Bourdel-Marchasson, I; Delmas-Beauvieux, MC; Peuchant, E; Richard-Harston, S; Decamps, A; Reignier, B; Emeriau, JP; Rainfray, M. Antioxidant defences and oxidative stress markers in erythrocytes and plasma from normally nourished elderly Alzheimer patients. Age Ageing. 2001 May;30(3):235-41.

20. Desnuelle, C; Dib, M; Garrel, C; Favier, A. A double-blind, placebo-controlled randomized clinical trial of alpha-tocopherol (vitamin E) in the treatment of amyotrophic lateral sclerosis. ALS riluzole-tocopherol Study Group. Amyotroph Lateral Scler Other Motor Neuron Disord. 2001 Mar;2(1):9-18.

21. Liu, J; Head, E; Gharib, AM; Yuan, W; Ingersoll, RT; Hagen, TM; Cotman, CW; Ames, BN. Memory loss in old rats is associated with brain mitochondrial decay and RNA/DNA oxidation: partial reversal by feeding acetyl-L-carnitine and/or R-alpha-lipoic acid. Proc Natl Acad Sci USA. 2002 Feb 19;99(4):2356-61.

22. Matthews, RT; Yang, L; Browne, S; Baik, M; Beal, MF. Coenzyme Q10 administration increases brain mitochondrial concentrations and exerts neuroprotective effects. Proc Natl Acad Sci USA. 1998 Jul 21;95(15): 8892-7.

23. Shults, CW; Haas, RH; Passov, D; Beal, MF. Coenzyme Q10 levels correlate with the activities of complexes I and II/III in mitochondria from

parkinsonian and nonparkinsonian subjects. Ann Neurol. 1997 Aug; 42(2):261-4.

24. Shults, CW; Oakes, D; Kieburtz, K; Beal, MF; Haas, R; Plumb, S; Juncos, JL; Nutt, J; Shoulson, I; Carter, J; Kompoliti, K; Perlmutter, JS; Reich, S; Stern, M; Watts, RL; Kurlan, R; Molho, E; Harrison, M; Lew, M; Parkinson Study Group. Effects of coenzyme Q10 in early Parkinson disease: evidence of slowing of the functional decline. Arch Neurol. 2002 Oct;59(10):1541-50.

25. Shults, CW; Oakes, D; Kieburtz, K; Beal, MF; Haas, R; Plumb, S; Juncos, JL; Nutt, J; Shoulson, I; Carter, J; Kompoliti, K; Perlmutter, JS; Reich, S; Stern, M; Watts, RL; Kurlan, R; Molho, E; Harrison, M; Lew, M; Parkinson Study Group. Effects of coenzyme Q10 in early Parkinson disease: evidence of slowing of the functional decline. Arch Neurol. 2002 Oct;59(10):1541-50

26. Parnetti, L; Amenta, F; Gallai, V. Choline alphoscerate in cognitive decline and in acute cerebrovascular disease: an analysis of published clinical data. Mech Ageing Dev. 2001 Nov;122(16):2041-55.

   Parnetti, L; Amenta, F; Gallai, V. Pharmacological treatment of noncognitive disturbances in dementia disorders. Mech Ageing Dev. 2001 Nov;122(16):2063-9.

27. Gamoh, S; Hashimoto, M; Sugioka, K; Shahdat Hossain, M; Hata, N; Misawa, Y; Masumura, S. Chronic administration of docosahexaenoic acid improves reference memory-related learning ability in young rats. Neuroscience. 1999;93(1):237-41.

   Gamoh, S; Hashimoto, M; Hossain, S; Masumura, S. Chronic administration of docosahexaenoic acid improves the performance of radial arm maze task in aged rats. Clin Exp Pharmacol Physiol. 2001 Apr;28(4):266-70.

28. Hadjiev, D; Yancheva, S. Rheoencephalographic and psychological studies with ethyl apovincaminate in cerebral vascular insufficiency. Arzneimittelforschung. 1976;26(10a):1947-50.

29. Yoshikawa, T; Naito, Y; Kondo, M. Ginkgo biloba leaf extract: review of biological actions and clinical applications. Antioxid Redox Signal. 1999 Winter;1(4):469-80.

   DeFeudis, FV; Drieu, K. Ginkgo biloba extract (EGb 761) and CNS functions: basic studies and clinical applications. Curr Drug Targets. 2000 Jul;1(1):25-58.

Diamond, BJ; Shiflett, SC; Feiwel, N; Matheis, RJ; Noskin, O; Richards, JA; Schoenberger, NE. Ginkgo biloba extract: mechanisms and clinical indications. Arch Phys Med Rehabil. 2000 May;81(5):668-78.

30. Winter, JC. The effects of an extract of Ginkgo biloba, EGb 761, on cognitive behavior and longevity in the rat. Physiol Behav. 1998 Feb 1;63(3):425-33.

31. Sastre, J; Millan, A; Garcia de la Asuncion, J; Pla, R; Juan, G; Pallardo, FV; O'Connor, E; Martin, JA; Droy-Lefaix, MT; Vina, J. A Ginkgo biloba extract (EGb 761) prevents mitochondrial aging by protecting against oxidative stress. Free Radic Biol Med. 1998 Jan 15;24(2):298-304.

32. Corrigan, FM; Horrobin, DF; Skinner, ER; Besson, JA; Cooper, MB. Abnormal content of n-6 and n-3 long-chain unsaturated fatty acids in the phosphoglycerides and cholesterol esters of parahippocampal cortex from Alzheimer's disease patients and its relationship to acetyl CoA content. Int J Biochem Cell Biol. 1998 Feb;30(2):197-207.

33. http://www.realhealthnews.com/fedup/enough.shtml and http://dream line.freeyellow.com

34. Borek, J. Antioxidant health effects of aged garlic extract. J Nutr. 2001 Mar; 131(3s):1010S-5S.

35. Reiter, RJ; Tan, DX; Cabrera, J; D'Arpa, D; Sainz, RM; Mayo, JC; Ramos, S. The oxidant/antioxidant network: role of melatonin. Biol Signals Recept. 1999 Jan-Apr;8(1-2):56-63.

36. Reiter, RJ; Tan, DX; Osuna, C; Gitto, E. Actions of melatonin in the reduction of oxidative stress. A review. J Biomed Sci. 2000 Nov-Dec; 7(6):444-58.

37. Abbott, RD; Ross, GW; White, LR; Nelson, JS; Masaki, KH; Tanner, CM; Curb, JD; Blanchette, PL; Popper, JS; Petrovitch, H. Midlife adiposity and the future risk of Parkinson's disease. Neurology. 2002 Oct 8;59(7):1051-7.

38. Stallibrass, C; Sissons, P; Chalmers, C. Randomized controlled trial of the Alexander technique for idiopathic Parkinson's disease. Clin Rehabil. 2002 Nov;16(7):695-708.

39. Miyai, I; Fujimoto, Y; Yamamoto, H; Ueda, Y; Saito, T; Nozaki, S; Kang, J. Long-term effect of body weight-supported treadmill training in Parkinson's disease: a randomized controlled trial. Arch Phys Med Rehabil. 2002 Oct;83(10):1370-3.

40. Mattson, MP. Existing data suggest that Alzheimer's disease is preventable. Ann N Y Acad Sci. 2000;924:153-9.

41. Fillit, H; Hill, J. The costs of vascular dementia. A comparison with Alzheimer's disease. J Neurol Sci. 2002 Nov 15;203-204(C):35-9.

42. Otsuka, M. Analysis of dietary factors in Alzheimer's disease: clinical use of nutritional intervention for prevention and treatment of dementia. Nippon Ronen Igakkai Zasshi. 2000 Dec;37(12):970-3.

43. Capurso, A; Panza, F; Solfrizzi, V; Torres, F; Capurso, C; Mastroianni, F; Del, Parigi. Age-related cognitive decline: evaluation and prevention strategy. Recenti Prog Med. 2000 Mar;91(3):127-34.

44. Lebowitz, BD; Pearson, JL; Schneider, LS; Reynolds, CF; Alexopoulos, GS; Bruce, MI; Conwell, Y; Katz, IR; Meyers, BS; Morrison, MF; Mossey, J; Niederehe, G; Parmelee, P. Diagnosis and treatment of depression in late life: consensus statement update. Journal of the American Medical Association. 1997;278:1186-90.

CHAPTER 8
1. Ostrowski, RP. Effect of coenzyme Q10 (CoQ10) on superoxide dismutase activity in ET-1 and ET-3 experimental models of cerebral ischemia in the rat. Folia Neuropathol. 1999; 37(4): 247-51.

2. DiMauro, S. Exercise intolerance and the mitochondrial respiratory chain. Ital Neurol Sci. 1999 Dec;20(6):387-93.

3. Kiss, B; Karpati, E. Mechanism of action of vinpocetine. Acta Pharm Hung. 1996 Sep;66(5):213-24 (in Hungarian).

4. Circulation, 1995.

5. Teucher et al., 1996.

6. Shigenaga, MK; Hagen, TM; Ames, BN. Oxidative damage and mitochondrial decay in aging. Proc Natl Acad Sci USA. 1994 Nov 8;91(23):10,771-8. Stevens et al., 1996. Deuther-Conrad et al., 2001. Van Dam, 2001.

7. Volpe, SL; Taper, LJ; Meacham, S. The relationship between boron and magnesium status and bone mineral density in the human: a review. Magnesium Res. 1993 Sep;6(3):291-6.

8. Nielsen, FH. Studies on the relationship between boron and magnesium which possibly affects the formation and maintenance of bones. Magnesium Trace Elem. 1990;9(2):61-9.

9. Marks, LS; Partin, AW; Epstein, JI; Tyler, VE; Simon, I; Macairan, ML; Chan, TL; Dorey, FJ; Garris, JB; Veltri, RW; Santos, PB; Stonebrook,

KA; deKernion, JB. Effects of a saw palmetto herbal blend in men with symptomatic benign prostatic hyperplasia. J Urol. 2000 May;163(5): 1451-6.

10. Konrad, L; Muller, HH; Lenz, C; Laubinger, H; Aumuller, G; Lichius, JJ. Antiproliferative effect on human prostate cancer cells by a stinging nettle root (Urtica dioica) extract. Planta Med. 2000 Feb;66(1):44-7.

11. Ishani, A; MacDonald, R; Nelson, D; Rutks, I; Wilt, TJ. Pygeum africanum for the treatment of patients with benign prostatic hyperplasia: a systematic review and quantitative meta-analysis. Am J Med. 2000 Dec 1;109(8):654-64.

12. Koscielny, J; Klussendorf, D; Latza, R; Schmitt, R; Radtke, H; Siegel, G; Kiesewetter, H. The antiatherosclerotic effect of Allium sativum. Atherosclerosis. 1999 May;144(1):237-49.

CHAPTER 9

1. Washington Post, Sept 4, 2001, p. A10.

   Spindler S. Proceedings of the National Academy of Sciences. 2001 Sept 11; 98:10630-10635.

2. Lane, MA; Ingram; DK; Roth, GS. Nutritional modulation of aging in nonhuman primates. J Nutr Health Aging. 1999;3(2):69-76.

   Roth, GS; Ingram, DK; Lane, MA. Caloric restriction in primates and relevance to humans. Ann N Y Acad Sci. 2001 Apr;928:305-15.

   Lane, MA; Mattison, J; Ingram, DK; Roth, GS. Caloric restriction and aging in primates: Relevance to humans and possible CR mimetics. Microsc Res Tech. 2002 Nov 15;59(4):335-8.

3. Zinna, EM; Yarasheski, KE. Exercise treatment to counteract protein wasting of chronic diseases. Curr Opin Clin Nutr Metab Care. 2003 Jan;6(1):87-93.

4. Schols, AM. Pulmonary cachexia. Int J Cardiol. 2002 Sep;85(1):101-10.

5. Chavannes, N; Vollenberg, JJ; van Schayck, CP; Wouters, EF. Effects of physical activity in mild to moderate COPD: a systematic review. Br J Gen Pract. 2002 Jul;52(480):574-8.

6. Wright, PR; Heck, H; Langenkamp, H; Franz, KH; Weber, U. Influence of a resistance training on pulmonary function and performance measures of patients with COPD. Pneumologie. 2002 Jul;56(7):413-7.

7. Vogiatzis, I; Nanas, S; Roussos, C. Interval training as an alternative modality to continuous exercise in patients with COPD. Eur Respir J. 2002 Jul;20(1):12-9.

8. Spruit, MA; Gosselin, R; Troosters, T; De Paepe, K; Decramer, M. Resistance versus endurance training in patients with COPD and peripheral muscle weakness. Eur Respir J. 2002 Jun;19(6):1072-8.

9. Lee, IM; Rexrode, KM; Cook, NR; Manson, JE; Buring, JE. Physical activity and coronary heart disease in women: is "no pain, no gain" passe? JAMA. 2001 Mar 21;285(11):1447-54.

CHAPTER 10

Recipes printed by permission of Marcus Guiliano.
The following juice recipes reprinted by permission of Penguin Putnam/Avery edition of JOY OF JUICING.

> Very Nutty Shake
> Iced Cinnamon and Spice Tea
> Date and Almond Smoothie
> Apple Strawberry Shake
> Cauliflower, Celery, Carrot, Beet Juice
> Honeydew Melon Shake
> Apple Grape Sprout Juice
> Lemon Apple Juice
> Celery Apple Carrot Juice
> Lemon Apple Cucumber Juice
> Grandma's Mixed Vegetable Juice
> Chocolate Walnut Shake

CHAPTER 11

Unless otherwise noted, all information is based on Gary Null's research.

Kaplan, Dr. Robert Michael. *The Power Behind Your Eyes.* Rochester, VT: Healing Arts Press, 1995.

Seaman, Barbara, and Null, Gary. *For Women Only.* New York: Seven Stories Press, 2000.

Seaman, Barbara. *Women's Health Solutions.* New York: Seven Stories Press, 2002.

Index